SAS AND ELITE FORCES GUIDE
UNARMED COMBAT

HAND-TO-HAND FIGHTING SKILLS FROM THE WORLD'S MOST ELITE MILITARY UNITS

WITHDRAWN FROM COLLECTION

D1069894

SAS AND ELITE FORCES GUIDE
UNARMED COMBAT
HAND-TO-HAND FIGHTING SKILLS FROM THE WORLD'S MOST ELITE MILITARY UNITS

MARTIN J. DOUGHERTY

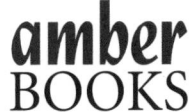

amber
BOOKS

First published in 2010 by
Amber Books Ltd
74–77 White Lion Street
London N1 9PF
www.amberbooks.co.uk
Appstore: itunes.com/apps/amberbooksltd
Facebook: www.facebook.com/amberbooks
Twitter: @amberbooks

Copyright © 2010 Amber Books Ltd

Reprinted in 2012, 2013

All rights reserved. No part of this work may be reproduced,
stored in a retrieval system, or transmitted in any form or by
any means, electronic, mechanical, photocopying, recording, or
otherwise, without the prior permission of the copyright holder.

ISBN: 978-1-906626-81-5

Project Editor: Michael Spilling
Design: Graham Beehag
Illustrations: Tony Randell

Printed in Malaysia

DISCLAIMER
This book is for information purposes only. Readers should be
aware of the legal position in their country of residence before
practicing any of the techniques described in this book. Neither
the author or the publisher can accept responsibility for any loss,
injury, or damage caused as a result of the use of self defence
techniques described in this book, nor for any prosecutions or
proceedings brought or instigated against any person or body
that may result from using these techniques.

CONTENTS

INTRODUCTION

Special forces are renowned for getting the job done fast and efficiently. This often requires the sudden and overwhelming application of violence, giving the enemy no chance to respond. The same tactics are used in special forces unarmed combat systems, which emphasize quick, simple and deadly responses to whatever threat may present itself.

Special forces soldiers are normally armed when carrying out their missions, enabling them to deal with opposition quickly and effectively. However, some circumstances require a more personal approach to combat. Weapons can jam or be dropped, sentries must be eliminated quietly, or a disarmed soldier may need to escape from his captors.

If a special forces soldier has to resort to unarmed combat, something has usually gone wrong. His personal weapon, sidearm, knife, grenades, entrenching tool and various heavy objects among his kit that could be used as improvised weapons are all either inaccessible or else he has been caught unprepared. In such a situation, the most useful tools in the soldier's armoury are his aggression, self-confidence and will to win. These are the weapons he carries with him everywhere.

Most of us will never be required to search a building for terrorists or to rescue hostages from gunmen, but ordinary people do find themselves in danger. The circumstances may be less extreme, but the threat is no less real. An effective response can literally save your life.

Assault team

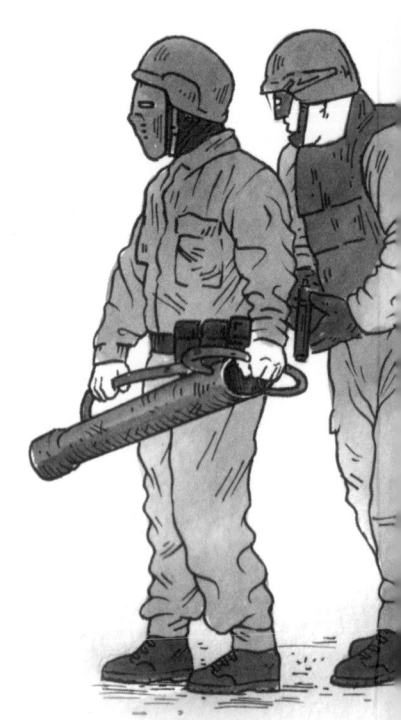

SPECIAL FORCES COMBAT TECHNIQUES

Most people do not have the time to undertake lengthy combat training and to find out what works and what does not. Fortunately, the techniques employed by special forces troops have been pressure-tested under the most difficult conditions possible. If a technique works for a wounded soldier outnumbered four to one by armed men, in the dark and in the

This heavily armed special forces team carries a range of weaponry, but none of it is any use unless directed with skill, courage and determination.

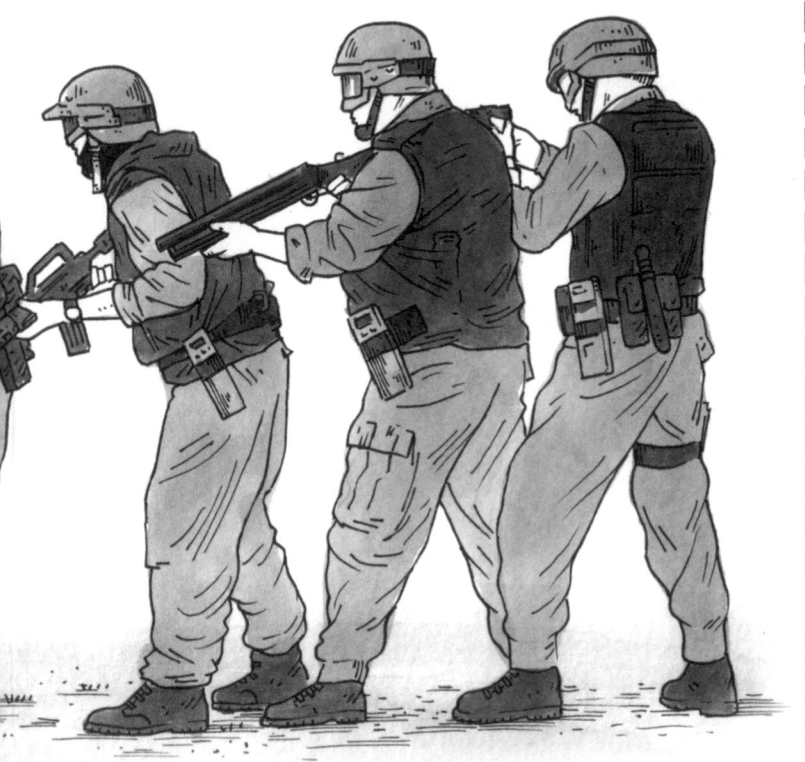

midst of a gunfight … it will work anywhere.

There are no real 'secret combat techniques' used by special forces troops. What there is, is a tried and tested body of technique which is both simple and deadly, coupled with determination to survive and win.

Most of us will never storm an airliner to free hostages, but we might fight for our lives against a drunk with a knife. The following chapters show how special forces combat techniques can help keep ordinary people alive in extraordinary circumstances.

Special forces in action

Sudden assaults from an unexpected direction are the hallmark of special forces operations. Once the attack begins, relentless aggressive action overcomes all resistance.

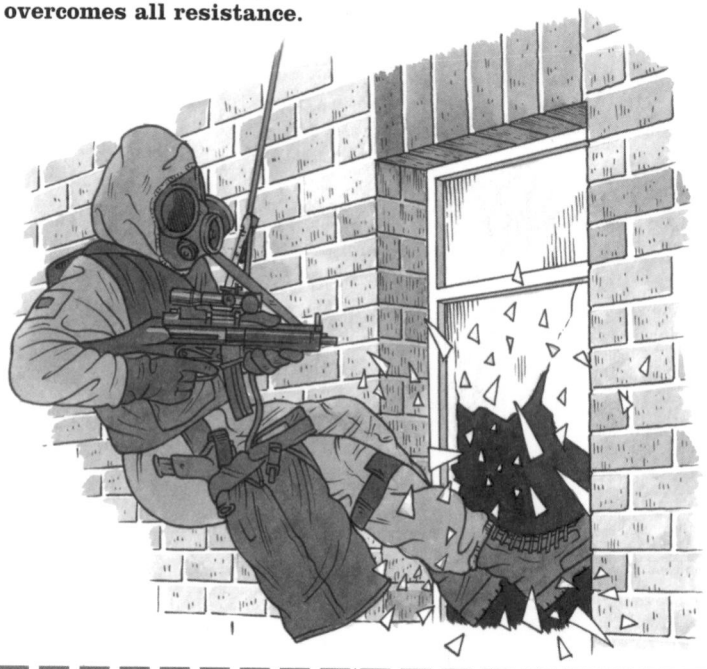

Chin jab

The upward palm shot to the jaw, or 'chin jab', was taught to World War II commandos. It is an extremely effective strike producing a fast knockout.

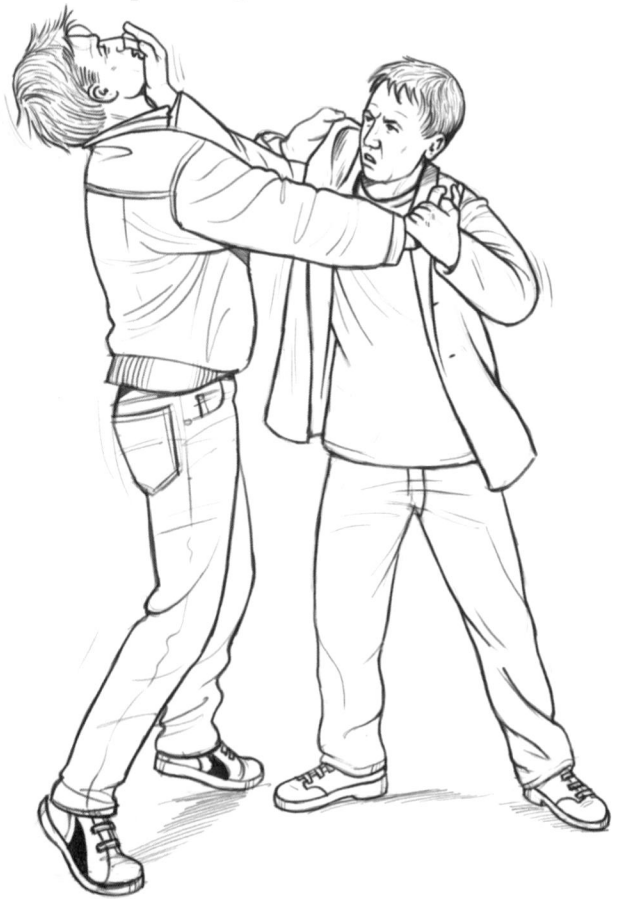

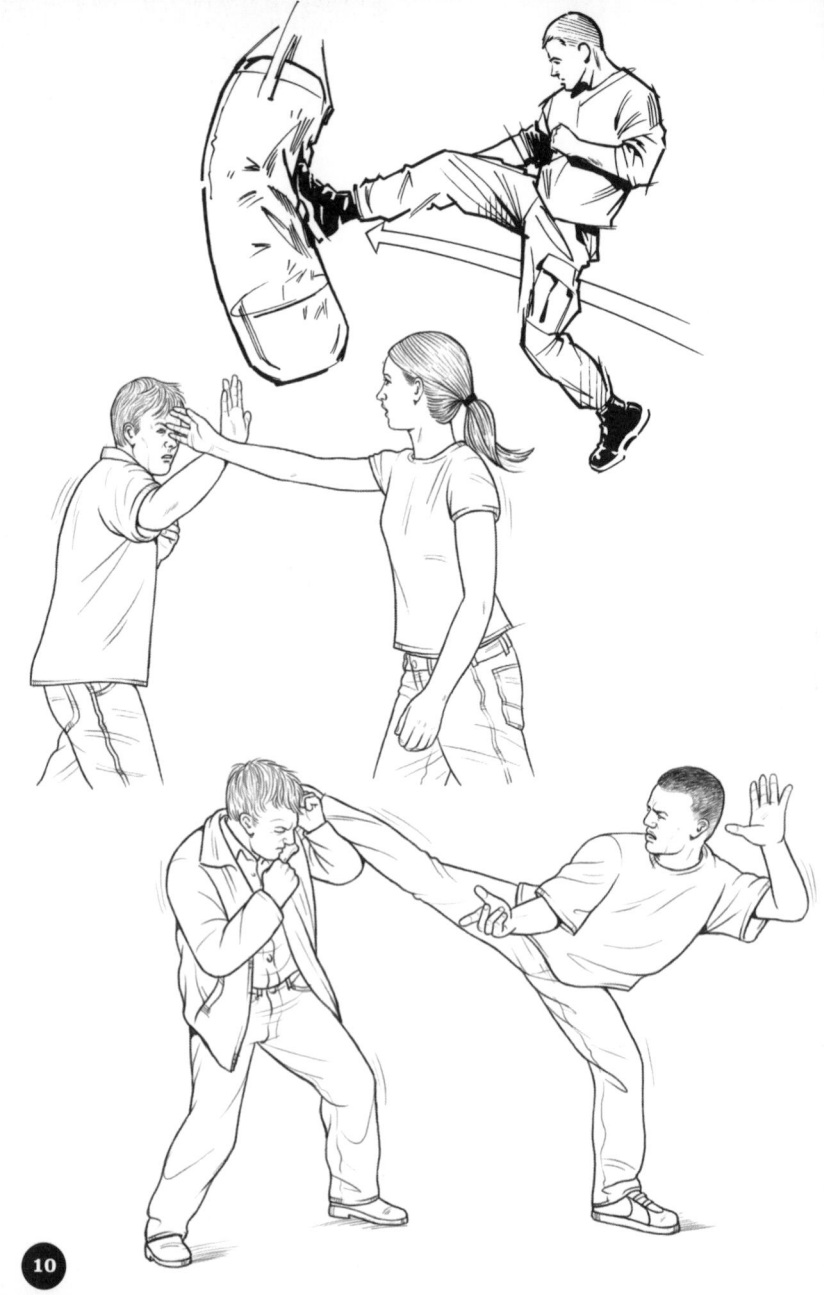

10

A key element in military planning is to make an assessment of the threat likely to be faced. This permits the correct equipment to be issued and a suitable plan to be put in place. For example, a team assaulting an oil rig seized by gunmen would not expect to encounter armoured vehicles and can probably dispense with antitank weapons. Combat will likely be at close quarters where sub-machine guns and shotguns are more useful than sniper rifles. No special forces team would ever be committed without at least some understanding of the threat to be faced.

The same philosophy applies to self-defence. In order to defend yourself effectively you need to understand the nature of the threat as it really is, rather than relying on an impression gained from movies and headlines. What sort of threat are you likely to face? What will an aggressor actually try to do? What are the odds of being faced with a weapon or a gang?

FALSE IMPRESSIONS

It may seem from a cursory look at the news that the streets are a battleground, a deadly arena of fists,

. . . .

Left: You must train for what is likely to happen – have a range of responses available, to deal with lower-level threats.

1

'Know your enemy' is a profound military maxim. It also applies to self-defence.

Preparation

The Threat

Extreme threats

Generally it is better to surrender property than to tackle weapons, but if you think you are going to be harmed anyway, fighting is your only option.

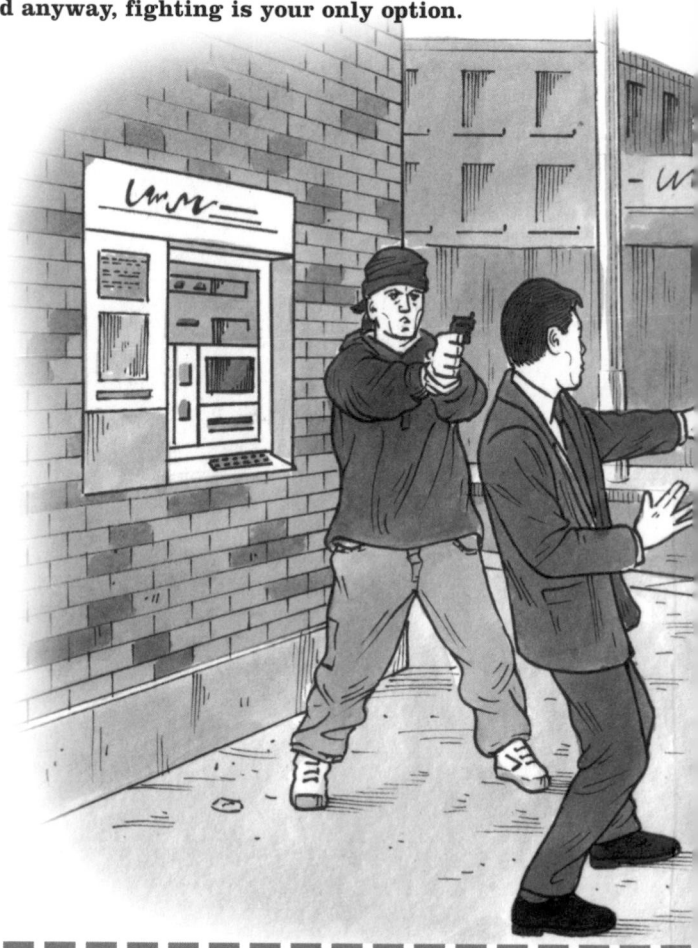

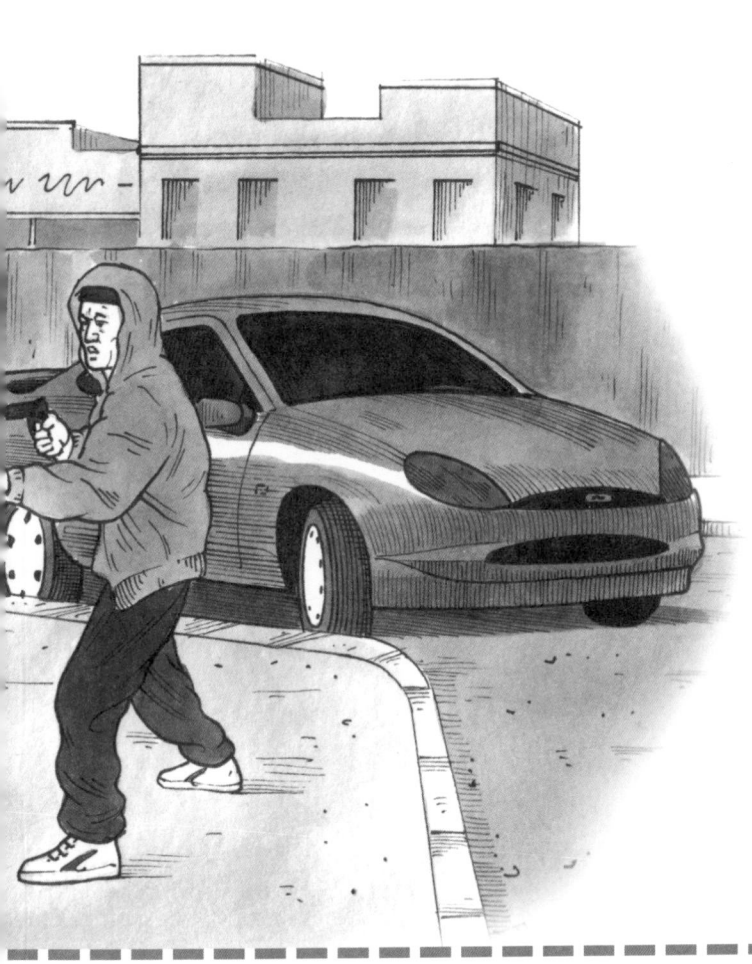

Be aware!

Most robberies and many assaults are opportunistic. Distractions such as phones and music can make you vulnerable.

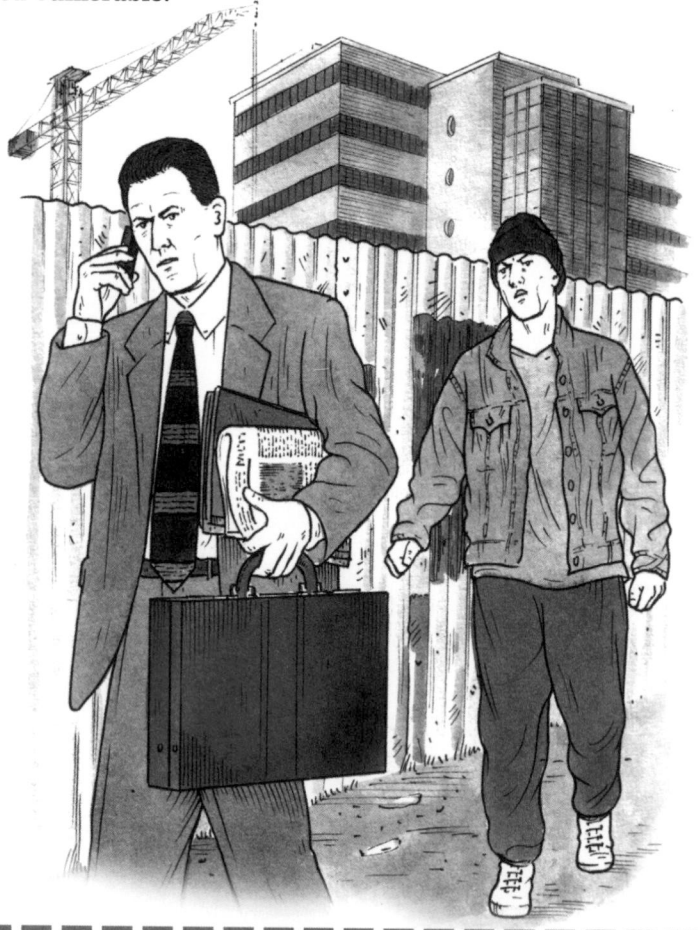

guns and knives. In fact armed attacks are not at all common, though they are serious enough to merit attention when they do happen. Lesser levels of violent assault are more frequent, but even these are not as likely as many people think.

The perception of constant street violence derives mainly from the fact that it gets reported while its absence does not. Headlines like 'nobody got stabbed today' would not sell a lot of newspapers, so we are told about incidents that do happen and never hear about the millions of people who go about their business unharmed. To illustrate that, look at this page. The words stand out but there is a lot more white space between and around them. You do not notice it because it is not brought to your attention. So it is with violence – a lot more people do not encounter violence than do. That said, if it happens to you then it does not matter how uncommon it is.

THE LIKELY THREAT

As a rule, civilians are most likely to face an unarmed threat. This does not mean the level of threat is trivial – anyone is capable of killing with their bare hands if they try hard enough, and being kicked while helpless on the ground can result in death or permanent injury. Attacks with weapons are less common. When they do occur they tend to involve

small, easily carried and concealed weapons, such as knives, or items that can be quickly picked up and used, such as glasses and bottles.

Blunt-instrument attacks are generally more premeditated, as the weapon has to be carried openly if it is large enough to be any use. Other weapons such as chains and samurai swords are quite rare. As to firearms, in Britain at least attacks are still relatively rare.

There are two likely forms an attack might take. The first is a sudden assault with no warning. This is almost always premeditated, and the aggressor might use deception or stealth to get close enough to attack. The other sort of assault gives you more warning, but there are other problems associated with it. This is an escalating confrontation that becomes violent.

Surprise Attack

Surprise attacks are very hard to deal with. Not just because you can be taken out by the first blow, but also because psychologically it is very hard to get into a combative mindset while you are shocked and hurt. Military training teaches troops to switch on their aggression instantly, and good self-defence training does too. In both cases the aggression is controlled and directed; there is no point in firing or flailing wildly.

However, it is better not to be caught by surprise if at all possible.

Knife threat

Any armed threat is extremely serious. It may be better to surrender property than to tackle a weapon, but be aware that some attackers will hurt you even after being given what they want.

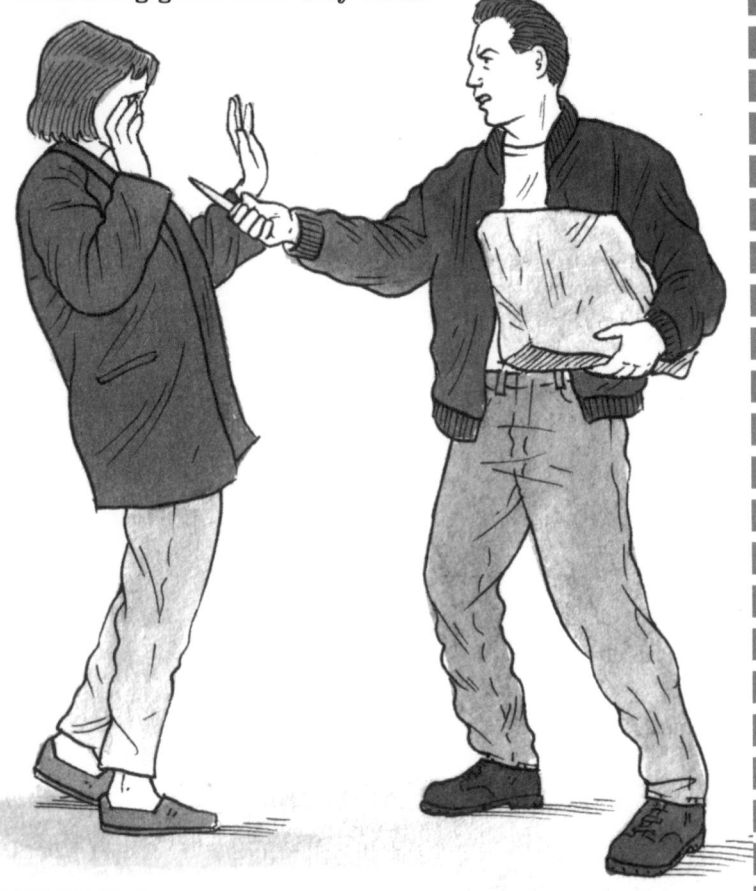

Stealthy attackers can be somewhat countered by:

- Staying in lit areas.
- Not walking close by blind spots such as corners.
- Not allowing yourself to be distracted by music or your phone.

Deceptive attackers often use distraction techniques such as asking you the time or for cigarettes. This allows them to get close enough to launch their attack without warning. If at all possible, you should not allow anyone you do not trust within arm's reach.

Confrontation

Confrontations erupt over all kinds of things, especially where alcohol is involved. Most do not lead to violence, and of those that do, many could have been prevented. The key is to remain calm and not allow yourself to be drawn into an escalating confrontation, and never to allow anyone to get close to you while they are in an aggressive, confrontational state.

The usual pattern for a confrontation is for it to begin with an exchange of words which become more abusive, aggressive and threatening. This is often accompanied by arm-waving and 'posturing', along with violence against objects. An individual who mouths off, inviting you to 'come here if you think you're hard enough' while remaining out of reach or backing away generally does not want to fight. Unless you say something that pricks his ego enough that he just has to attack you, he will normally satisfy himself with a barrage of insults and go off to tell his mates he won. That is not very pleasant but it is a better outcome than a fight.

Escalation

Sometimes, but not always, a confrontation escalates. Someone who starts getting closer and pushing or grabbing you is a very serious threat. He will probably keep on escalating the situation until something makes him stop – something you do or perhaps an outside intervention – or until he gets what he wants. You might be lucky; he might just want to rag you about a bit to show how tough he is. But you cannot predict how much violence he wants to do to you, so hoping for the best is not a great strategy.

Some confrontations go straight to blows of course. There is no set pattern that must be observed. Likewise, the assailant may be satisfied with hitting you a couple of times, but equally he might be willing to stamp on your head while you are helpless on the ground. Bystanders might also join in – it can and does happen. The point is that once a

Wrist grab

Wrist grabs are normally a factor in domestic situations or arguments rather than full-blown fights. All the same, you must yank yourself free immediately in case the aggressor decides to follow up with a blow.

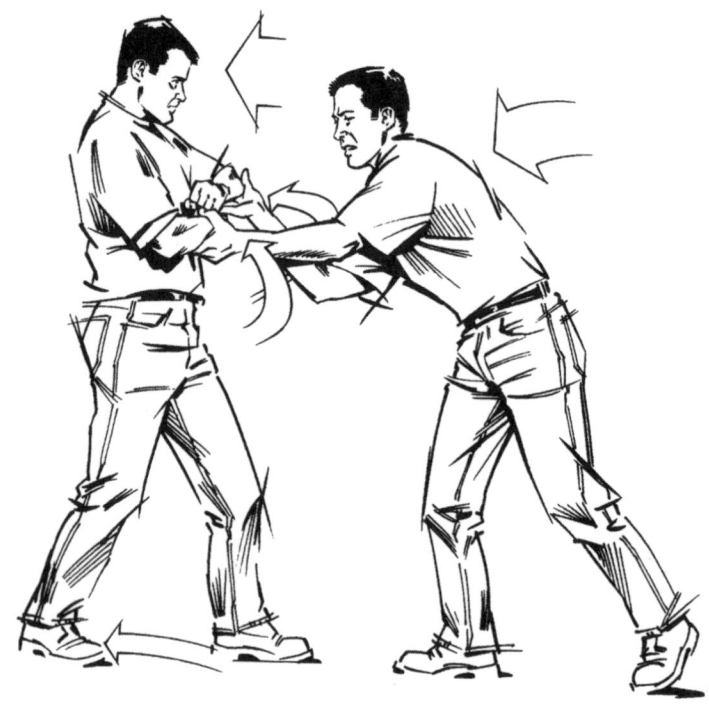

Open hand threat

Posturing with splayed hands is a classic sign of aggression. The woman cannot say for sure whether the man is about to become violent. She has adopted a 'fence' posture to keep him at a distance.

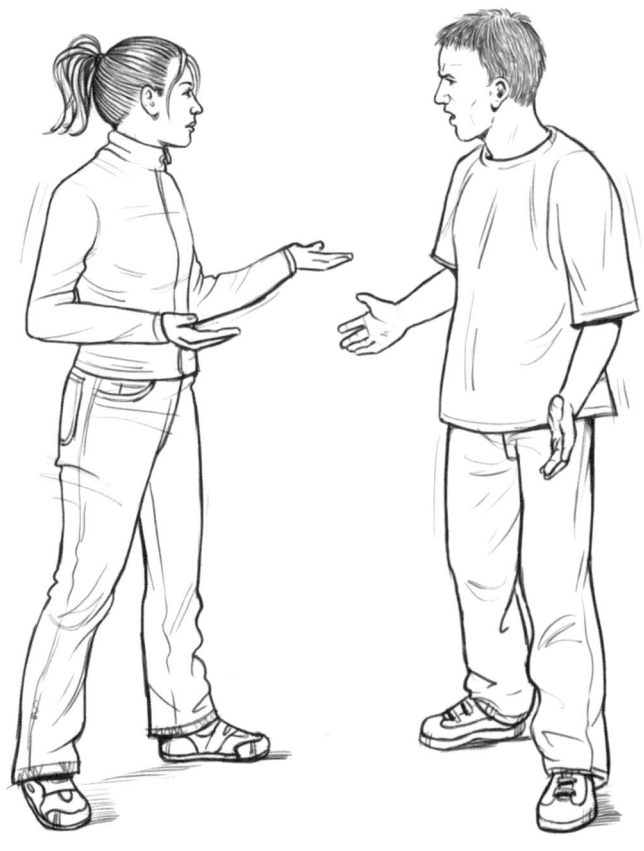

confrontation becomes physical you have no way to know how bad it is going to get, and the outcome of even an unarmed attack can be life-changing or even life-ending.

Real Fights

Whilst almost anything can happen in a fight, an analysis of vast numbers of altercations shows that the same things tend to come out over and over again, whilst others rarely happen at all. Most situations involve at least some 'posturing' and threats, which we term the open-hand threat. Once matters get past this stage, physical violence ensues.

By far the most common gambit in a street fight is the big swinging punch with the strong hand. Over 80 per cent of injuries resulting from street violence are caused by blows to the head. Grabbing and wrestling are also common. Real fights never look like a Kung-Fu movie; they are a desperate blur of aggression and brutality. You must be prepared for this reality if you want to survive.

TIP:
STREET FIGHT FACTS

- Most aggressors will simply wade forward swinging, and grab once they get close enough. Even people with some training are prone to behave like this under the stress of combat.
- Complex strategies are uncommon and do not work very well. Fights are not chess games where moves and subtle countermoves are played out. Simple movements performed with confidence and aggression work best.
- Distance tends to decrease rapidly. It is instinctive to close with an opponent, so unless there is a conscious decision to keep the range open, e.g. to use superior boxing skills, most fights close in fast, at which point grabbing and grappling takes place.
- Going to the ground is common in fights that go on for any length of time, often because the combatants simply fall over something or each other. However, by the time most fights reach the ground someone is winning and what happens on the ground is often a beating rather than a fight. It is relatively rare for a fight to go to the ground while both combatants still have a decent chance to win.

Facing Aggression

Fortunately, most of the people who start fights are not very skilled. They rely mainly on picking fights with people they think they can beat (or restricting themselves to posturing

Aggressive body language

We recognize aggressive body language instinctively. Snarling, shouting, 'pecking' the head forward and so forth are all part of 'posturing' intended to cause fear and intimidation.

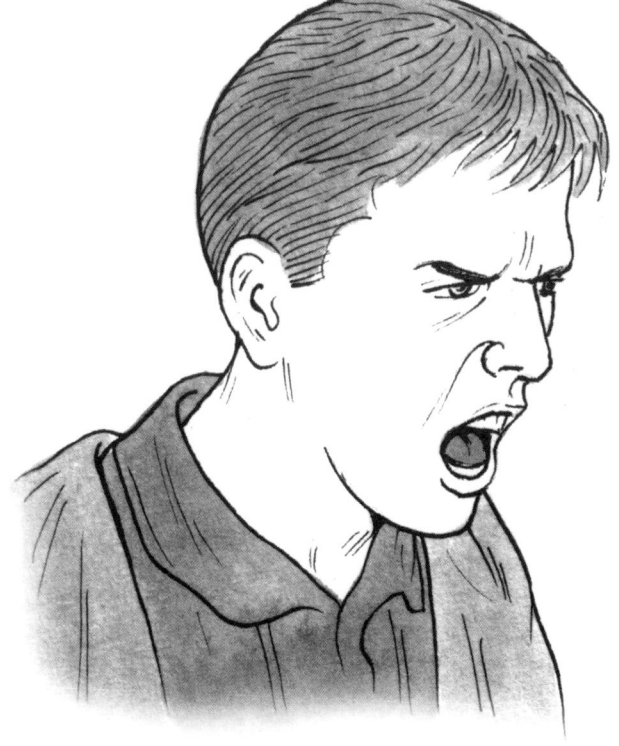

and threats if they are not sure) and using sheer aggression to defeat their victim. This can work very well, since most ordinary people are unused to raw aggression.

As a result, most 'fights' are not really fights at all. What they are, is someone picking a victim, establishing dominance by posturing and threats, and then unloading a barrage of blows once they are sure the fight can be won. More than anything else, good training must teach the student to overcome their fear and react intelligently and effectively. Without this, you are beaten before the fight has started.

MARTIAL ARTS vs UNARMED COMBAT AND SELF-DEFENCE

There is a difference between unarmed combat and self-defence. Unarmed combat is all about killing or incapacitating an opponent as quickly as possible. For a soldier on

TIP: COMMON ATTACKS

- Big swinging punches are the commonest attack by far. Usually the first attack comes from the strong hand – the right in most people.
- Jabs and other lead-hand punches are very uncommon. An aggressor might swing right-left-right, but is very unlikely to open with a lead-hand shot.
- Kicks are normally used against downed opponents but are occasionally directed at the legs and lower body. High kicks, and any sort of trained martial arts kicks, are very rare in real fights.
- Knee strikes sometimes follow a grab. This is an instinctive movement and is thus fairly common where a fight has become a wrestling match.
- One-handed grabs are common. The usual pattern is to grab clothing with the weak hand and hit with the strong one. Grabs with the strong hand are normally used to exert dominance in domestic violence situations. They are not common in fights.
- Two-handed grabs may be used to exert dominance or to set up for a headbutt.

Idiotically high kicks

This sort of thing is incredibly rare in the real world, for the very good reason that it does not work. Kick low if you kick at all.

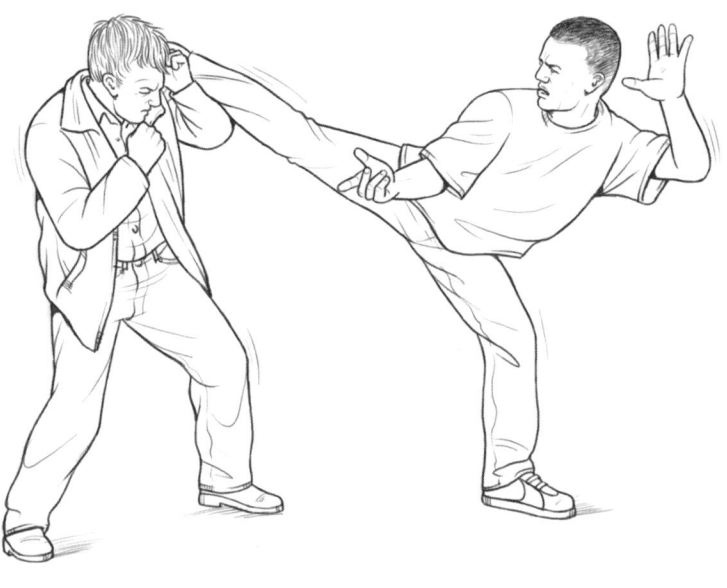

a mission, that is exactly what is needed. However, for civilians there are other considerations, most notably laws governing the use of force against other people. There are circumstances when a civilian is entitled to injure or even kill a person, but in order to avoid legal trouble the use of force must be appropriate to the circumstances. Thus, while unarmed combat skills can be used for self-defence, not all unarmed combat is self-defence as such.

Any responsible instructor will ensure that his students understand the relevant law governing self-defence, just as military instructors ensure that troops understand when it is acceptable to use their weapons or unarmed combat skills, and when it is not.

Martial Arts

A great variety of martial arts and self-defence training is available for anyone who cares to look. However, care should be taken when selecting a class. Almost any martial arts instructor will say that their art is excellent for self-defence, and in some cases they are correct. However, most martial arts contain a large amount of material that is not really useful to someone looking for pure self-defence. Some teach 'self-defence' techniques that simply will not work and might get the user killed or seriously injured.

The commonest reason for this deficiency is lack of knowledge. Most martial arts practitioners train against other martial arts people, usually from the same system. They get to be very good at dealing with their own style. It should also be noted that many martial arts teach defences specific to their own system. For example, Karate blocks are great for dealing with Karate attacks, but not so good against wild hooking blows thrown by the typical 'street' aggressor.

Martial Arts and Sports for Self-Defence

- **Boxing** – Some of the best striking skills you can get, also stance, footwork and strike defences.

Sparring to build skills and fighting spirit.
- **Brazilian Ju-Jitsu** – Teaches mainly groundfighting skills. Excellent for 'positional' skills, i.e. learning to get an assailant off you. Also joint locks, chokes and strangles.
- **Kickboxing** – Similar to boxing but also with kicks. Note that many kickboxing kicks are not really suitable for self-defence.
- **Mixed Martial Arts (MMA)** – Teaches all-round fighting skills. Also excellent for fitness and conditioning.
- **Judo** – Probably the best 'standup' grappling training available. Teaches throws and takedowns, and how to avoid being taken to the ground. Also some groundfighting and an excellent fitness workout.
- **Ju-Jitsu** – Teaches all-round fighting with kicks, strikes and grappling skills including groundwork.
- **Muay Thai, or Thai Boxing** – Probably the best striking art of all, with some grappling and clinching skills too.

Just because an art is not listed here does not mean it is worthless for self-defence. These arts were chosen because they are widely available and tend to be the same wherever the class is found. Quality can of course vary from class to class.

Close-in grappling

Many fights become a close-quarters wrestling match. A martial art that does not prepare you for this is not a good choice for self-defence.

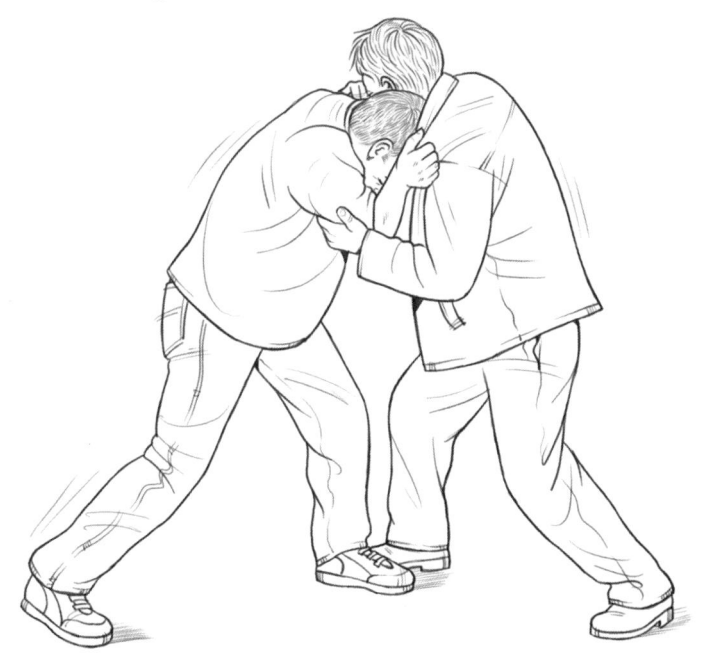

Self-Defence Training

There are plenty of self-defence courses on offer, but they can vary considerably. Some are simply 'applied martial arts', offering what amounts to a watered-down martial arts syllabus which in come cases can be entirely divorced from reality. Others are decent enough in some areas but do not deal with a wide enough spectrum of threats. Examples include courses on 'breakaway techniques' which are designed to release the user from a

TIP:
SPECIALIZED MARTIAL ARTS

If you decide to learn a martial art, keep in mind what it is intended for.

As an example, Taekwondo is a striking-only art with rules against certain strikes. Taekwondo fighters often become very good at fighting one another in a formal sparring match, but can develop 'blind spots' regarding many of the things that are not permitted in their competition rules. This does not make Taekwondo bad. Far from it – it is an excellent sport for building fighting spirit, developing balance and fitness, and learning some powerful kicks. What it is not is a complete self-defence system.

Similarly, Judo teaches awesome grappling skills, is excellent for fitness, and allows players to develop a deep understanding of how to keep their footing while sending others crashing to the floor. But it does not teach how to deal with strikes, because these are not allowed in a Judo match.

grab. So far so good, but the range of threats is much wider than that.

Good self-defence training teaches students to deal with all of the likely threats, and concentrates on a small number of highly flexible skills rather than enormous numbers of specialized and complex techniques. It also includes as much realism as is practicable, simulating the stress and fear of an assault. In the military, battlefield skills are practised under conditions that are as realistic as possible, so that troops do not panic under stress and forget their training.

Good self-defence trainers have learned this lesson and adopted the concept, if not the exact same methods.

Going Your Own Way

If it is not possible to find a self-defence instructor who can provide suitable all-round training, it is possible to find the necessary components from what is on offer and essentially build yourself a set of skills. For example, a boxing or kickboxing class will teach good striking skills plus sparring and fitness work while Judo or Ju-Jitsu will provide excellent grappling skills. This is not an ideal solution as it does mean taking part in activities that are not all that relevant to self-defence, but some of those activities are good fun and/or useful for fitness, so the time is not entirely wasted.

It is also possible to obtain some training equipment and do some work with a friend. Care is necessary here – formal classes have insurance

Deflecting a grab

The aggressor's attempt to grab has been knocked aside, but this has not ended the situation. What's to stop them trying again?

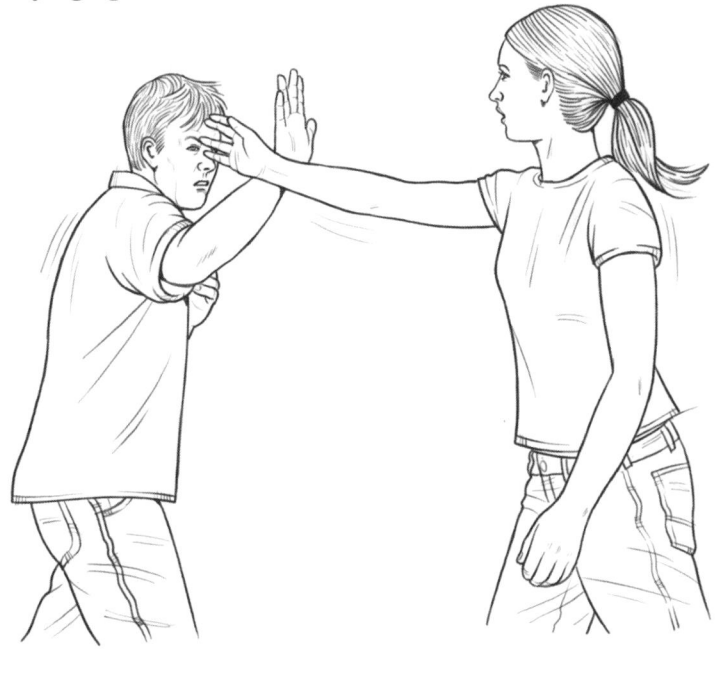

TIP: EVALUATE WHAT YOU ARE TAUGHT

It is worth evaluating what is on offer in the light of the information in this book. Different answers to the same threat may be equally valid ... but they may not. The techniques in this book have been pressure-tested in real combat against someone trying to cause injury or even death. Others may not have.

in place and qualified instructors to ensure that risks are kept to a minimum. It is better to find a class if at all possible, backing this up with some fitness training or relatively low-risk activities such as bag work or striking focus pads.

In particular, practising choking and strangling techniques without proper supervision is not a good idea at all.

Finding a Good Class

It is hard to say exactly what makes a good self-defence or martial arts class. However, there are certain warning signs that can help you avoid wasting your time in a poor one. You can still get a lot out of a class that exhibits some or all of these traits, but generally speaking the quality of self-defence training suffers when these things happen:

- **Air-punching** – You cannot learn to deliver force with a strike without hitting something. Good training involves hitting focus pads, punchbags or other resilient objects.
- **Overcomplication** – Complicated techniques simply do not work under pressure. Good training emphasizes simple, reliable tools that work under a range of circumstances.
- **Excessive 'martial-artyness'** – Long lectures about 'samurai spirit' and philosophy, excessive time spent bowing and performing obscure rituals. Good training is simple and to the point.
- **Wild claims and secret techniques** – Elite Ninja Death-Touch techniques do not exist. A class that promises to reveal unknowable secrets of the elders after years of training is probably just trying to retain members for financial reasons. Effective techniques are simple and quite mundane.
- **Excessively formal, neat and tidy techniques** – Good training looks a bit scruffy because students are

pushing their limits and responding to a range of threats rather than simply working through neat set-pieces.

• **Too many grades** – Some martial arts have a great many belts and grades, often as a way to generate revenue. Not only is this expensive but it usually results in vast numbers of techniques being taught, many of which are of dubious usefulness at best.

Working a bag

A wildly swinging bag may impress ignorant onlookers, but a good strike or kick dents it and causes it to shudder rather than swing.

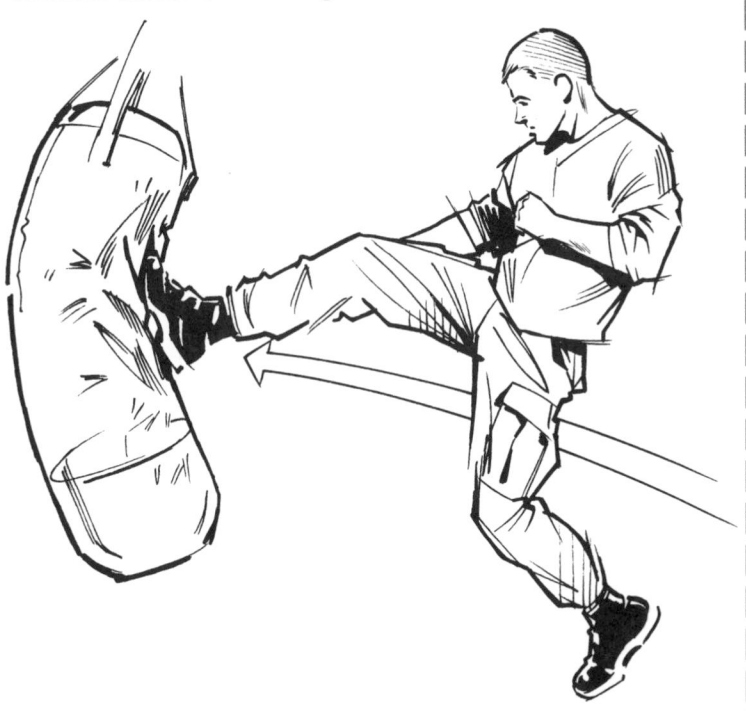

Striking post training

Martial arts striking posts (*Makiwara*) can be used to train a range of blows including punches and hammerfists. The latter use the base of the hand and not the knuckles.

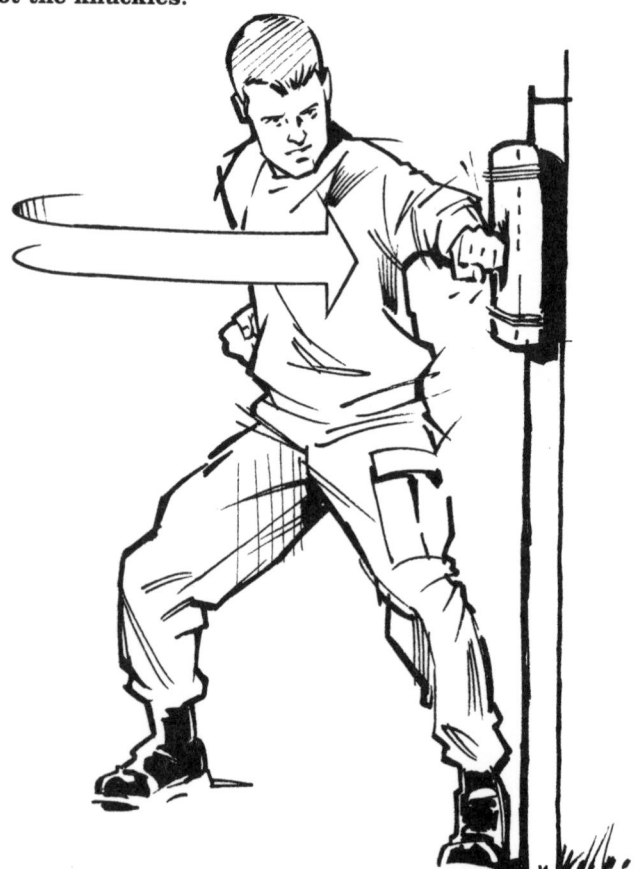

LEGAL CONSIDERATIONS

Soldiers carrying out a legitimate mission against an enemy force need not worry too much about legal considerations as their use of force has already been sanctioned by their superiors. Obviously, there are still some considerations regarding civilian casualties, surrendered enemy personnel and the like, but overall soldiers in wartime are free to engage the enemy as necessary. Indeed, they are expected to do so.

Military personnel also encounter dangerous circumstances where the situation is not entirely clear. Troops are often deployed on peacekeeping operations or to protect humanitarian aid workers in a lawless environment. In such situations, soldiers have to follow Rules of Engagement that indicate what actions are lawful and which are not.

Rules of Engagement

Civilians, too, are subject to rules of engagement. The law on self-defence varies from one country to another, and it is wise to check on the local circumstances when travelling. The general situation tends to be that there are specific laws against doing violence (or even threatening violence) against other people, but self-defence makes these actions permissible if the circumstances necessitate them. Thus if, for no good reason, you punched some random person you just met, you would be committing a crime. However, if that person took a swing at you, you would be entirely within your rights to use force to stop them.

Your Right to Self-Defence

You have the right to use force to protect yourself or someone else from violence or crime, but your response must be proportionate to the level of threat you face. Your use

TIP: THE LEGAL ISSUE

The whole legal question can all be summed up like this: if, after you have dealt with the threat, someone asked you 'did you really need to do that?' and you can honestly answer 'Yes, and here are the reasons ...', then you will not have committed a crime if your answer seems reasonable. You might have to explain yourself to the police, but if you can show that you genuinely perceived a need to defend yourself, then you will have remained within the law.

Imminent attack

Clenched fists are a clear indication of violent intent. The aggressor here has 'chambered' his right hand to strike – you will need to act fast or get hit.

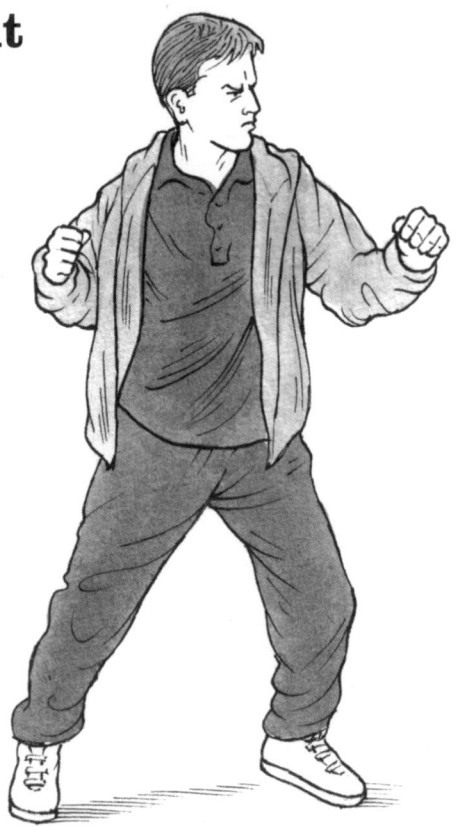

of force is only self-defence as long as there is a threat – if you have to hit someone 92 times to make them stop attacking you, then there is nothing wrong with that if they were still a threat after 91. If you then continue to beat on them after they are helpless, you become the aggressor and can be prosecuted.

Note that your opinion of how much the person deserves a good kicking for hitting you does not count – self-defence applies only while there is a threat. If you want to get some payback after the threat is nullified that's your choice, but you will answer for it.

Use of Force

You do not have to wait for someone to hit you before you 'fight back'. Not only is this not necessary, it is also undesirable as you could be taken out of the fight by that first blow. You are entitled to use an appropriate level of force as soon as you recognize a threat.

Note the use of the word 'appropriate', not 'minimum'. The law does not require a person to carefully work out exactly what level of force is required to stop an attack, nor to match a given threat with a textbook response. So long as your actions are reasonable under the circumstances you are justified in law. Thus someone who uses a weapon against an unarmed but physically superior individual is probably not committing a crime.

Perception of Threat

The level of force used must be appropriate to the threat as you perceive it to be – and you have to be able to justify your perception. Hitting someone because 'they looked a bit dodgy' is not acceptable, but if you can explain what signs of aggression you saw and why you feared for your safety, then so long as your response was proportionate to the threat you

thought you faced, your actions are justified in law.

This does mean that an honest mistake can still constitute self-defence. If, for example, someone gave you reason to believe they were about to hit you and you knocked them out, they might claim your actions were unreasonable because they were 'only having a laugh'. However, if you can show that you genuinely thought there was a threat

TIP: SELF-DEFENCE AND THE LAW

Self-defence law is in fact very much as common sense would suggest:

- You are entitled to use force to deal with a threat.
- You are entitled to use as much force as you need.
- The amount of force you use must not be excessive.
- Once the threat is nullified, you must stop fighting.
- You can strike first if the circumstances warrant it.
- You may arm yourself if the threat is severe enough to justify this.

Crossing the line

There is no doubt about the threat here – the aggressor has made an attacking move and needs to be dealt with decisively.

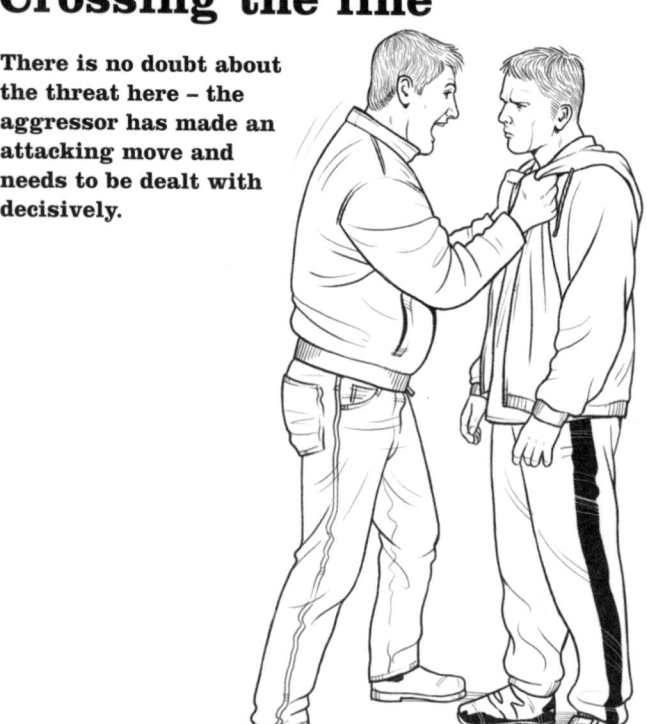

that justified knocking the 'aggressor' out, then doing so would be legal.

When It's Over, It's Over

Once the threat is nullified, you must stop because further violence is not self-defence at all. You are entitled to ensure your safety by making sure the attacker is unable to continue, but once that is obvious then you are expected and required by law to cease using violence.

Much the same comments apply to military personnel. If someone ran at an armed patrol waving a weapon, they would be entitled to shoot in order to stop him. Even if the weapon later turned out to be a realistic replica, they would still have acted lawfully because a lethal threat was perceived – and a lethal threat justifies a lethal response such as opening fire.

If the aggressor was hit but still kept on charging, the troops would be justified in continuing to fire. If the aggressor went down but kept pointing his weapon at them, they would still be justified. There is a possibility that the target might be disabled but the troops might not yet have realized it. They would be justified in making sure the threat was nullified during this time. But if he was lying helpless and disabled, then further shooting on their part would be excessive.

Extreme Measures

There are circumstances where extreme force is justified. There is no tit-for-tat 'he's got a knife so I can kill him' principle, but if your only course of action to stop an attacker from doing something extremely serious to you resulted in his death or very serious injury, then so long as your actions were warranted by the circumstances, they would be lawful.

Note that you are not required by law to try to escape from a situation or to surrender property rather than fighting for it. However, if you do claim self-defence then you will need to show why you could not have used other means to end the situation without violence. For example, if you chose to fight someone when you had a clear opportunity to escape, you would be required to explain why you did not take it. There may be a good reason of course, which is fair enough. But if there is not, then this might undermine your assertion that you only did what you had to in order to protect yourself.

TIP: STAYING OUT OF LEGAL TROUBLE

As a general rule, your claim to have acted in self-defence will be greatly strengthened if you can show that you did not want to fight and took steps to end the situation without violence. You are not required by law to do any of these things, and indeed the aggressor might not give you the chance to, but if you had the opportunity and instead chose to bash his head in, your claim of self-defence might be weakened.

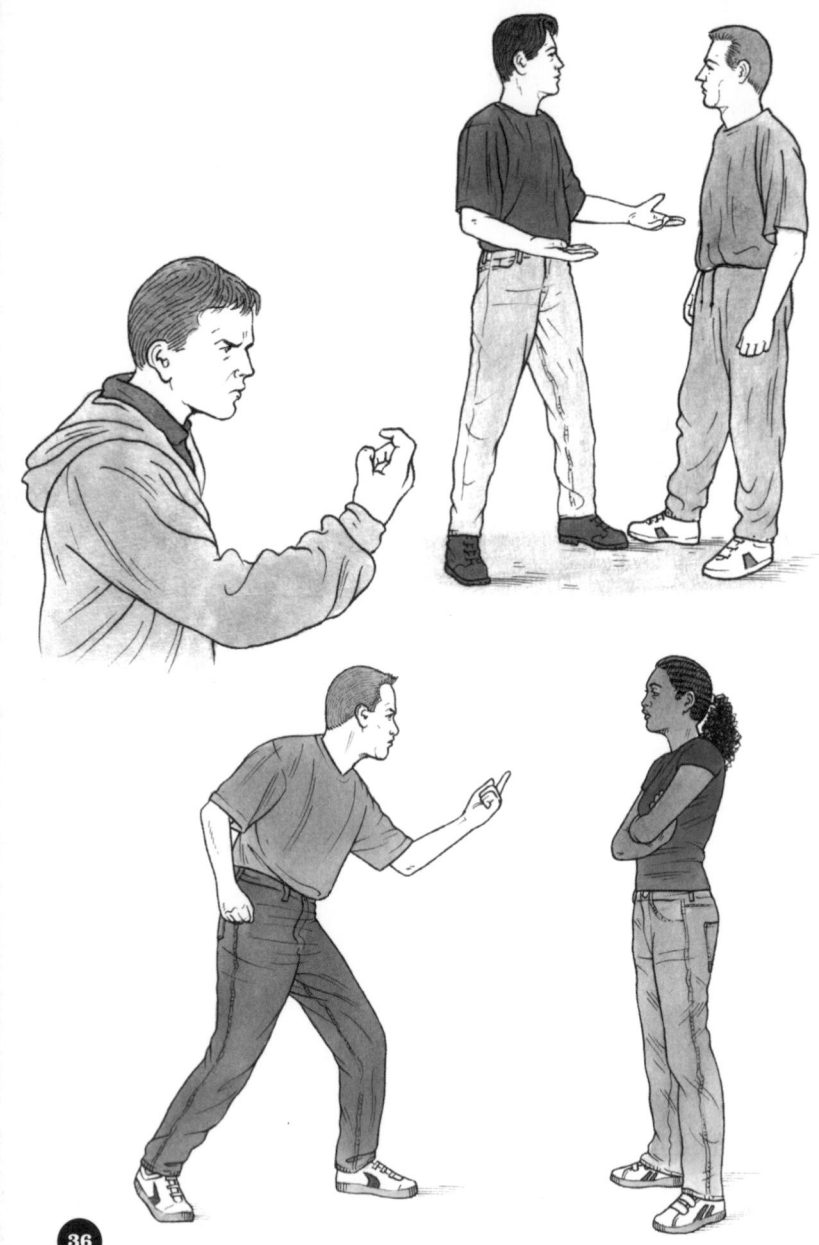

2

If you know how, you can defeat someone without laying a hand on them.

Special forces troops are very, very good at fighting. However, this is not their primary function. They exist to carry out their missions as efficiently as possible. If this can be done without contact with the enemy, so much the better. Indeed, the motto of the British Special Boat Service is 'Not by Strength, By Guile', reflecting their ability to get the job done without the enemy even knowing something was happening a lot of the time. Special forces troops fight when they have to, and use other means to accomplish their objectives whenever possible.

There is nothing new in the concept of winning without fighting. The ancient Chinese general Sun Tzu wrote that the pinnacle of brilliance was to defeat the enemy without actual combat. In a military context, he suggested that misdirection, deception, stealth and all manner of other tricks could be used to accomplish the defeat of the enemy or at least to make the fight easier.

SELF-DEFENCE WITHOUT FIGHTING

The goal of self-defence is not actually to defeat or destroy the enemy, any more than eliminating

. . . .

Left: If someone is being aggressive but has not initiated violence, then non-violent measures may be your best option.

Preparation

Win Without Fighting

Standing firm

Most people who start confrontations do not actually want to fight. If you can remain calm and do not show signs of giving in, they will often be deterred.

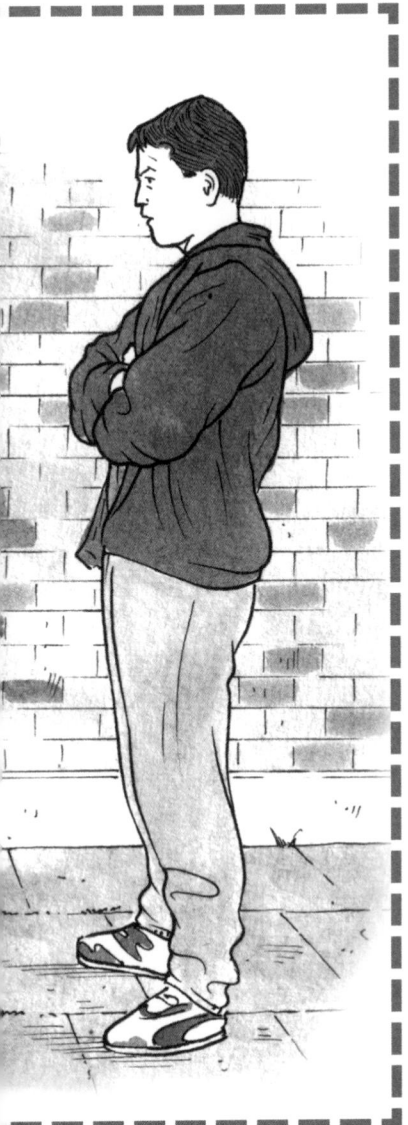

the guards is the primary mission of a special forces team sent to rescue hostages. The goal is to preserve your own safety and to get out of the situation with as little damage as possible. If that means fighting then so be it – you must fight and win. But there are other methods that can work just as well.

Sometimes, of course, violence finds you no matter what you do to avoid it, and sometimes it is better to enter into a confrontation on your own terms than to let an ongoing problem continue. For example, there is often no point in getting into arguments over trivial matters, but sometimes it is necessary to take a stand here and now rather than allow someone to get away with bullying you.

Pick your fights wisely. If you draw a line you must defend it, or else you will simply get pushed around even more. But do be aware that any confrontation or argument can escalate into violence. It is usually unlikely, but it is still wise to be mentally prepared in case things go wrong. Violence, when it happens, happens fast.

AVOIDING CONFLICT

Soldiers sent to carry out a mission against the enemy will almost certainly have to engage in combat at some point. But special forces in particular are extremely good at avoiding fights they do not need to

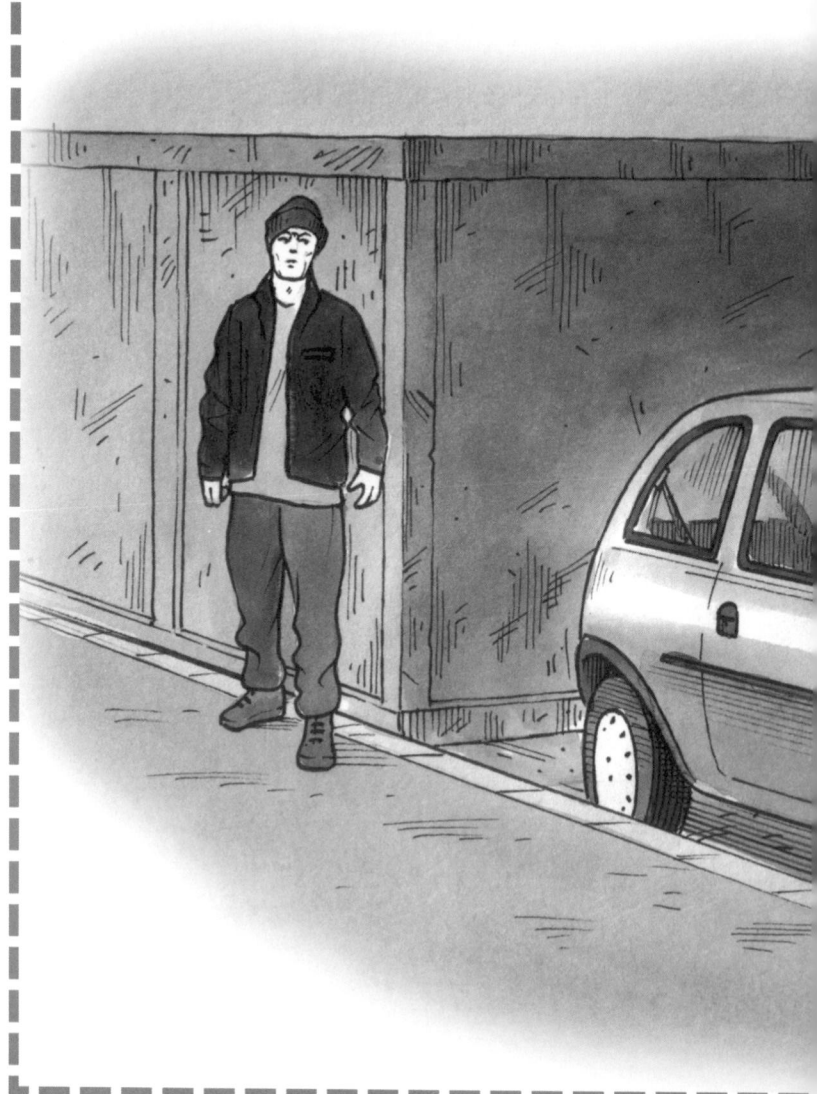

Avoiding dangerous places

Many situations can be avoided by using common sense. For example, park somewhere that does not offer concealment to a potential attacker to lie in wait for your return.

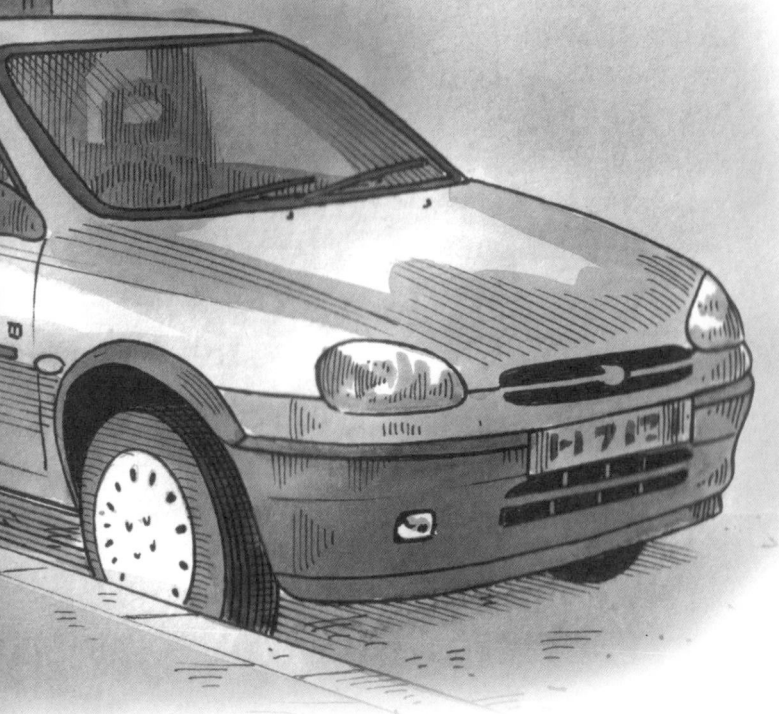

get into. They evade enemy patrols wherever possible, sometimes hiding from enemies that they could easily 'take out'. These people are the absolute best warriors on the planet, but they still pick their fights with care. This philosophy carries over into self-defence. It makes good sense to avoid unnecessary conflict, and this is entirely in keeping with the goal of self-defence – you cannot possibly get hurt in a fight that did not happen.

There is nothing cowardly about threat avoidance, although some people find that their ego gets in the way. They want to show everyone how tough they are and consider threat avoidance to be a sign of weakness. That is a choice we all have to make, but if an SAS squad armed with grenades and automatic weapons is willing to hide from a lone sentry, then surely it is acceptable for the rest of us to avoid unnecessary conflict.

THREAT AVOIDANCE

Everyone knows about shortcuts down dark alleys and talking to strangers in cars, yet a surprising number of people cheerfully disregard advice they have been hearing since childhood and put themselves in unnecessary danger. Victims of assault often say afterwards that they could see it coming. The problem, then, is not being able to spot danger but being willing to act on this information and avoid it.

There is not that much to threat avoidance except common sense. Fast-food outlets and taxi ranks are obvious flashpoints for violence just after the bars close. Poorly lit or lonely places are hazardous at night. Some areas have a bad reputation and some are just obviously unsafe. Yet people blithely wander through these places with a shrug and the statement that 'it'll be all right'. And actually, it usually is, but you can reduce your chances of becoming a victim by staying away from such places.

Quite often, a gang of teenagers or young men hanging around are doing just that and do not mean anyone any harm, but if you do not like the look of someone, it is best to remove yourself from the vicinity. It is often obvious when someone is looking for trouble – your instincts will pick up clues from their attitude and demeanour. If you can leave, or stay away in the first place, it is probably wise to do so.

WHAT AN AGGRESSOR WANTS

If someone is looking for trouble, whether it is to do violence just for the sake of it, or for robbery, rape or any other purpose, they may come to you. You cannot always know what a potential aggressor is looking for, but one thing you can be sure of – it is

Reading aggressive behaviour

Generally, a person who is behaving aggressively but keeping his distance is 'posturing' and probably does not intend violence. If he wants to get close to you, he does intend to get physical.

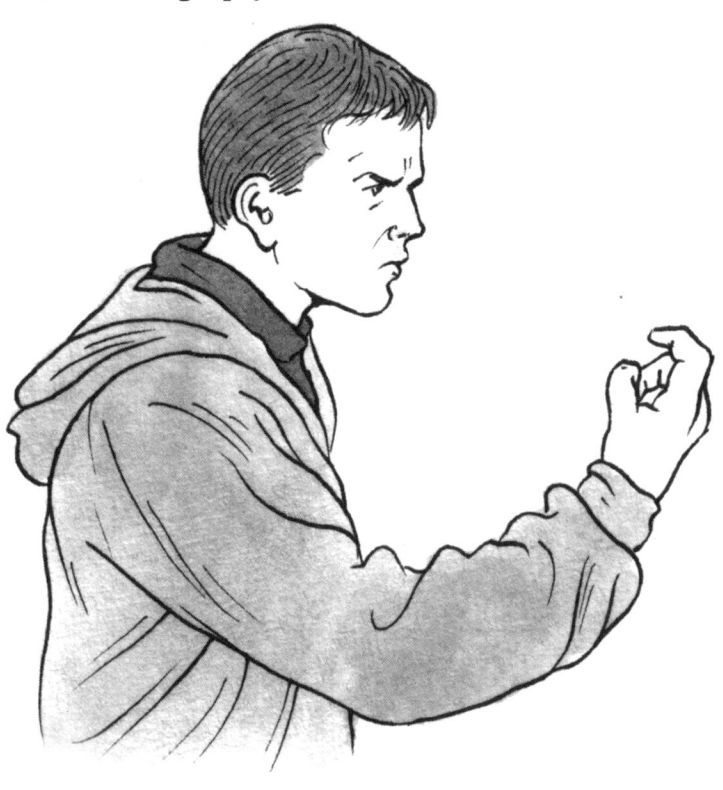

not a fight. That might seem odd, but the truth is that an aggressor wants a victim, not a struggle.

Aggressors, even the ones who just want to hurt someone, are out to get what they want at a minimal cost to themselves. You cannot predict how high a price the aggressor is willing to pay in terms of risk or pain from your efforts at resistance, but you can make sure he knows the price will be high. He will weigh the gain against the risk and if you seem like more trouble than you are worth he will look for another victim.

TIP: SERIAL KILLERS AND THEIR VICTIMS

To take a fairly extreme example, as a rule serial killers select victims that they think they can control. Thus someone who comes across as lacking in self-esteem and who displays submissive behaviour is a more likely victim than someone who is assertive, for the very simple reason that the latter is likely to be far more difficult to control.

ATTACK-PROOFING YOURSELF

You cannot make yourself 100 per cent attack-proof, but you can be an obviously expensive target. This does not necessarily mean acting tough and aggressive – indeed, doing so can actually trigger confrontations rather than deterring them – but there are some simple measures that will make most potential aggressors leave you alone in favour of an easier victim.

Firstly, do not make yourself a really easy target. Someone who is wandering along with their hood up listening to music on headphones, or totally absorbed in a phone conversation, is very easy to sneak up on. Someone who places themselves in a lonely, dark place is making it easy for an aggressor and runs a higher risk than a more cautious individual. You do of course have every right to go where you please and to listen to whatever you like, but it is worth being aware of the risks.

Don't Look Like a Victim

Your posture and demeanour are extremely important in avoiding being selected as a victim. A slouched or defensive posture with arms crossed, looking at the ground, makes you look like an easier victim than someone who is upright, alert and businesslike. If you appear confident and in control of your surroundings, you are much less likely to be chosen as a victim.

Too close!

The defender (right) has let an aggressive or agitated person get far too close. At this distance, it is virtually impossible to stop a punch or grab in time.

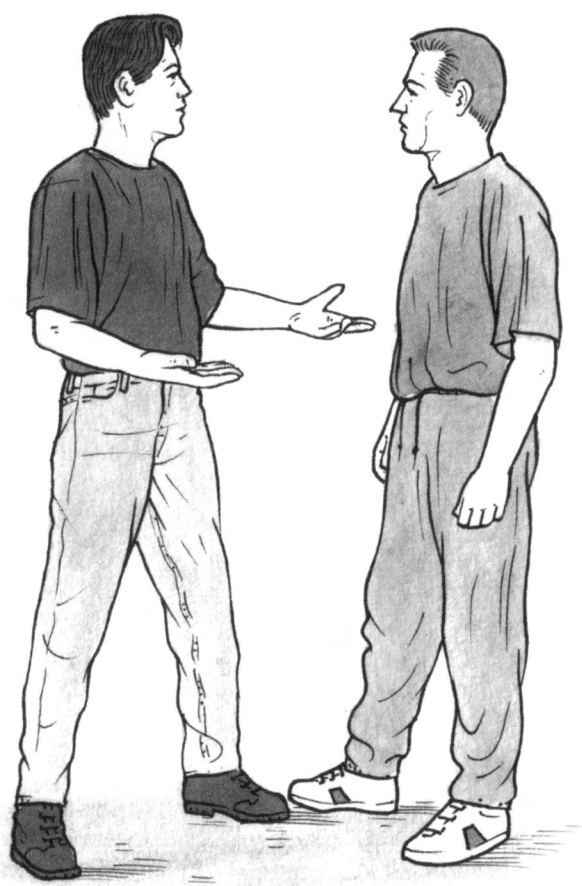

Keep your distance

If the aggressor remains this far away, it may be possible to de-escalate the situation. He would find it difficult to launch an effective surprise attack from here.

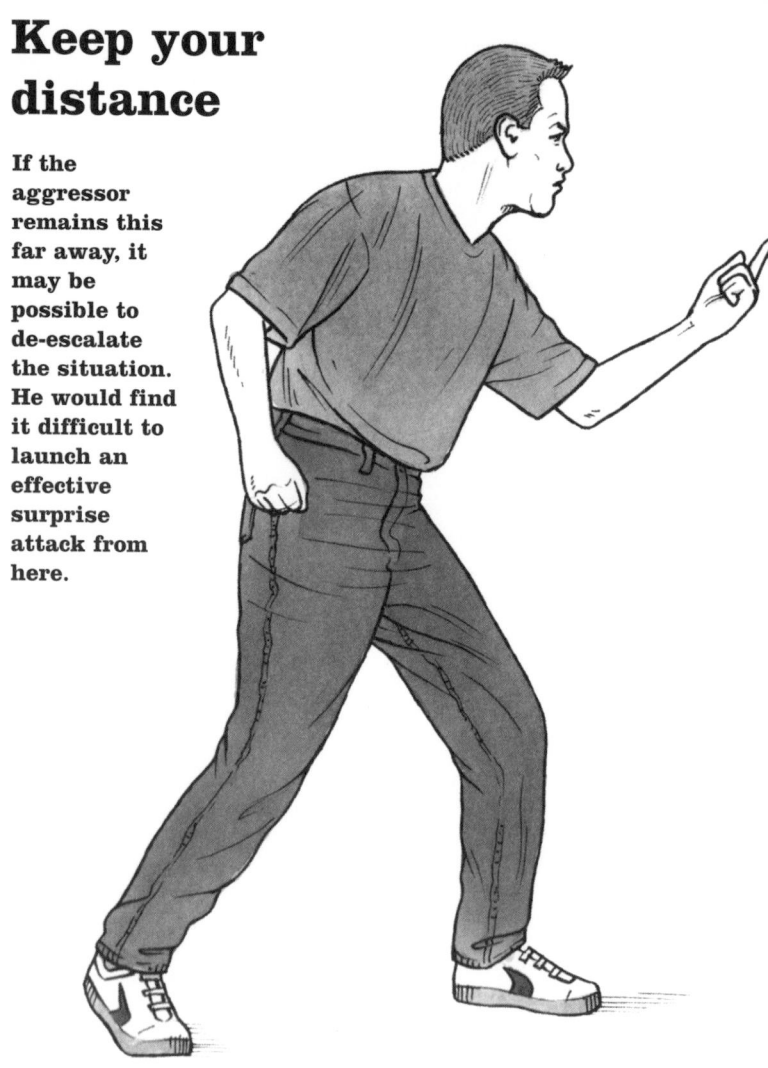

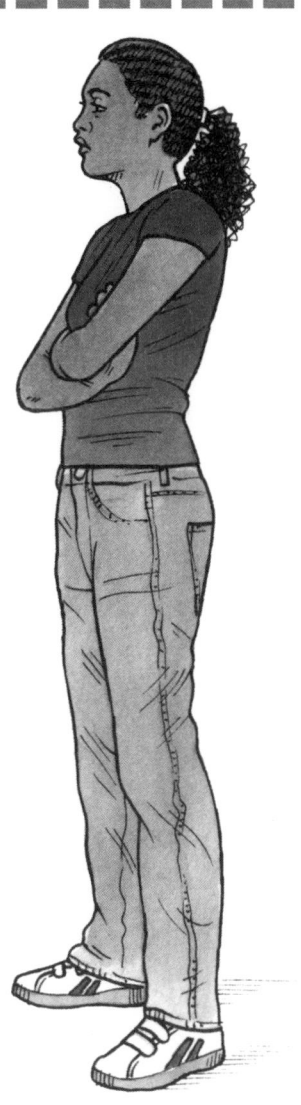

Don't React Like A Victim

How you react to a developing situation is also critical. There is nothing wrong with being polite and considerate, so long as it is clear that you are choosing to be civil rather than being coerced by the aggressor. It is possible to head off many potentially serious problems by taking a stand early and making it clear that you will not accept the situation.

This stand can take one of two forms, which are best described as deterrence and de-escalation. Deterrence is a fairly 'hard' response, though it does not have to be rude or aggressive. Essentially, you are saying something like 'hey, no more of that' and making your displeasure very clear. This can work well if you are physically a reasonable match for the potential aggressor, but it can also lead to escalation.

De-Escalation

De-escalation is the opposite approach to deterrence. Instead of making a harsh response you try to calm things down or make an excuse to cover your withdrawal. This can mean apologizing for something that is not your fault. If it ends the threat then it is still a victory. De-escalation is often a good strategy as it allows the aggressor to go away without losing face. Many confrontations are fuelled by ego as much as anything else, so trying to back the aggressor down may push him into a position in which his ego forces him to attack you. One problem with de-escalation is that it does allow the aggressor to think he has won. In a one-off confrontation with someone you will never see again, this is not a problem and is probably the best strategy. However, in an ongoing situation de-escalation may not always be the best solution.

DOMESTIC SITUATIONS

The domestic environment is somewhat different to a confrontation between strangers outside a fast food outlet at 2.00 a.m. on Saturday morning. 'Domestic' in this context does not just mean between partners but any situation where there are social rules in place. That can include workplaces, social groups, family events such as weddings and so forth. If the other party thinks that they 'won' a given confrontation, this may validate their behaviour. They have no real reason not to do the same things again.

Under such circumstances the only real solution is to make sure that the other party knows that their conduct will not be tolerated. This can precipitate a very unpleasant confrontation, but it is the only chance to sort out a deteriorating domestic environment. If this fails, you will have to accept being bullied, perhaps the victim of violence, or get out of the situation altogether – which is easier said than done.

JUST RUN AWAY, MAYBE?

There are still far too many people who subscribe to the 'oh, just run away' school of thought on self-defence. Running is an option under some circumstances, but it is more often impractical. For example, there is no point in an overweight 50-year-old trying to outrun a 19-year-old who plays football all day, and running at all when you have a toddler with you is an exercise in pointlessness.

If you do need to run, then blindly fleeing is not a good idea. Special forces troops receive extensive training in Escape and Evasion techniques, and for good reason. They are taught to seek safety and to lose their pursuers rather than just

TIP: RUN, OR STAY?

Running is an option, but you should only run if it offers a decent chance of escape, or if there are simply no better options. Make an opportunity to flee and take yourself to safety if you can. If it is not practical, you will have to deal with the situation where you are.

legging it across the countryside. You can do likewise, running towards safety rather than away from danger. Public places with lots of people are a good bet, but any area covered by CCTV cameras offers a reasonable second option. An aggressor may be deterred by the possibility of video evidence for a conviction, though this is by no means guaranteed.

Making a Break

Before you can escape you must make the initial break. If you simply turn to run, an aggressor who is facing you and within about 3–4m (9–12ft) will almost certainly catch you before you have gone a few steps. You must make an opportunity to escape. One option is to 'bash and dash' – hitting the aggressor hard enough that he is unable to chase you for a moment. If you hit him hard enough, he may not be able to come after you at all, or may not want to!

Another option is to use deception and distraction. For example, if someone is demanding your wallet, handing it over may not guarantee safety – some muggers will brutalize or even kill their victims after being given property. So instead of passing it over you might toss it at his feet and take off. Given the choice between picking up the money or going after you, he will normally take what he is given, which grants you a chance to be some distance away by the time he is ready to give chase.

TIP: WHAT YOU MUST NEVER DO

The one thing you must never do under any circumstances is allow yourself to be taken elsewhere. Once you are in an aggressor's chosen location, your chances of escape diminish enormously and you can be certain that he has something very grim in mind.

IF ALL ELSE FAILS

If avoidance, deterrence, de-escalation and escape have all failed, then you will have to resort to physical means. At this point, your mindset and will to win are more important than any fighting skills you may have. People have successfully defended themselves with nothing more than biting and scratching, and skilled fighters have been beaten because they gave up.

Strength, physical toughness and knowledge are extremely useful tools, but they are worth nothing if you are already beaten in your own mind. So long as you do not give up, you still have a chance.

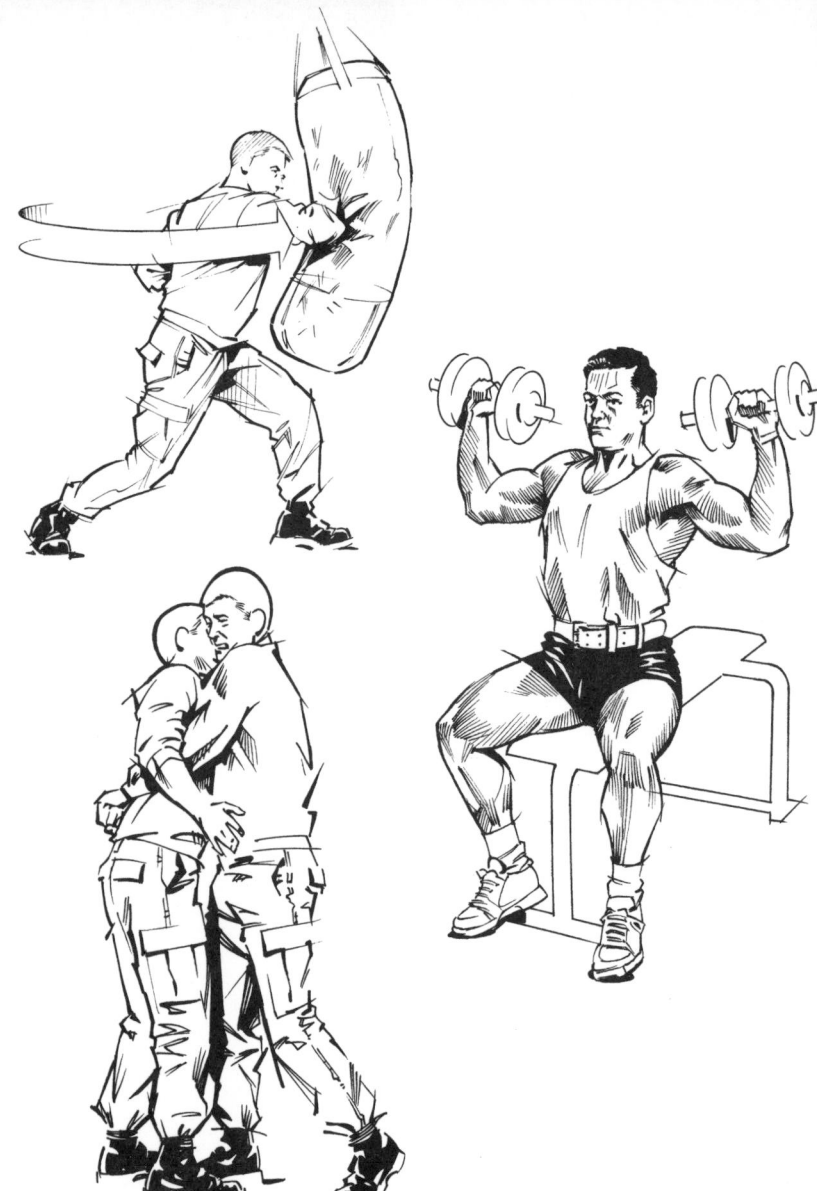

Military personnel are trained to win. Much of what goes on in training is related to fitness or specific skills like weapons handling, survival or communications, but threaded through everything the soldier does is a common theme; his training is designed to increase his confidence and mental toughness.

Military forces very rarely fight to the death. Normally one side loses confidence and either negotiates a surrender or tries to retreat. Some attempts to withdraw are conducted with skill and determination; others collapse into a rout. Here, too, the deciding factor is morale, i.e. confidence in the ability to get the job done.

MENTAL TOUGHNESS

Napoleon Bonaparte, one of the greatest generals in history, recognized this factor when he said 'the moral is to the physical as three is to one'. In other words, the man who led his armies to conquer all of Europe knew that while tactics and equipment were important, the key factor was the willingness of his troops to keep fighting when things looked bad.

. . . .

Left: You can train to defend yourself in many ways. Technique training with a partner can be complemented by fitness work whenever possible.

3

Once a situation kicks off, you fight with what you have. Good preparation can literally save your life.

Training to Win

Preparation

Front cover

Sometimes your only option is to cover up and 'ride' a blow. However, this is not a winning strategy. If you panic and stay covered up, all you will do is make the beating take longer. If you want to win, you will have to take the fight to the enemy.

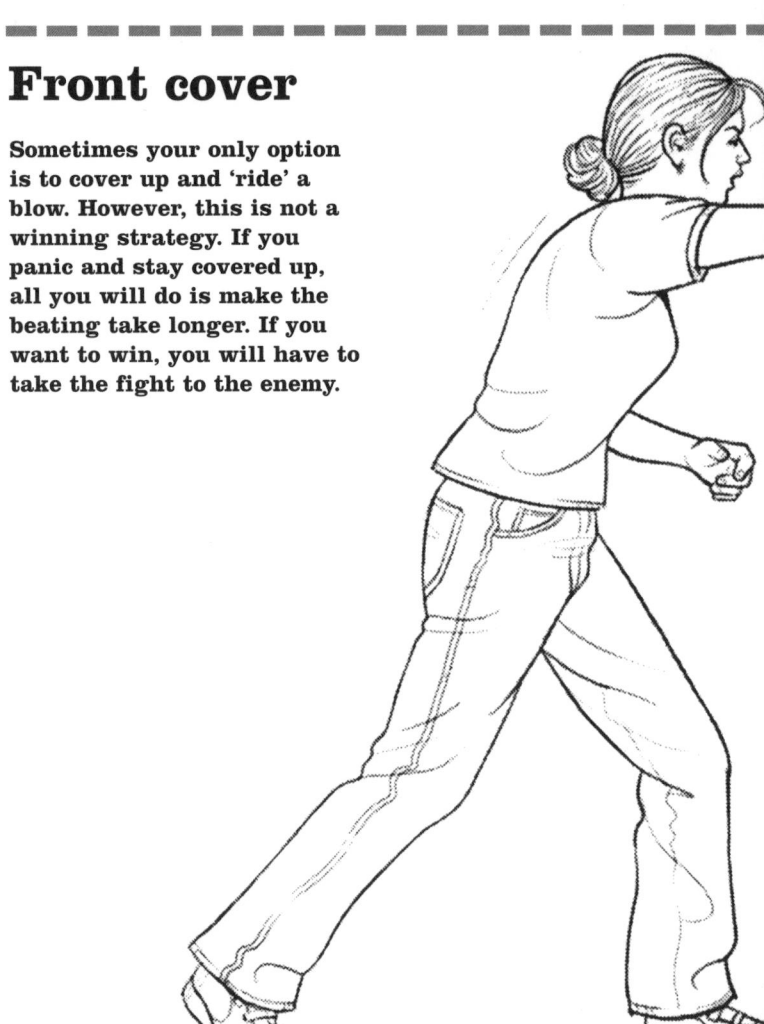

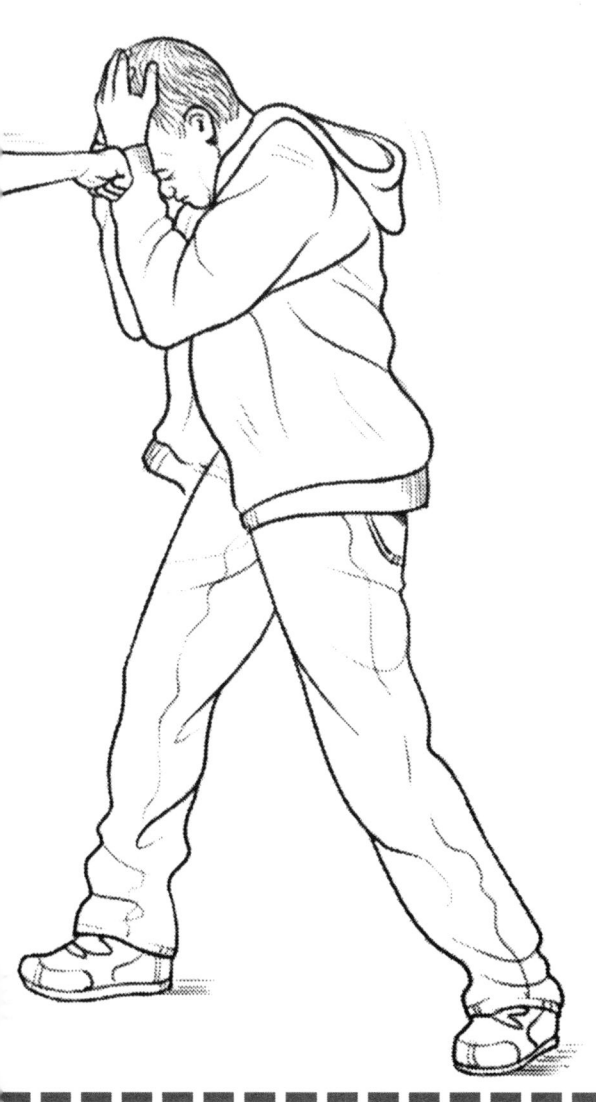

TIP: FEAR OF FAILURE

Many people never attempt the things they would like to do because they are afraid of failing. Say you want to learn to fly a helicopter ... does it matter that you cannot because you tried and failed, or because you never tried? The result is the same. On the other hand, if you try you might succeed.

This is where training yourself to win begins – with being willing to try.

It cannot be stressed enough that the ability to function in the fight environment is the most important skill you can develop, and that ability is entirely mental. No skills or physical strength will save you if you panic and fold up in the face of aggression – you have to meet the problem head-on and do something about it.

That means you have to be able to make the decision to fight for your survival when your instincts may be telling you to curl into a ball and hope it all goes away.

A Winning Attitude

Many battles have been won by forces that would have been considered beaten in any rational analysis, but who just refused to give up. Others have hung in the balance and been won by the side that refused to quit no matter how bad the situation got. It is this determination to win that allows small groups of special forces troops to carry out apparently suicidal missions and emerge not only victorious, but often unscathed.

It is possible to gain some of these advantages for yourself. True, no civilian has the benefit of elite forces training, but some of the methods can be adapted. For one thing, success becomes a habit. It begins with the realization that you can win; you can succeed. Maybe you will never be the best in your field, but you can achieve. You can beat your chin-up record, or lose a couple of pounds, or shave a couple of seconds off your time for three laps of the park ... or whatever goals you set yourself.

Building Self-Confidence

There are three aspects to training to defend yourself: skills, fitness, and the confidence you achieve through both of the others. This is developed by setting yourself a realistic, sensible goal and beating it. Be conscious of success; if you perform an excellent takedown or land a really massive shot on the heavy

Close-in grapple

One way to protect yourself from blows is to get in close and hang on. A range of powerful takedowns can be set up from this position.

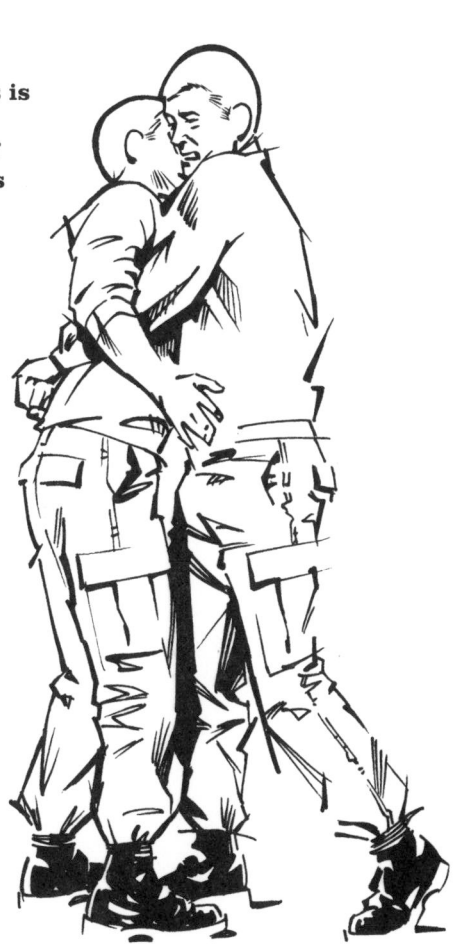

Wide chamber

This is one of the commonest 'street' attacks. Seeing a fist drawn back like this often frightens the victim into immobility. Good training helps you overcome this fear and act to protect yourself.

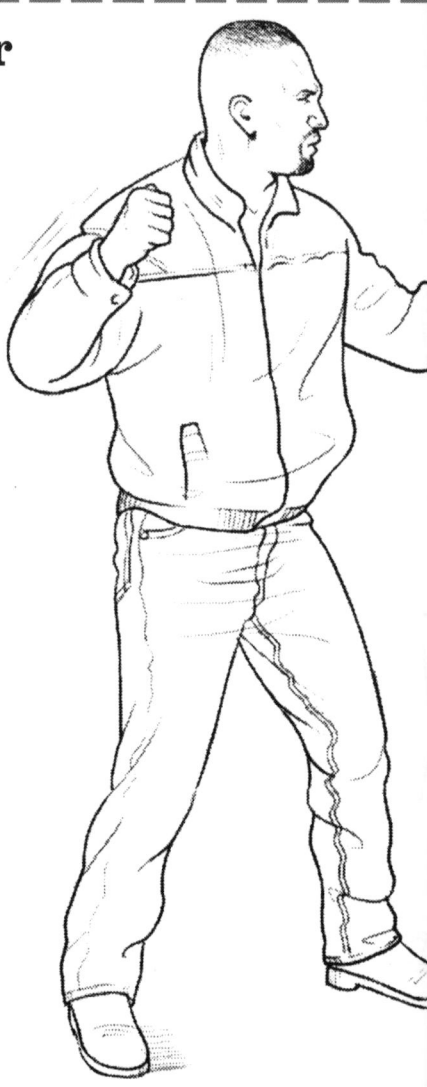

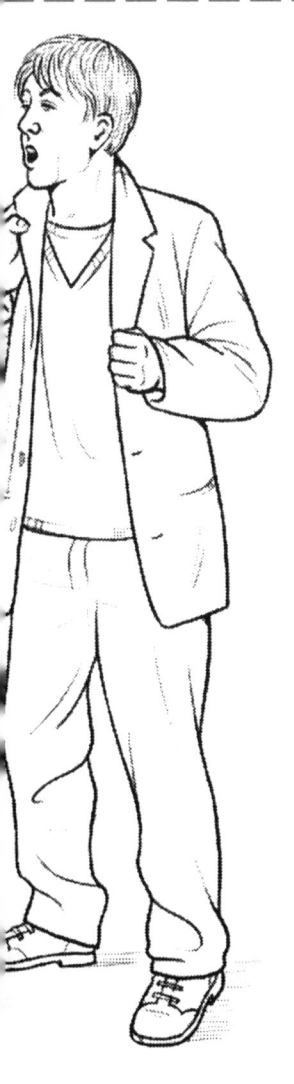

bag, savour the feeling. Likewise, if you beat your press-up record or best time, that is an achievement you can rightly feel proud of. It is almost as if you can create a 'bank balance' of confidence this way. Setbacks and fear reduce the balance, but so long as you are in credit then you are still in the fight.

Knowing that you can hit hard and grapple well helps overcome the fear you will inevitably feel in a confrontation. So will familiarity with the 'fight environment' and with what assailants might actually do. The unknown is frightening, but by learning what might happen in a fight and knowing you can deal with it, you will gain confidence in your ability to win.

Benefits of Training

There are real benefits to be gained from sparring, standup wrestling and 'rolling' (i.e. groundfighting with a partner) that go beyond the obvious fitness and skill-practice. Someone who has never had a punch thrown at them might not recognize what is about to happen, or might be intimidated into immobility by the intent to strike them. Someone who has sparred a lot is more likely to think 'oh look, a right hook. What else have you got?' – not only will they have well-developed skills to deal with a right hook, but also it is well within their experience and therefore not as

TIP: TRAINING FOR SUCCESS

You should approach your training with a clear understanding of the mental side to it all. Remember that giving up becomes a habit, as does success.

frightening. For example, we all know that being run over by a bus would be serious and possibly fatal, but we do not cower in fear every time one goes by. Instead we recognize the hazard and treat it with respect, but we also know how to deal with it. Thus we cross the road carefully but without quaking in stark terror.

Mental Preparation as You Train

Mental preparation should run right through any training you do. Any physical skills you might learn should be practised in a way that builds confidence as well as capability. For example, many martial arts teach striking and kicking techniques by hitting the air. This is only going to be useful if you are attacked by a cloud! The mechanics for delivering force have to be learned by actually hitting something.

In addition, you have to feel something work in order to have confidence in it. Imagine you are facing an attacker and you are trying to decide whether to gamble on a pre-emptive strike. Are you really going to bet your safety on something you have never actually done for real? If you have felt a bag shudder under the impact or seen a partner's eyes widen as your shot hits the focus pads he is holding, then you will have confidence in your shot. If all you have ever hit is air, you will probably lack the confidence to throw the strike, and thus miss an opportunity to end the matter before you get hurt.

Effective Training

When training in unarmed combat skills, the pattern is simple. Learn the technique by 'walking through it' carefully and slowly, with compliance from a partner if you are learning something like a takedown or throw. Then do it properly and remove the partner-compliance. Then, when you are confident in the technique, try it out in sparring or an attack drill where the opponent tries to make things as realistic as possible. If it still works under those conditions, the technique is combat-worthy.

When training general fitness, train with a view to mental preparation as well as physical improvement. Set goals you can beat with some effort, and work at beating them. And do not give up! If you go for a run, finish it unless there is a pressing reason not to, such as an injury. It does not matter if you have to walk the route you thought you could run; finishing at all is better for your confidence than gaining a habit of giving up when things get tough. If you plan to do three one-minute rounds on the bag, do them feebly if that is what you have to do, but do them.

The Gameplan

One of the best ways to avoid panic in a desperate situation – and, not coincidentally, to win – is to have a gameplan. There will not be time to think through a coherent strategy, but you should quickly form an almost instinctive gameplan. This will be something very simple like 'Door is over there. Attacker between me and it. Knock him down and run for the door.' It does not sound like much but it will really help.

People are often debilitated by confusion, because they just do not know what to do for the best. Once you have decided on a gameplan, that problem goes away. If things get desperate, having a plan of action can help you avoid panic.

As an example, suppose you fell into the sea and were getting very tired. Would it help you find the strength to struggle on if there was a lifebelt floating just a few metres from you? A gameplan gives you something to focus on and aim at.

Be Willing to Reset Your Goals

You must be willing to revise your plan if it is not going to work, rather than fixating on something that you cannot achieve. The disappointment when a plan fails can also be debilitating.

One trick used in special forces training is to send a soldier off on a long march, telling him that he is to walk until he reaches the vehicle sent to pick him up. Of course, it drives off as he approaches. This can be repeated several times, forcing the solider to deal with the disappointment of getting to the end of his arduous march, only to find that it is not the end at all.

Those with the right mental attitude reset their goals and continue marching. The same applies

> ### TIP:
> ### RUNNING ON EMPTY
>
> It has been rightly said that 'exhaustion makes cowards of us all', but even after your body has run out of steam you can sometimes keep going on courage alone.

here; your gameplan is what you intend to do. If it fails you make a new plan and continue. There is thus a danger that a failed plan will cause you to give up, but on balance the benefits of having a plan to start with greatly outweigh the risks.

Scenario Training

'Scenario' training is useful in learning to form a plan quickly. Training partners play the part of one or more aggressors, forcing you to quickly decide what to do depending on their actions. It is important that scenarios are realistic of course; scenario training is not the same as sparring, nor do assailants march up and throw a single attack before standing around waiting for you to perform a 17-move sequence on them.

Good scenario work also includes aggression, with the assailants pushing, grabbing, swearing … and sometimes not attacking at all. Good scenario work includes developing the ability to determine if a situation is about to explode or if the suspicious person in front of you is actually just agitated because he has missed his bus.

By building aggression and uncertainty into the situation, students are taught to analyse what is going on, make a decision and act upon it. This ensures that whatever happens, the student has seen it before and knows how to deal with it – and

perhaps more importantly, knows that he does.

Benefits of Mental Preparation

If you know how to quickly form a plan and have the confidence to act decisively to implement it, you have an excellent chance to defend yourself. Add in as much physical fitness as you can manage, some skills and techniques, and your chances are very good indeed. You cannot know how serious the threat you will face will be, nor if you will ever face one, but you can make sure you know how to deal with whatever happens.

Ironically, that makes it less likely that you will be attacked. As already noted, aggressors pick their targets and if someone is mentally prepared to defend themselves, it shows. Mental preparation makes it likely that an aggressor will find someone else to pick on, or that someone you get into a confrontation with will decide to posture and threaten rather than piling into you. And if it does happen, well, at least you are prepared for it.

PHYSICAL TRAINING

Physical training can be divided into two components: combat skills and fitness. Skills include things like striking techniques, takedowns and joint locks, as well as more general training in how to use these skills. The usual pattern is to learn a single technique in isolation, then add it to your repertoire, and

Stretching routine

Warming up and stretching your muscles is crucial before beginning any training routine. These two stretches cover the main muscle groups in the legs.

- **Quadricep stretch (right):** Standing facing a wall, lift your foot behind you and hold at the ankle. Hold the stretch for 10 breaths, then repeat with the other leg.

- **Seated hamstring stretch (below):** Sit with your legs stretched out before you. Keeping your back as straight as possible, lean forward, reaching your hands towards your ankles. Hold for 10 breaths, then repeat on the other side.

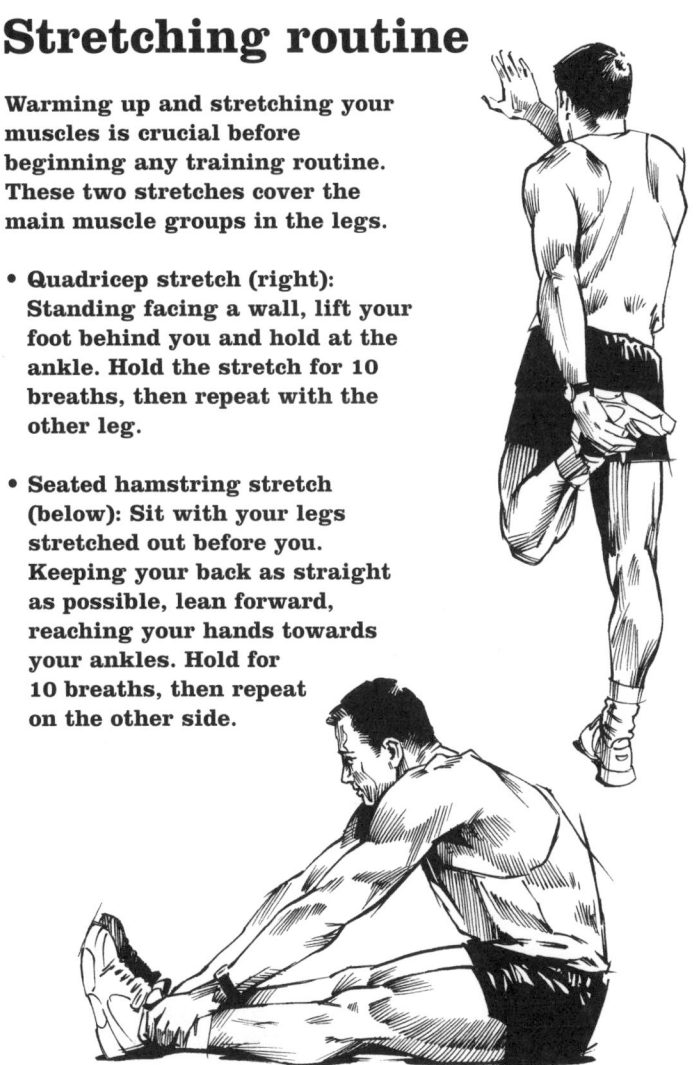

finally hone it as part of your total fighting system.

As an example of this process, you might spend some time on a specific strike such as a right cross, developing it into an effective tool. Then you would spend more time working the bag or pads with combinations incorporating your right cross, and finally use it in sparring along with all your other striking, footwork and evasion techniques.

Fitness and Conditioning

While you are drilling your techniques, you are also developing fitness and conditioning. Conditioning is, among other things, a measure of how used you are to a given activity. No matter how fit you are, doing something you are not used to is more tiring than an activity that you do all the time. Conditioning also helps your body deal with being hurt; if you are well conditioned you will recover faster and suffer less than someone who is not.

Fitness has many benefits beyond fight survival, but when under attack your fitness level is of paramount importance. You cannot know how fit you will need to be in order to meet a given challenge.

However, the rule is simple – the fitter you are, the better. That goes for life in general, but in a fight it can mean the difference between escape and a severe beating. Even if you cannot achieve much in the way of fitness, every little helps. The other

Exercise 1: Parallel bar dips

- **To perform parallel bar dips, stand between the parallel bars.**

- **Holding them with each hand, lift your body off the ground until your arms lock.**

- **Cross your legs, then lower your body until your upper arms are parallel with the bars.**

- **Repeat 10 times or until tired.**

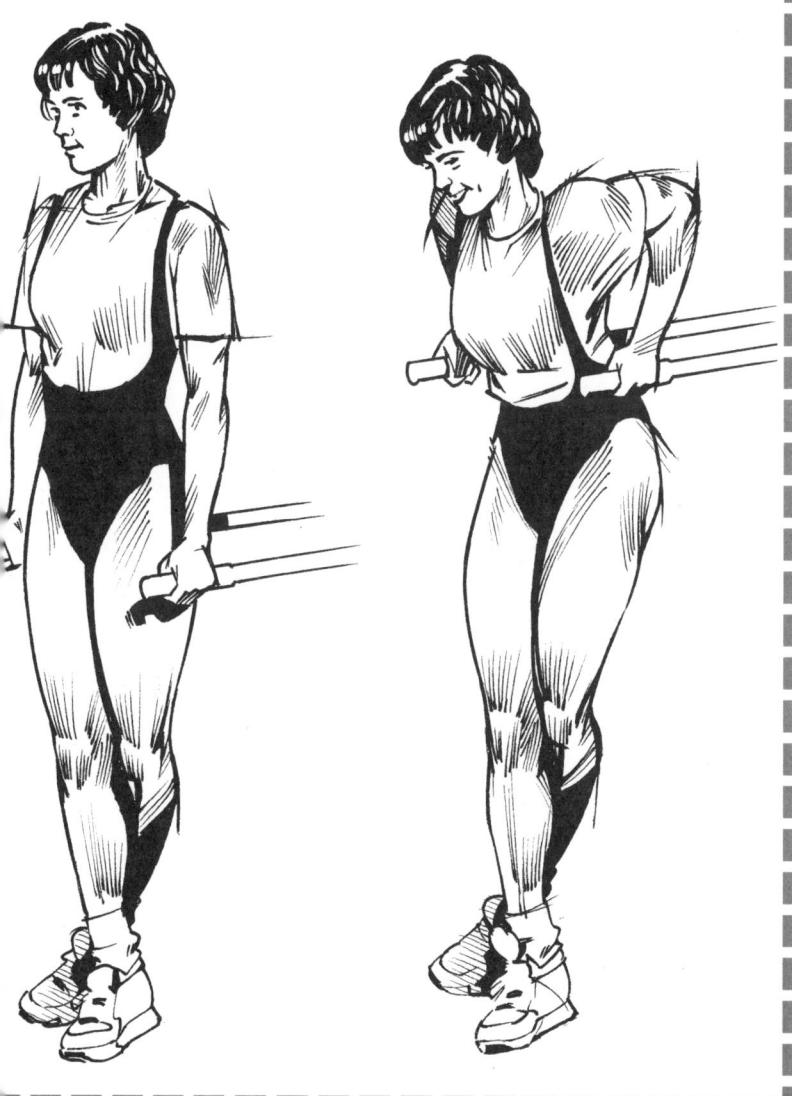

guy might be getting tired too. If he has five seconds' worth of fight left in him and you have 10, you will win.

Fitness Training

Before embarking on a programme of fitness improvement, it is worth considering your health in general and any limitations you may have. Be realistic and do not push yourself too hard. Gaining injuries in training is counterproductive, and it is possible to make yourself ill just by overtraining.

Rest is as important as exertion when training, especially when recovering from injuries or strains. When making the decision whether to train around an injury or illness, consider the longer term. Sometimes a week or two off and then a return to training when you are ready is more useful than struggling through and making yourself worse. On the other hand, you will need to decide whether you need to stop or you just want to. Be sensible and build up gradually, and you will achieve greater long-term benefits than by bulling your way through an insane training regime and then having to take time out to recover.

General Fitness

General fitness can be subdivided into three parts: flexibility, strength and cardiovascular fitness (also known as CV, or 'cardio'). Of these, flexibility is the least of your worries. Many martial arts require high levels of flexibility, but practical military unarmed combat relies mainly on natural movements. Provided you have a normal range of movement and are in generally good health, you will possess sufficient flexibility already.

Strength is useful, but there is no need to take this to extremes. Improved muscle tone is always beneficial, and it looks good too, but huge bulging muscles are unnecessary. Body-building for its own sake is not relevant to unarmed combat; it is better to have a modest amount of functional muscle mass well conditioned to combat movements than the sort of physique that wins contests. That said, it is a myth that huge muscles will slow you down; if you have that sort of build, it will be of benefit. If not, there are more useful ways to spend your training time than developing it.

Cardio is King

Cardiovascular fitness is extremely important. Cardio is all about getting air in and out of your lungs, transferring oxygen from it into your blood and getting it to the muscles and organs that will use it. Combat uses up oxygen at an incredible rate, mainly due to adrenaline. As your body gets short of oxygen it does not function as well. Not only does this make you slower and weaker but it can affect your judgement too; your brain can be deprived of the oxygen it needs by the exertion of your muscles, leading to mistakes that can get you killed.

Good cardio fitness offsets this by ensuring that your body is highly efficient at getting oxygen to where it is needed. This is perhaps the most important aspect of training. Unfortunately, it is one of the most boring as well. There is no substitute though; hours of preparation are needed for a few seconds of fighting. Those seconds can have life-changing or life-ending consequences though, so it is well worth putting the time in.

The Basic Exercises
It is not necessary to invest in large amounts of complex equipment in order to train effectively. Bodyweight exercises can be done anywhere, with an absolute minimum of equipment, or even none at all.

This list is by no means exhaustive, but it will provide a starting point. It is always a good idea to warm up before beginning any heavy exertion. Start light and increase the pace or intensity when you feel you are ready.

Work through a series of 'rounds' on the bag, using different strikes and remembering to breathe. For variety and a tougher workout, you can add in elbows, kicks and knee strikes. Depending on what you are trying to achieve, rounds can be anywhere from 30 seconds to three minutes in length, with rests in between of one to two minutes. Start

> ### TIP: THE MOST IMPORTANT EXERCISE OF ALL
>
> The most important thing you can train yourself to do is to remember to breathe. That might seem odd, but people tend to hold their breath while fighting or exerting themselves. Train yourself to breathe out on each action (e.g. each punch, each press-up). Once the air is out, your body will bring more in without conscious effort. If you forget to breathe, no amount of training or skill is going to help you.

with a light warm-up round before you begin to push it.

The weight of your strikes can be varied, from very light to extremely heavy. A 30-second 'blast' of shots thrown as hard and fast as you can will really take it out of you. This could be done as a peak in a longer round, easing off before and after, or could be an entire round.

You can work preset combinations with a heavy bag or just pound on it.

Exercise 2: Seated barbell press

- For the barbell press, sit straight with your feet set slightly apart so that your weight is distributed evenly.

- Holding a barbell at the level of each shoulder, raise them above your head on the 'in' breath, then lower them on the 'out' breath.

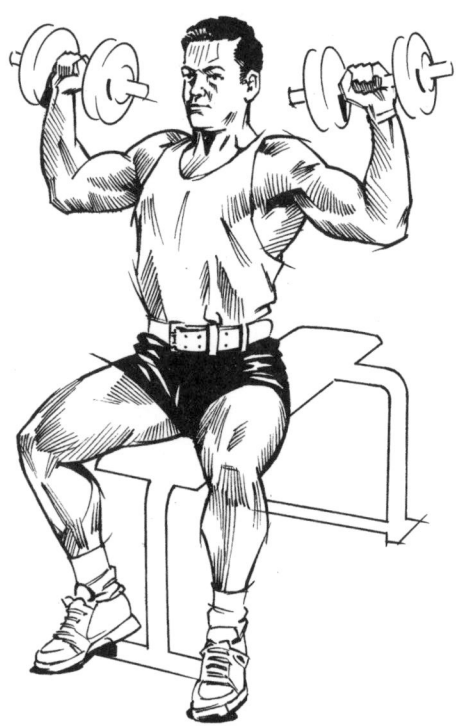

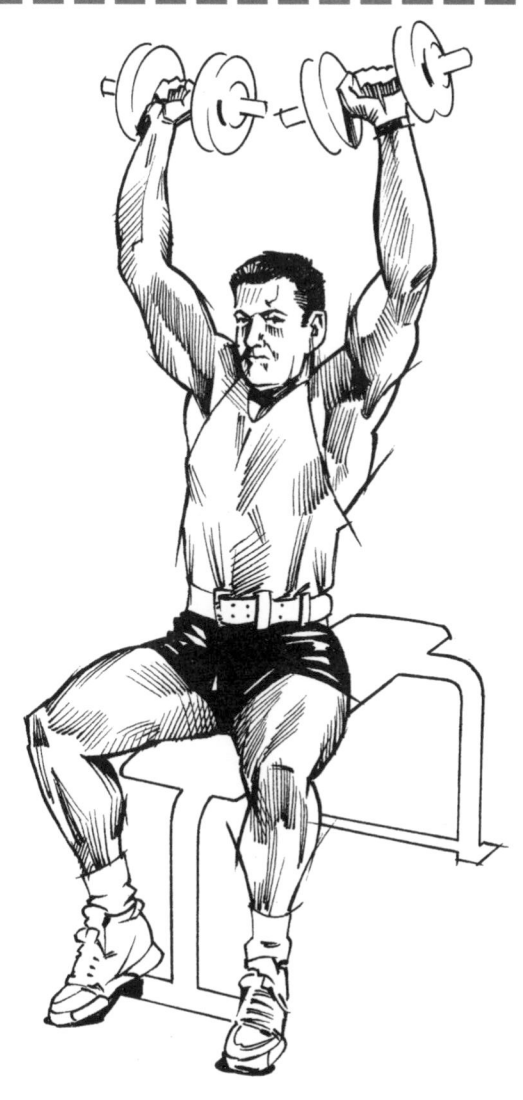

Exercise 3: Quad lifts

- To work your quadriceps, sit with your back straight and arms locked to your side.

- Raise the weight with your shins, until your legs are straight.

- Lower slowly and smoothly, and repeat.

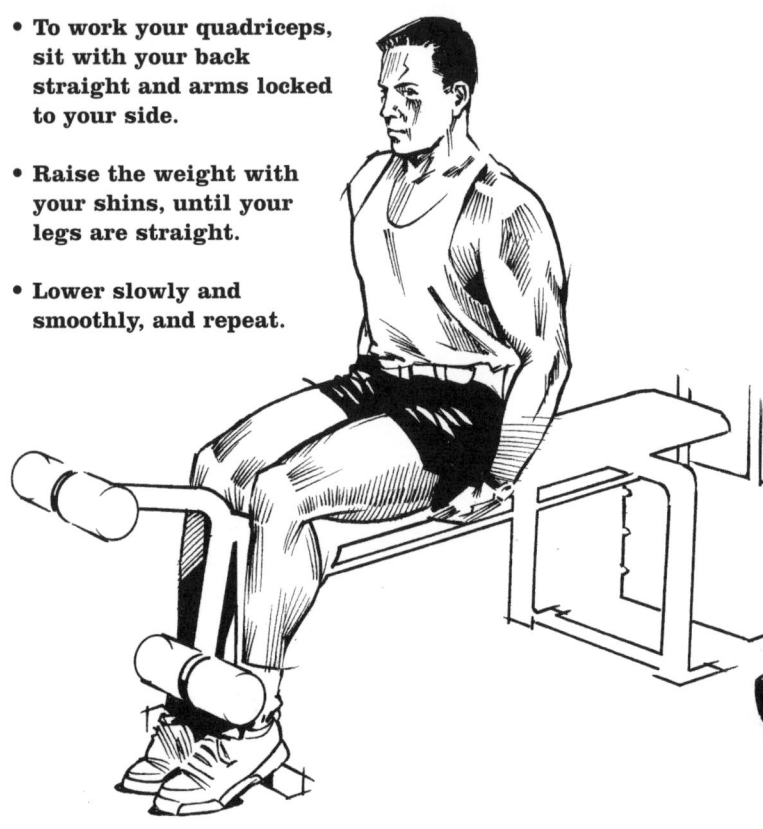

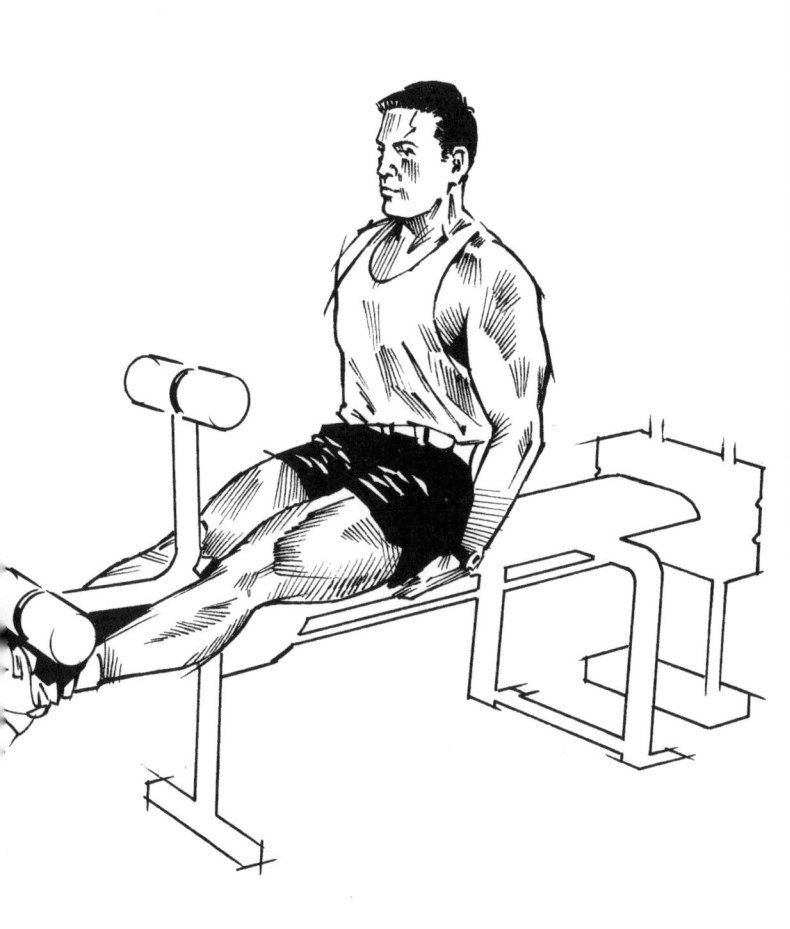

Exercise 4: Squats

Squats work your legs and build endurance.

- Keep your back straight and make sure your knees do not go past 90 degrees as this puts excessive strain on the joints.

- Slow, deliberate squats give the best results.

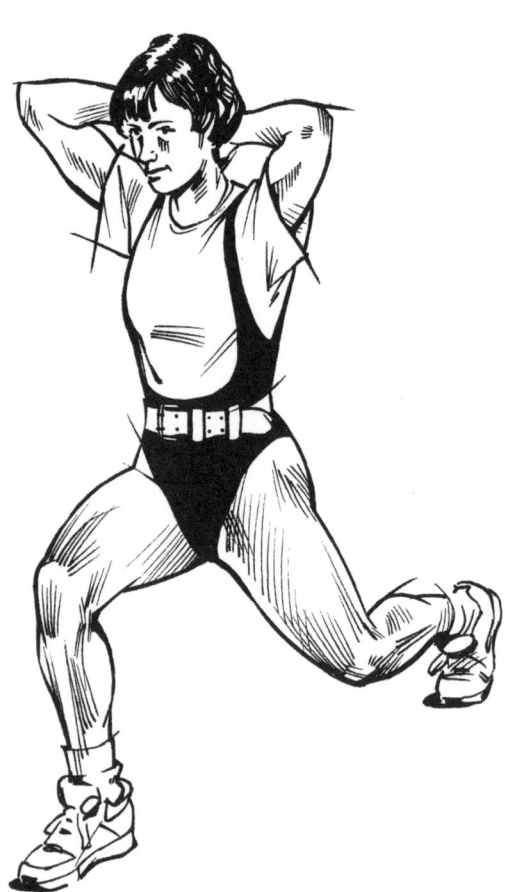

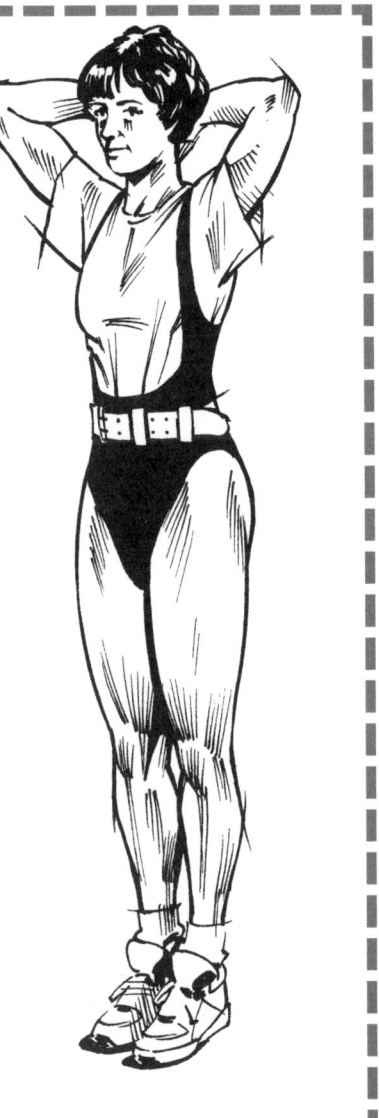

For added variety, practise moving and dodging as you strike. You can also suddenly lunge in and clinch the bag to throw knee strikes or wrap one arm around it and attack with the other arm … plus headbutts and knees. This might get you some funny looks down at the gym but it is an excellent way of learning to focus aggression and to deliver hard shots from extreme close quarters.

TIP: USING THE HEAVY BAG

The heavy bag can be used for more than general pounding practice.

One good drill is to throw either an all-out onslaught for a set time or number of strikes, or a single shot as if your life depended upon it. In either case, stand calm and relaxed, then launch your assault upon a 'trigger'. This can be a training partner suddenly barking 'GO!' or you can do it yourself, which helps teach you to go to 'fight mode' instantly and whenever you need to.

Exercise 5: Press-ups

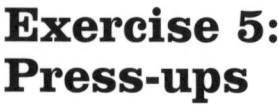

Press-ups work your upper body.

- Lower yourself by bending your arms until your nose is close to the floor, hold, then straighten your arms to return to your starting position.

- Doing your press-ups slowly and holding at the bottom is harder than just pumping away.

- Women should do press-ups from their knees rather than the toes as this can lead to internal complications.

- Do not do press-ups on your knuckles.

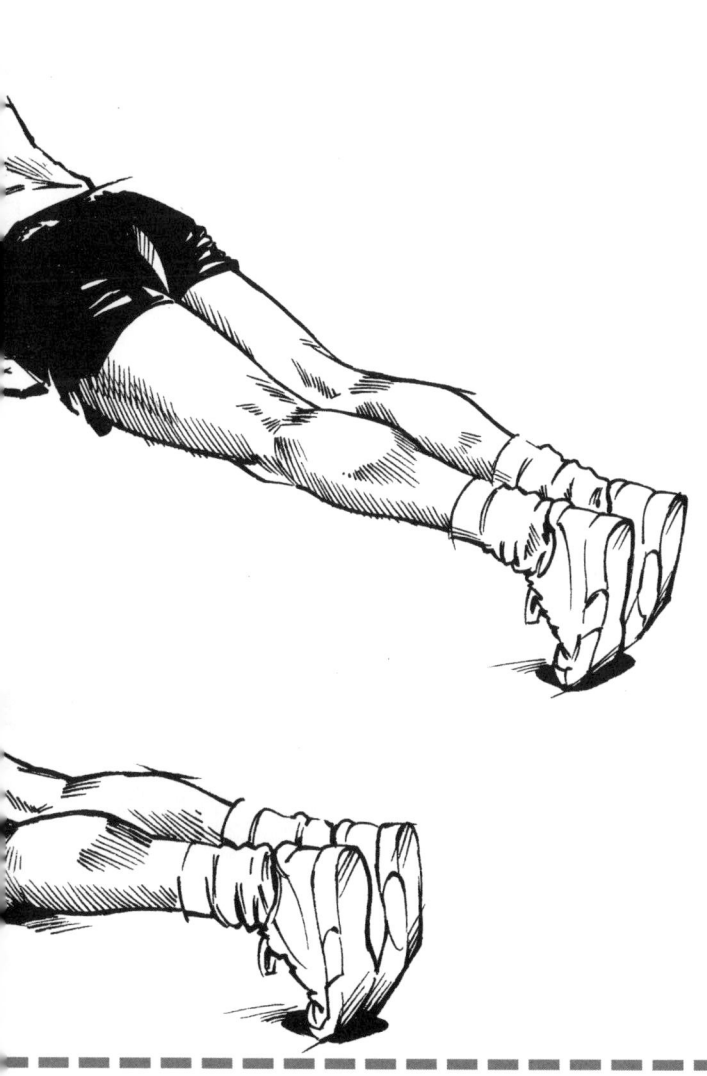

Exercise 6: Abdominal crunches

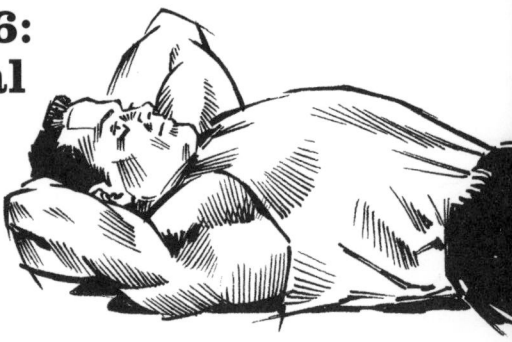

Crunches work your abdominal muscles, strengthening your core, which in turn supports everything you do.

• Slow, deliberate crunches are best.

• Do not try to yank yourself up by the back of your neck; pull yourself up from the abs.

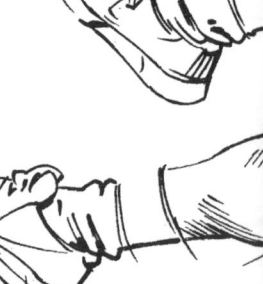

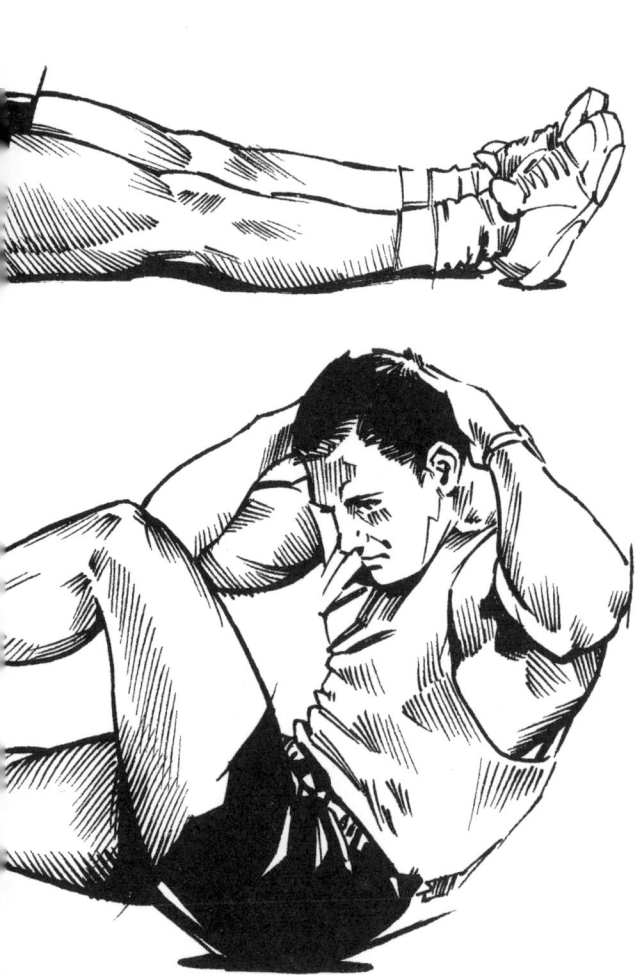

Exercise 7: Running

Running is the absolute best way to build all-round cardiovascular fitness, and requires only a place to run.

- A steady jog can be interspersed with short sprints or uphill runs to build endurance.

- As an alternative, an elliptical trainer (cross-trainer) machine can be used. This takes some of the impact out of the running action and is better for the joints.

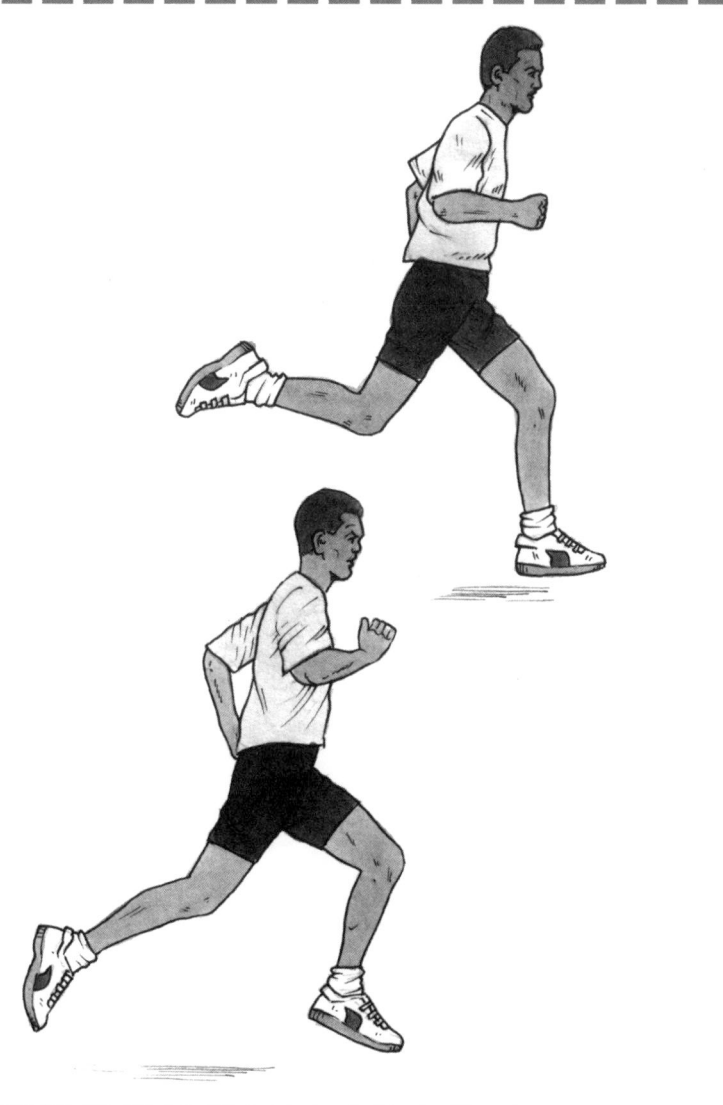

Exercise 8: Heavy bag

Working a heavy punchbag is excellent for stamina as well as skills training. In fact it is the best combination of cardio and skills work available. If you can only have one piece of kit, get a heavy punchbag.

- A hard shot on the bag should make it dent, not swing. You want your shots to crumple the opponent, not shove him around.

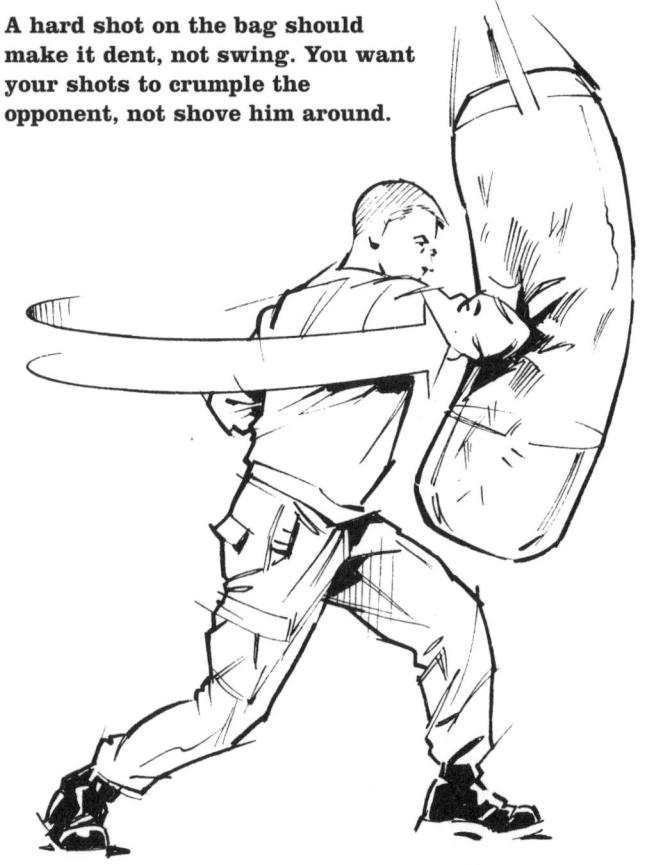

TIP:
FOCUS PAD DRILLS

There are many possible pad drills in addition to just banging away. If the pad-man moves around and occasionally takes a swipe with the pad, fairly realistic training is possible. It is also extremely tiring and thus good cardio training.

The following pad drill is just one of an infinite number of possibilities.

- Pad-man sets the pads straight and close together, making sure they do not shoot back into his face when hit. Striker throws a lead-hand shot followed by a cross. Punches should cross over into the opposite pad.

- Pad-man takes a wide hooking swipe at head height with his left pad. Striker covers his head and ducks or bobs out to the side the strike came from.

- Pad-man sets his right pad for a hooking strike. Striker straightens up and throws a hard right hook.

- Striker lunges forward and clinches pad-man around the head, pulling him in for a knee strike. Pad-man pushes the pads down to absorb the strike.

Repeat the drill for three to six repetitions, remembering to breathe out on each strike and to throw good, hard shots each time rather than rushing through the sequence.

Exercise 9: Focus pads

Focus pads (also called focus mitts or hook-and-jab pads) require a partner. 'Setting' the pads is a skill in and of itself – and surprisingly tiring.

- The pad-man must keep his arm springy rather than rigid when holding the pads to avoid injury.

- Pads can be used square-on for straight shots, side-on for hooks, and can also be brought down horizontally for knee strikes. They are not really suitable for taking full-on kicks and knees, so a measure of control is needed to avoid hurting your training partner – and remember that it is his or her turn next!

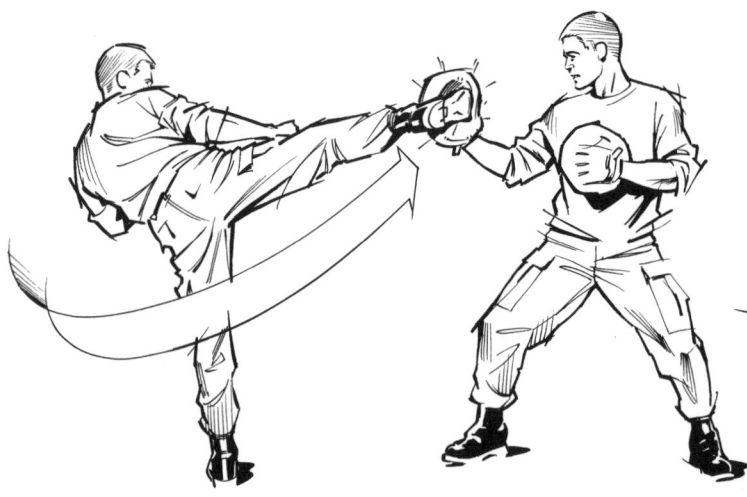

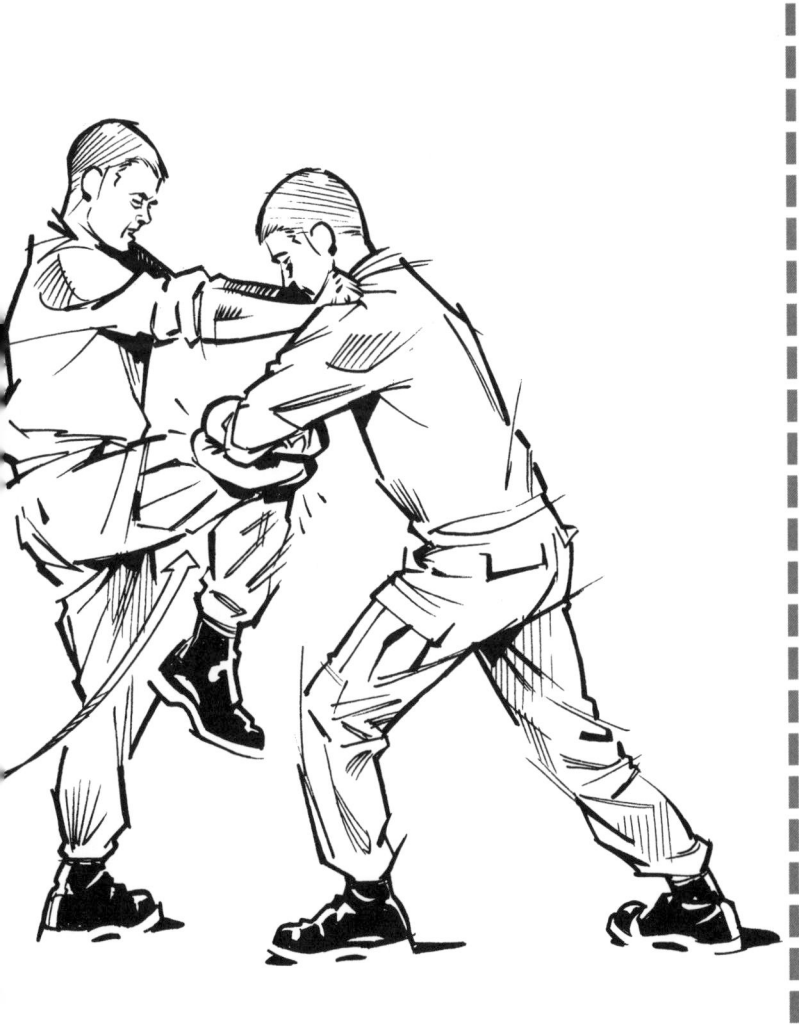

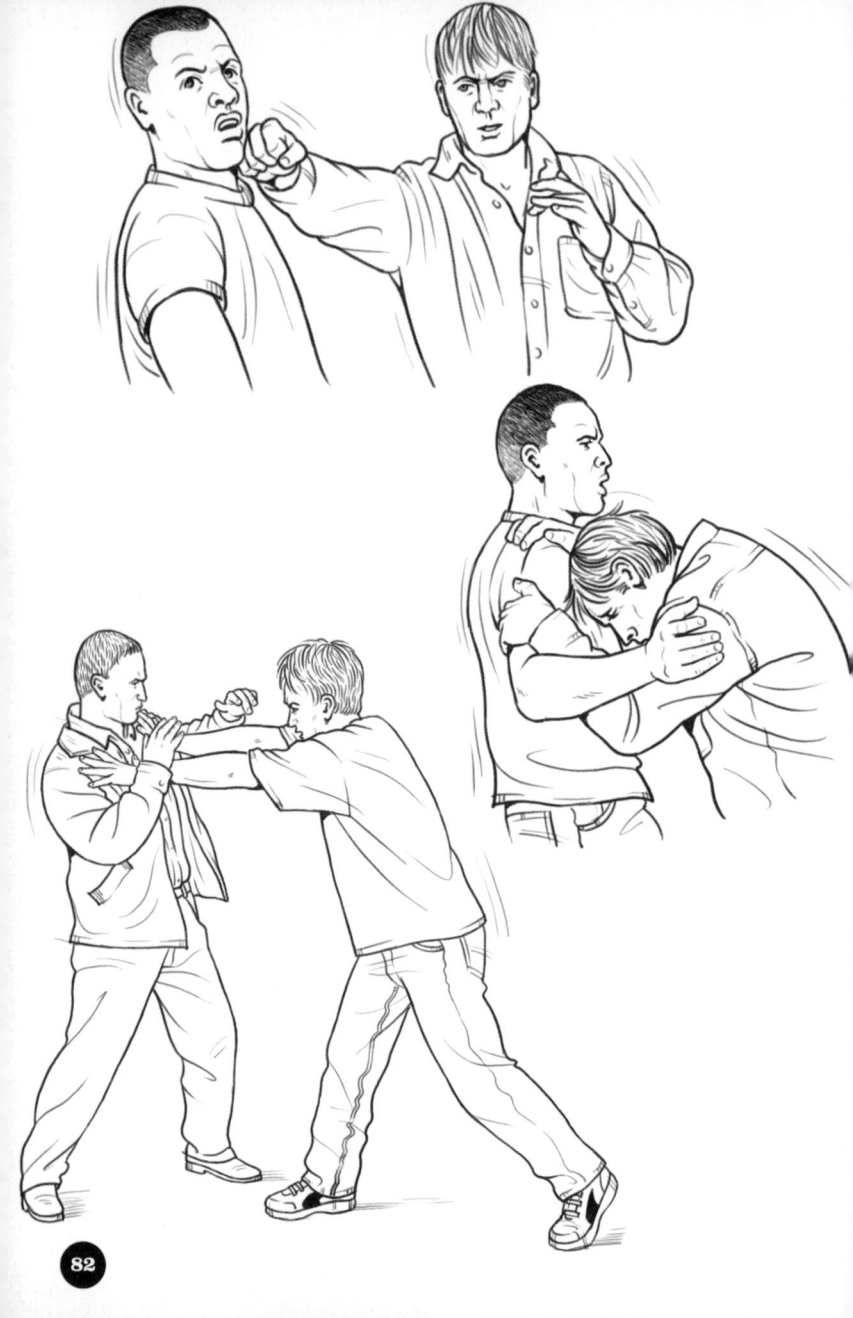

Military unarmed combat systems are not concerned with flashy, complex techniques or over-specialized moves designed to counter things the typical assailant will not do anyway. Instead, military combat systems rely on simple, highly effective concepts coupled with aggression to quickly demolish any opposition.

Many martial arts teach dozens, possibly even hundreds, of techniques and variations on them. This is reasonable enough if the student has years to study and train, but military forces need to achieve a good standard of combat capability in a short time. Thus military training seeks to turn the soldier into a good fighter and give him some flexible tools to use, rather than providing a vast array of knowledge and hoping that this will translate into combat efficiency.

This is not to say that all martial artists cannot fight; far from it, many are extremely effective combatants. However, others are technicians rather than warriors, who can perform their art well but who would struggle to handle a real situation. The military cannot afford this, and so focuses on the soldier rather than his skills.

. . . .

Left: A solid guard, good posture and effective movement are the foundations for everything else with self-defence tecxhniques.

4

No matter how much technique you know, none of it works without good basics.

Tools of the Trade

The Basics

TRAIN TO FIGHT, NOT TO PERFORM TECHNIQUES

Obviously, knowing some good, effective combat moves is extremely useful, but all the technique in the world is worth nothing to someone who panics or hesitates and thus never gets to use his training. Keep this in mind when training – a sloppy, badly executed and generally poor technique done with guts and determination will get you a better result than beautiful form in the class which falls apart under stress.

TIP: BREAKING THINGS

Many martial artists use 'breaking' techniques to demonstrate their skills. Boards, bricks, and even concrete blocks can be broken with hands, feet and elbows. But there really is no need to train this way. It takes a long time to build the relevant skills and you are unlikely to be attacked by a fence or wall. Concentrate instead on techniques for dealing with human opponents.

Thus, it is not enough to be able to perform the following techniques neatly and tidily. You must be able to use them to demolish an attacker. Good form and technique is a means to an end – for example, your punches will be more powerful if done right – rather than the objective itself. Thus, when training, you should bear in mind the object you are trying to achieve. It is one thing to 'perform a right cross' and entirely another to 'knock the other guy out by hitting him in the head with a right cross'.

Understand What Techniques Are For

This mentality of focusing on the outcome rather than the technique should pervade your training. It will also help you remember the techniques. You may find it hard to recall exactly what an 'outer reap takedown' is, but 'dump the other guy on his back with an outer reap' provides a clue. This is also, perversely, good from a safety perspective. If you abstract techniques you can become complacent and careless. 'Performing an arm lock' sounds quite harmless, but 'breaking his arm with an arm lock' is a good reminder of both what you would try to achieve in real combat, and also what might happen by accident in training if you are not careful.

It cannot be stressed enough that everything in the following section is dangerous – that is the point. Used well, it can save your life. However, it could also be misused to hurt people who do not deserve it, or carelessly to hurt a training partner. So train carefully while you train hard, and use what you know responsibly.

THE BASICS

Before you start trying to learn complex throws, takedowns and strikes, there are some fundamental concepts that you must understand. If you have a firm grasp of the basics, everything else will slot into place and you will be able to flow seamlessly from one technique to another. Without the basics, you might learn dozens of techniques but you will have no real idea how they fit together. This is not necessarily crippling, but it will impair your ability to adapt to changing circumstances in a fight.

The 'basics' consist of an understanding of your body's weapons; how they work, what to target with them and what will make your strikes most effective, coupled with a knowledge of how to move and keep your balance. With all this at your disposal you can often figure out the most effective thing to do mid-fight; indeed, many techniques will seem obvious once you understand how and why they work.

The basics are extremely important. A big, strong man who throws a punch with just the muscles of his arm may hit pretty hard, but a

TIP: HURTING PEOPLE

There are several ways to hurt someone. In very general terms these are categorized as:

- Striking them with hands, feet, elbows, knees, headbutts.
- Locking their joints so that they cannot move easily and applying enough force to disable the joint.
- Throwing them to the ground or making them fall on something hard.
- Choking or strangling them to cut off their air or blood supply.

small, light woman who can put her entire bodyweight behind a blow can cause more damage. Obviously, size and strength still matter, but there is nothing much you can do about your stature. You cannot get any taller and there is only so much muscle you can add in the gym, but good basics will enable you to get the most out of what you have.

Off balance

Getting shoved might seem to be a minor hazard, but once you are off balance you become an easy target. An assailant might also shove you to put you on the defensive and assert dominance over you.

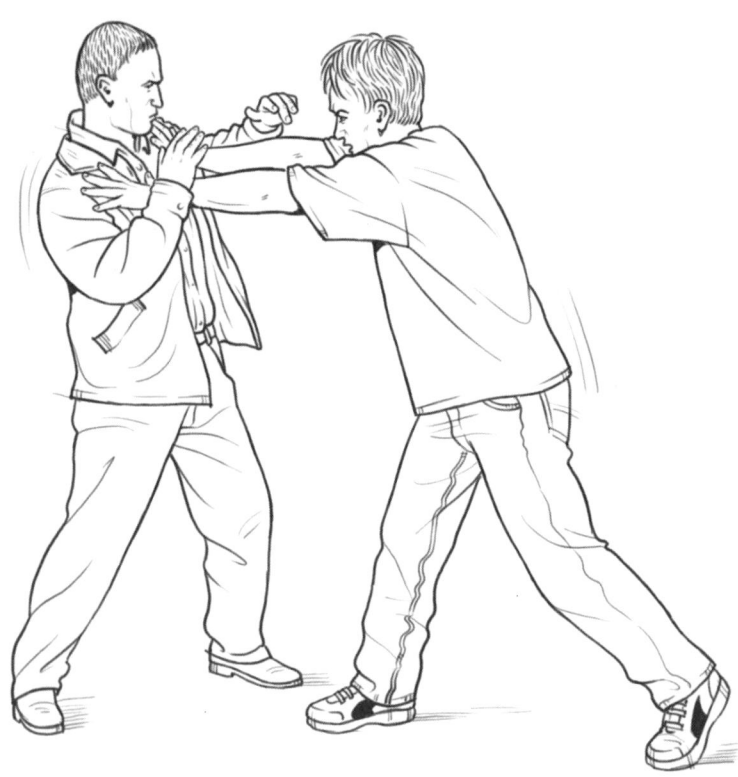

STANCE AND POSTURE

In the words of a very eminent self-defence expert, 'you can't fire a cannon out of a canoe'. In other words, nothing you do is going to work properly unless you have a good base. This does not imply that you have to learn unnatural and often just plain strange stances you might have seen in Kung-Fu movies; it simply means that you must maintain good body structure and balance while you are fighting.

Balance is instinctive – most people can walk across a room without falling over. If you try to walk on a moving bus or train, you will naturally flex your knees a bit and perhaps widen your stance, i.e. put your feet further apart. We all know that this helps us to keep our balance and to adapt to forces trying to make us overbalance, such as when the bus hits a bump in the road.

Try standing with your feet very close together and leaning this way and that. Repeat with your feet a bit further apart. Try it with your feet lined up, toe to heel. You will quickly find that there is a range of positions that you can remain upright in, and if you go beyond it you need to put a foot out to support yourself. The range of positions is greater when you have a wider stance. You will also note that you have the best all-round balance when your feet are not in a line.

The Boxer's Guard

This is the most basic and useful of all combat stances. If you are right-handed then you will use an 'orthodox' or left-side-forward stance, to get the best power from your strong hand. Feet should be about shoulder-width apart and both turned roughly 45 degrees to your right, knees slightly flexed. Your body will turn to the right somewhat, which helps protect your internal organs.

Hands are up, with the right about chin height and close to you, the left a little lower and about halfway extended. Hands can be closed into fists or kept open, whichever suits you best. Tuck your chin in a bit to protect your jaw and throat.

From this position, you can strike easily and can protect your head, which is vital. If anything comes in lower than your hands, it is easy to drop them down to counter it. Conversely, if your hands are too low then gravity makes it harder to raise them up to defend your head, which can lead to being knocked out.

Left-handed fighters sometimes choose to use the orthodox stance, or to reverse it and fight 'southpaw', i.e. with their right hand forward. Experiment with both and see which suits you best.

The Grappler's Guard

If you expect someone to try to tackle or grapple you, or you want to launch a grappling attack of your

The guard position

It is not necessary to have a perfect 'boxer's guard', but your hands need to be up, body turned about 45 degrees and your knees slightly flexed for movement. Do not expect to spend a lot of time in this position, though. Once a situation has developed to the point where you need a guard, you should be doing something rather than standing about.

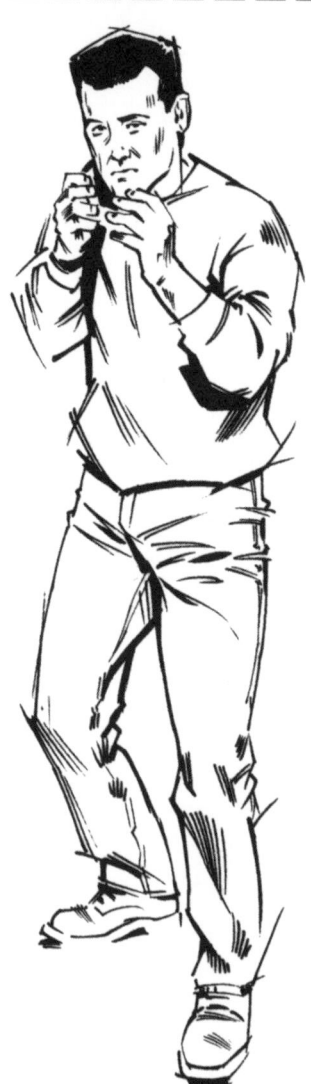

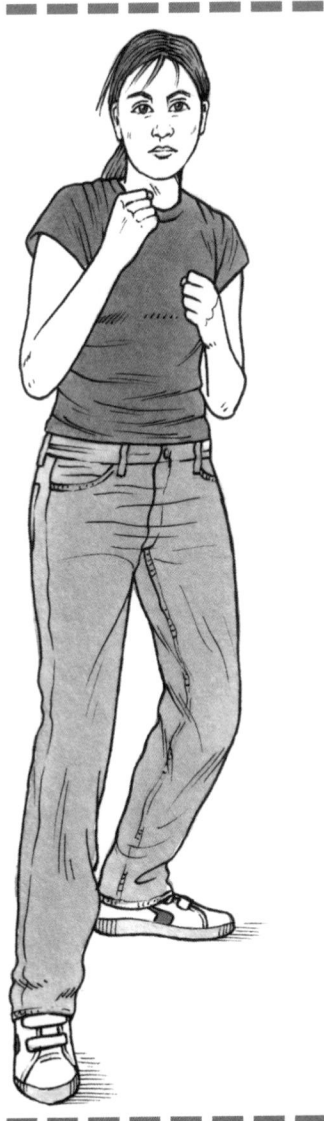

own, then a more square-on stance is sometimes useful. Crouch down a bit, to keep your centre of gravity low. This will enable you to avoid being overbalanced and to get under your opponent's centre of gravity to throw him.

This is not a position you should spend much time in – it is a launch platform for an attack or a starting position to receive and defeat a grappling attack. If you are not imminently expecting to grapple, a boxer's guard is usually a better choice of position.

The Fence

The 'fence' is not actually a fighting stance at all. It is very similar to a boxer's guard, and indeed it offers most of the advantages of the boxing stance, but it is used before a fight starts, i.e. when you think there is a chance that the matter can be ended without violence.

There are many variations of the fence. Among its advantages are that the open hands do not give away to an opponent that you are getting ready to fight, and the extended lead hand creates a barrier that may be enough to deter his approach.

Using the Fence

As already noted, the fence is not so much a fighting stance as a situational control tool. It is combined with a verbal gambit to try to deter the attacker or 'talk him down'.

The fence posture

The 'fence' is not a fighting stance; it is more of a way to control the distance as you try to find a way not to have to fight. There are many variations on the basic fence. The one on the left is assertive while the one on the right is quite subtle, disguised as 'talking with your hands'. Both work well in the right circumstances.

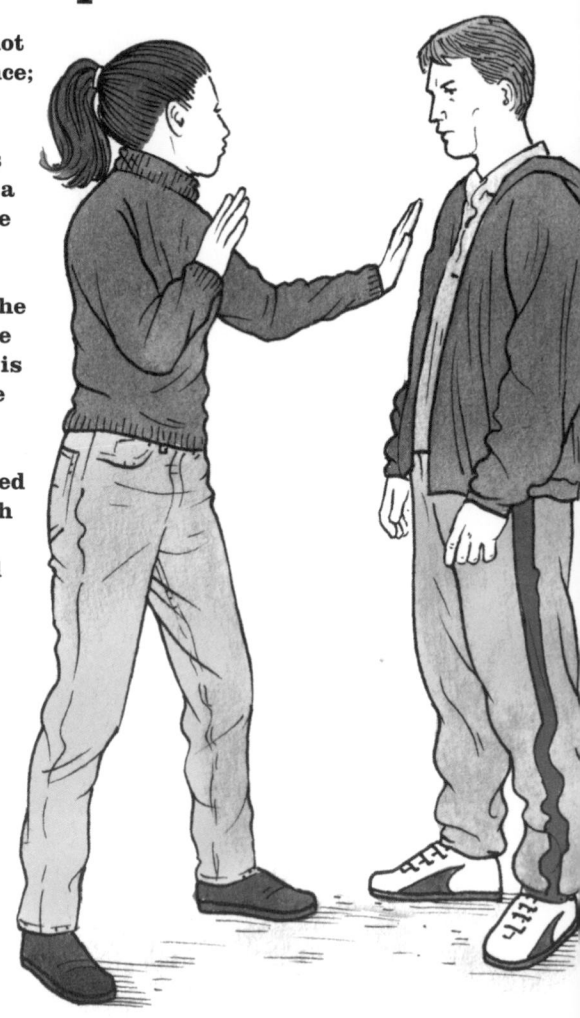

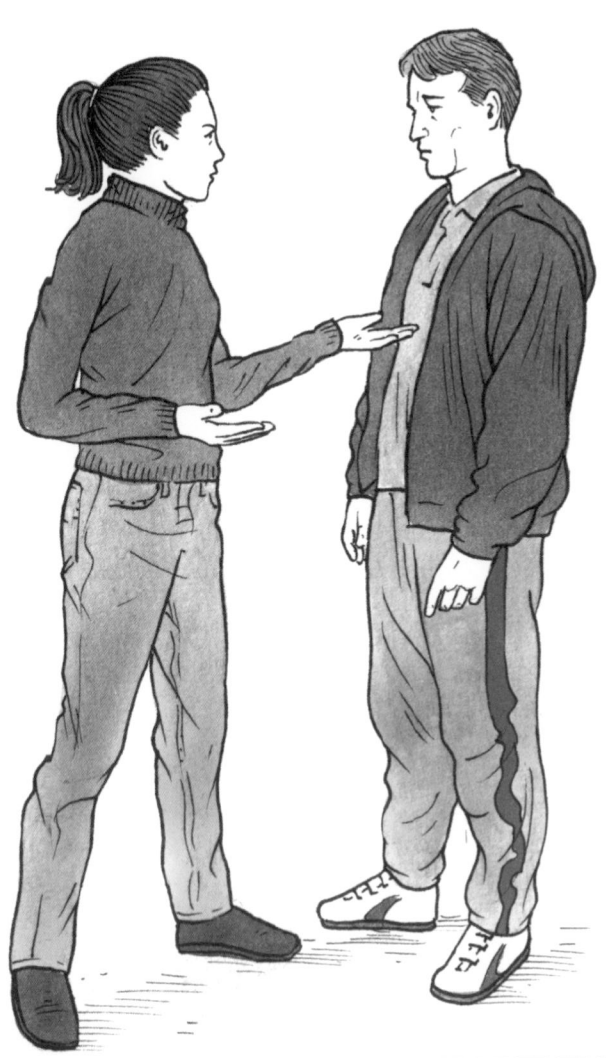

The grappler's guard

If you intend to launch a
grappling attack or defeat
one, you will need to drop
your weight a bit and
take up a wider stance.
Seeing someone in this
position is a clear
indication that they
intend to rush in
and tackle you.

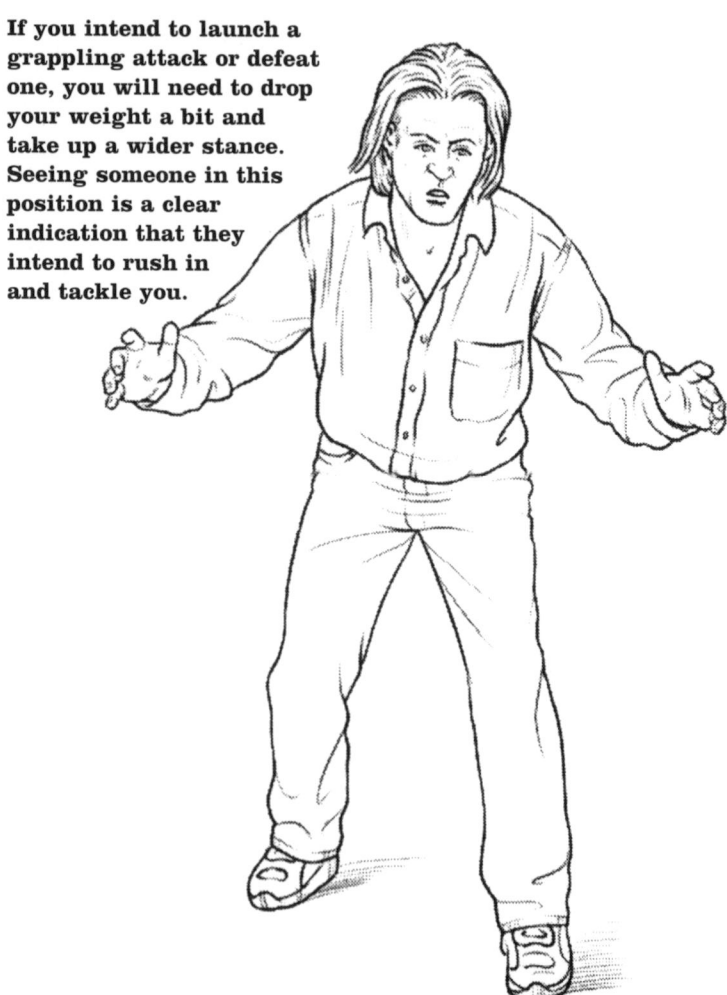

What you say depends on how you judge the situation. You might try a fairly passive approach or be quite aggressive. There is no guarantee that any given approach will work, but it can be worth a try if you think you can avoid violence.

The fence acts as a barrier while you use whatever verbal gambit seems most appropriate. Sometimes the fact that you have a hand up and in the way can be enough of a deterrent to make an aggressor look elsewhere for a victim but often your choice of words and demeanour is critical. Exactly what you say depends on how you judge the situation. The following approaches are examples only; you must tailor your response to what is happening at the time.

- **The Passive Approach:** 'Woah, easy pal, sorry about that … I'm just in a hurry to meet some friends …', said in a friendly and semi-apologetic tone as you withdraw and remove yourself from the situation. This approach can be seen as an invitation for the aggressor to posture a bit and act the big man, but that is not a bad thing. It gives him a reason to think he 'won', so he may not feel the need to push the matter. Your ego might not like being seen to 'back down', but if it gets you what you want (i.e. an end to the matter without a fight) then it is a win.

- **The Assertive Approach:** 'Okay, no closer. Now, what do you want?' Said in an even and calm, but commanding, tone this approach can dissuade someone who is looking for an easy victim. It is not inflammatory, and someone who responds aggressively was probably going to attack you anyway. It may seem a bit rude to behave like this, but if you are not sure about someone then they have no business being any closer to you than you permit them to be.

- **The Aggressive Approach:** 'Get Back! Leave me the **** alone!', accompanied if necessary by a shove. Swear as much as you like; it is a useful tool in projecting aggression, and that is what is necessary here. An aggressive approach is best used as a last-ditch attempt to deter someone who seems intent on attacking you, or who you think can be shocked into backing down. This works best if it is a surprise – if the 'victim' turns out to be a bit more of a fighter than expected, some potential assailants will look elsewhere. However, an aggressive approach can escalate a situation so should be used with care.

If the Fence Fails

If your use of the fence goes well, you may be able to take control of the situation and end it without violence taking place. However, if the assailant tries to push through your fence or grab your arm, then this is not going to be possible. At least you have clarified the situation though – anyone willing to use force to enter your personal space means you harm.

There is one last service your fence can do at this point. It identifies the optimum striking range for your strong hand. An assailant pushing through your fence will walk right onto a pre-emptive strike, which can end the matter then and there. And of course, if you later have to justify your actions, you can show how you tried to talk him down, push him away, and generally attempted to use means short of violence.

In short, a fence gives you a chance to avoid being attacked, to deter or talk down an attacker, and forces him to show his hostile intent when he is still at arm's length … and also allows you to know as you throw your first shot that you really are justified in hitting the aggressor because he has had fair warning. But once a fight begins, the fence is not useful. Use a boxer's guard for those instants when you are not doing something to bring the altercation to a successful close.

MOVEMENT

Much of the time, natural movement such as walking or running works fine in a confrontation, but when in close proximity to an opponent it is important to move in a way that gives you advantages whilst maintaining good balance.

Tactical movement is extremely important in a fight. You might want to keep the distance between you and an opponent open, put an obstacle between you, or manoeuvre so that you can make a dash for the door. Generally speaking, you will tend to circle to your right wherever possible since this takes you away from a right-handed opponent's strong hand. However, you are unlikely to win by manoeuvres alone, so whatever movement you make must fit in with your plan to end the situation. That generally means moving to a point where you can attack most effectively.

Hit–Move–Hit

Imagine you realize that a bad guy is about to hit you. You step in and strike him with a hard right cross. Ideally, he goes down and the situation is over. But if not, he is going to come right back at you. So, during the instant you gain while he is recovering from your first blow, you sidestep to your right. If he comes back with a wild swing, it will miss you. If he takes a second to orient himself and turn towards you, you still have time to strike him again. This concept is sometimes referred to as 'move–hit–move'.

The fence (front and side view)

The moment you feel threatened, the fence goes up. Once it is up, it stays up until the threat is removed or a fight begins. The fence should be accompanied by appropriate 'language', ideally something simple like 'Stay back. Leave me alone.'

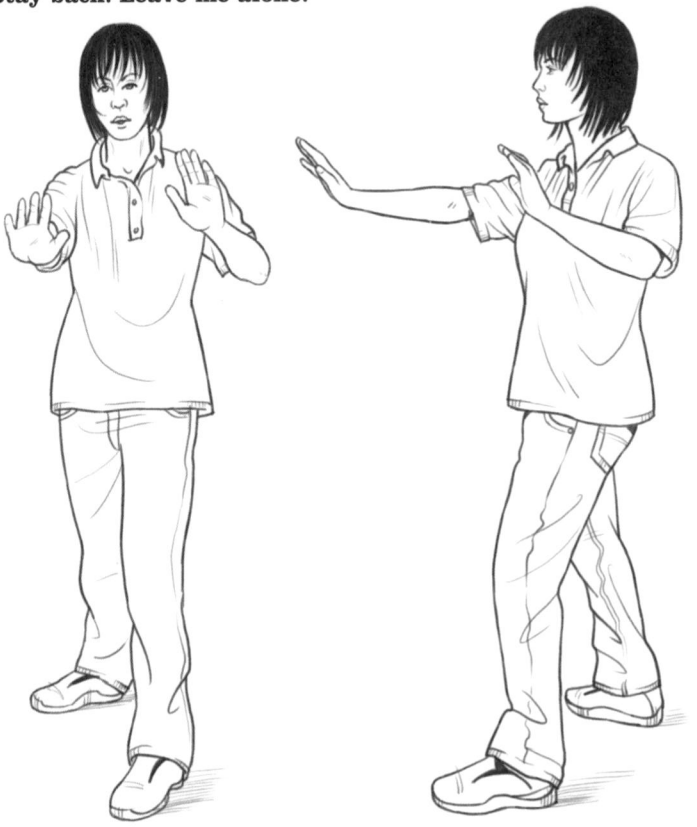

Hit–move–hit

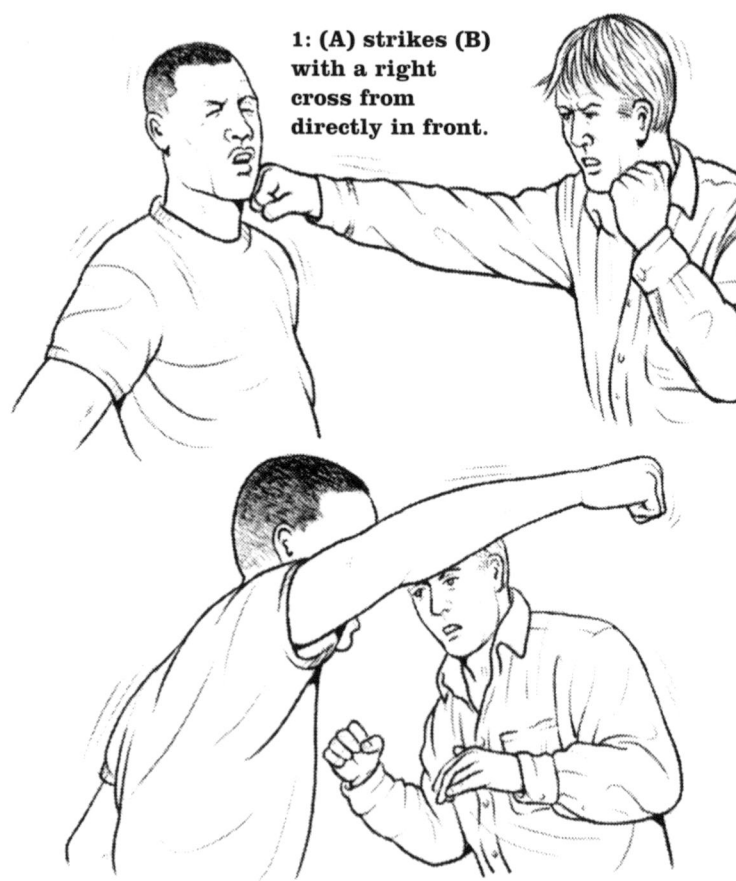

1: (A) strikes (B) with a right cross from directly in front.

2: (A) sidesteps to the right while (B) retaliates with a wild swing, missing.

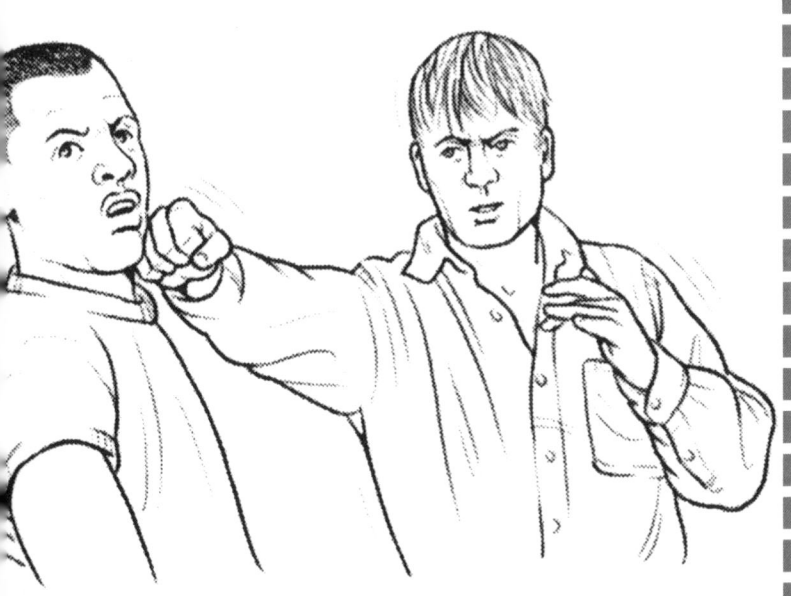

3: (A) strikes again from the side.

Grab and hit

One of the commonest of all attacks is to grab with the weak hand (usually the left) and hit with the strong one. Fiddling about trying to deal with the grab is pointless if there is a punch on the way.

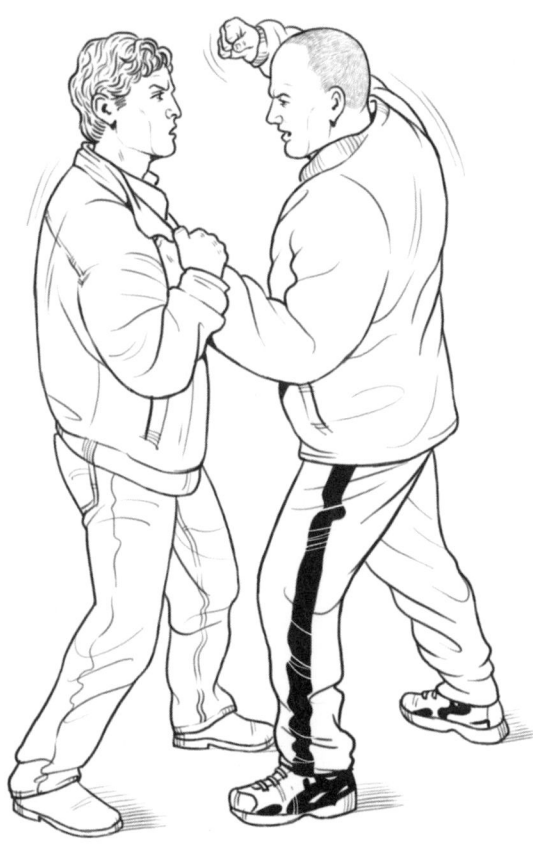

The Shuffle

Most of the movements you might make are variations on what is known as a push-shuffle, or just a shuffle. When shuffling, you never cross your feet and thus you retain a good 'base' even when moving.

You can shuffle at an angle or turn simply by stepping a bit to the side as you move forward or back. If you need to circle an opponent or avoid an attack, step to the side instead of forward or back. If you go right, step with your right foot and follow with the left, and vice versa. Again, you do not cross your feet. Keep your hands up as you move and face the opponent at all times.

If you need to change leads, you can 'step through'. This is about the only time your feet will be crossed. A step-through is basically a normal step – your back foot moves through and becomes your lead foot if you are going forwards, and your front foot moves back to become the rear one if you need to move backwards. Your lead hand swaps over as you change lead, i.e. if your left foot is forward, your left hand should be the lead hand.

The Drop-Step

The drop-step is used to deliver extra power on a blow, putting your body weight behind it. It is essentially a variation on the push-shuffle. Push hard with the back foot while taking a fairly long step forward towards the target with your front foot. Your blow should land just as the front foot hits the ground, so that your weight is moving forwards into the target. Do not take a huge step like a fencer's lunge; the timing is more important than the distance travelled.

Crashing In

The crash-in has several uses. You may want to get close enough to grapple, or to get inside the reach of a taller opponent. It is also useful if you have been hit and dazed but not put entirely out of the fight. If you allow yourself to take more shots you will eventually be demolished. Moving back is no good; the opponent will simply follow up. Ironically, the safest place to be while you collect your wits is in close.

Forward Drive

Most fights are very short, with little time for complex movement. As a rule you should attack as soon as possible and keep driving forward to retain the initiative. This does not preclude sidestepping or dodging an attack, but as with all combat it is generally better to be on the offensive than to allow the enemy to pick and choose where and how to attack. In short, the best approach is often that used by special forces teams – avoid the fights you can, but if you have to fight then get stuck in and take the opposition out before they have a chance to hurt you.

The shuffle

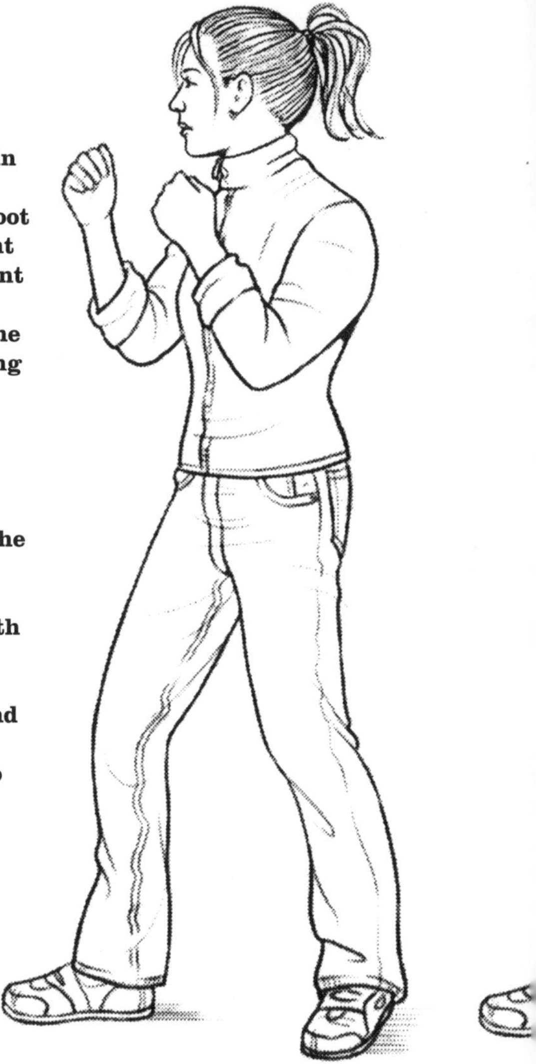

- To step forward in a shuffle, push with your back foot and lift your front one. Put your front foot down and bring the back one forward, returning to your basic 'boxer's guard' position. Do not take big steps.

- Moving back is the opposite way around; push yourself back with your front foot, reach back with your back foot and then move your front foot back to return to your starting stance.

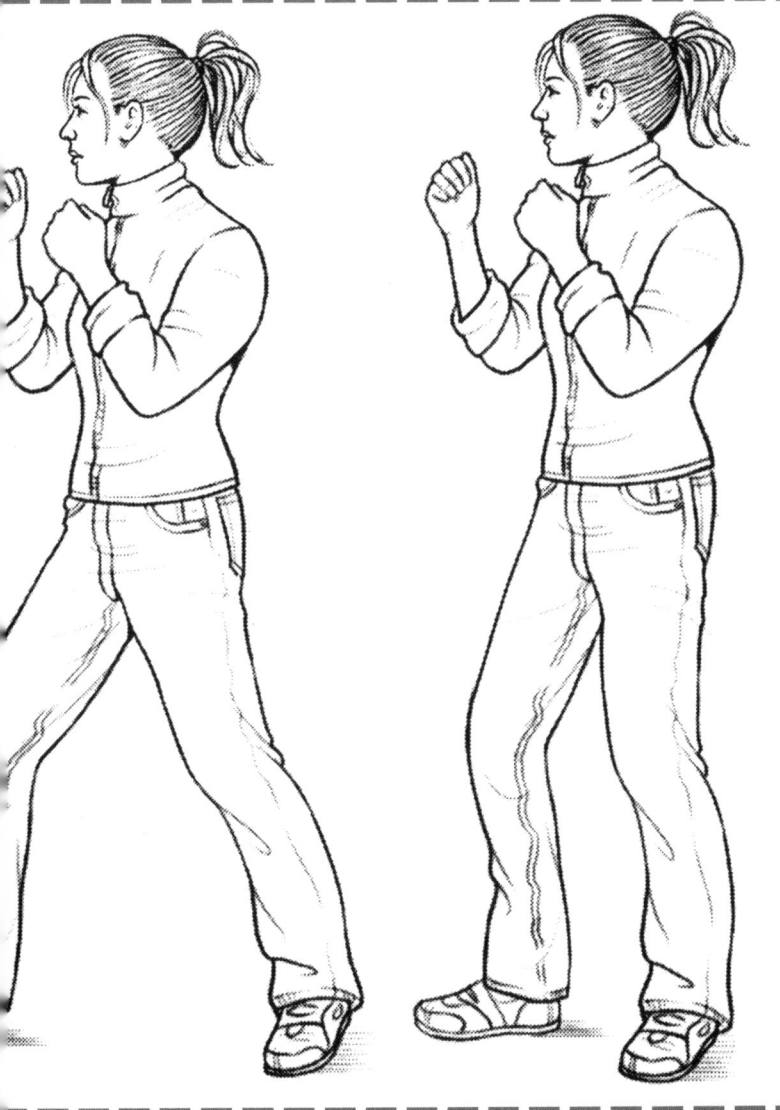

Crashing in

To crash in, simply cover your head and drive forward off the back foot, crashing into the opponent. Grab hold any way you can and stay in close until you can reorient yourself and begin fighting intelligently again. This is not a good situation to be in, but it is better than reeling backwards under a barrage of blows.

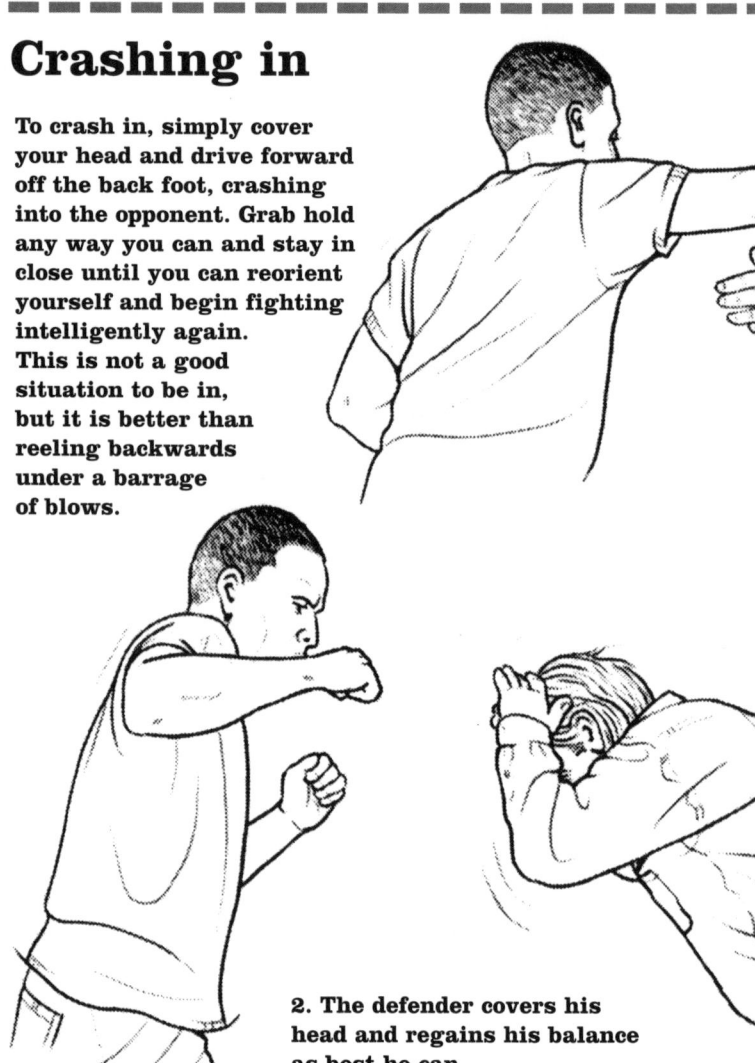

2. The defender covers his head and regains his balance as best he can.

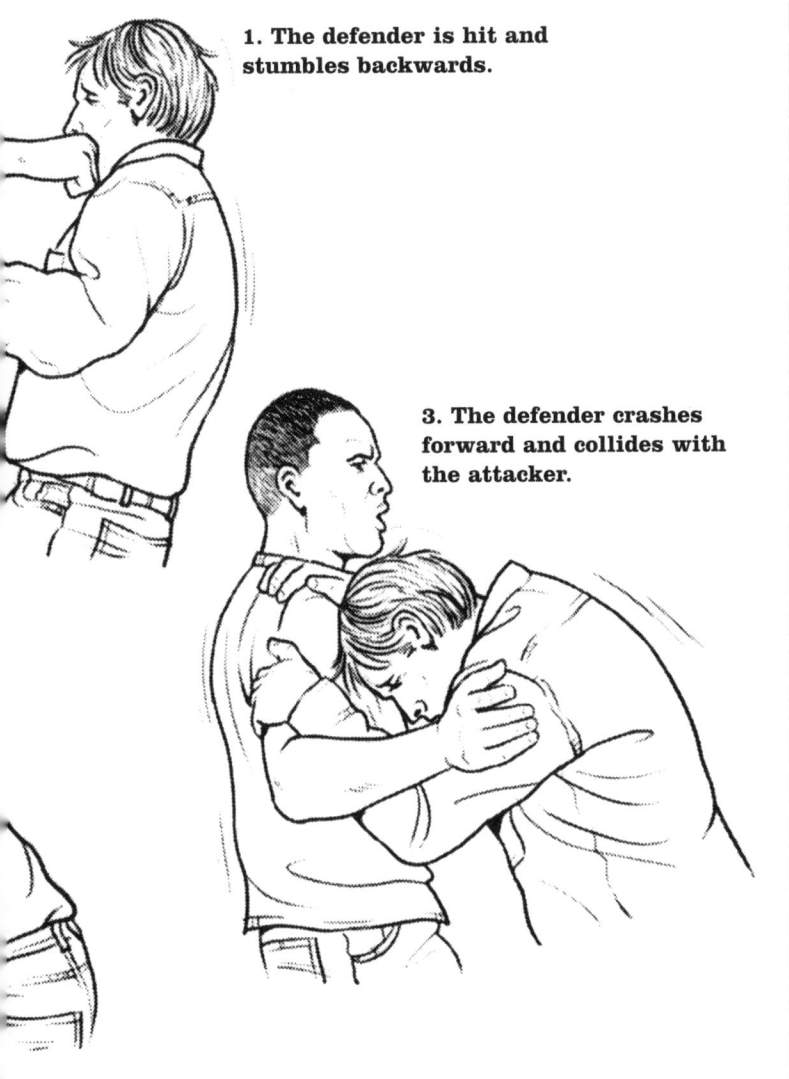

1. The defender is hit and stumbles backwards.

3. The defender crashes forward and collides with the attacker.

TARGETS

The human body is a strange thing. Racing drivers sometimes walk away from 321km/h (200mph) crashes, yet a relatively minor fall can result in broken bones or even death. It all depends on where and how the damage occurs.

The structure of the body is designed to protect the vital organs and critical functions as much as possible, but in order for it to operate it has to have weak areas. Rather than just flailing away at an opponent and hoping for the best, special forces soldiers are taught to attack the critical points of an opponent as efficiently as possible.

Taking Out an Opponent

There are three ways to take someone out of a fight:

- 'Switch them off' by rendering them unconscious.
- Cause sufficient damage that they cannot do you any harm even if they want to.
- Make them not want to fight any more by either convincing them to leave you alone or else hurting them enough to take the fight out of them.

The first option is best achieved with a knockout blow, usually to the head. Chokes and strangles also work well. Failing that, it may be possible to cause so much pain and damage that the aggressor loses consciousness, but this tends to require a prolonged beating. Most aggressors would become incapable of harming you long before they passed out.

Convincing someone not to attack you is really a pre-fight option. Once combat has started you are unlikely to be able to do this. However, there are sometimes opportunities for negotiation. If you can get a painful restraint on someone, you might be able to convince him that it is in his best interests to just leave you alone. However, this should only be attempted if you are very sure it will work. There is little to stop an aggressor from begging for release then attacking you again.

The upshot of all this is that unless you can achieve a knockout blow, it is more than likely you will have to strike the aggressor several times in order to subdue him. Most attempts to change an attacker's mind (i.e. convince him that he should go away and stop attacking you) require that you cause him pain and perhaps injury. Thus you should expect to have to strike blows if you engage in combat. You may be able to apply a choke, strangle or joint lock, but it can be difficult to get into the right position. As a general rule, strikes are the simplest and most effective option.

Target Areas

The human body has many vulnerable areas, and other points

where it is extremely resilient. There is some truth behind the concept of 'nerve points' or 'pressure points' – areas that can cause intense pain if poked just right – but in the middle of a fight you are unlikely to be able to target these points precisely. It is better to hit hard and aim for a fairly big target than to try for precise nerve strikes.

Generally speaking, it is fairly pointless to strike at large muscles such as the pectorals, thigh muscles and the upper arms. However, a suitably heavy blow with a weapon or with a hard striking surface (fist, knee and so forth) can damage a muscle or cause a 'dead leg/dead arm' that will impede use of the limb. A really heavy blow could break bones under

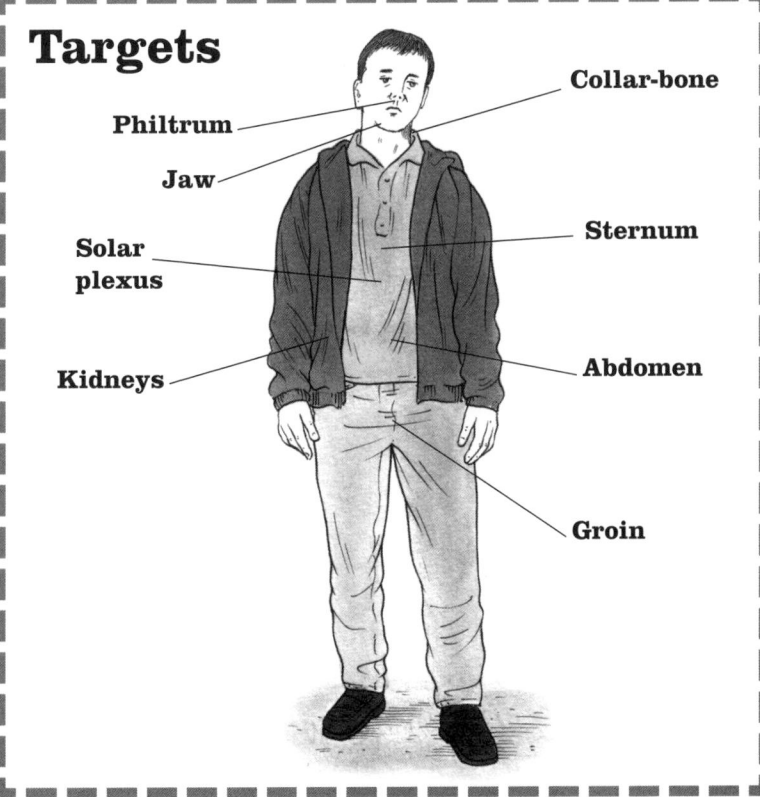

Targets

Philtrum

Jaw

Collar-bone

Solar plexus

Sternum

Kidneys

Abdomen

Groin

the muscle, but this normally requires a weapon such as a baton or stick.

The Head

Untrained people instinctively know to strike at the head. A hard enough blow anywhere on the head can cause unconsciousness due to 'brain shake', but some areas are more vulnerable than others.

- **The Skull** is very hard and is not a good striking area under most circumstances. Striking with a hard enough object can cause a skull fracture and/or death.
- **The Eyes** are one of the few areas of the body that cannot be protected by thick muscle. Poking or gouging at the eyes tends to produce a defensive reaction even if it does not cause much actual harm, so is useful in distracting an assailant from whatever you do next.
- **The Nose** is very sensitive. A blow to the nose can cause the eyes to fill up with tears, blinding the assailant for a moment.
- **Under the Nose** (the Philtrum) is also very sensitive to a blow or pressure.
- **The Jaw** can be struck from the front or side. This is the very best chance of causing a knockout, but the jaw is hard and can break your hand if you connect badly.
- **The Ears** can be grabbed and yanked or bitten to cause pain.

- **The Throat and Neck** can be struck from the side or front, or constricted to apply a choke or strangle. This can be lethal.

The head can be used in other ways. Where it goes, the body follows. Thus it is possible to turn someone or make them fall by twisting their head, pushing it backwards or pulling it down towards you.

The Torso

Unless you can deliver force well, striking most of the torso is somewhat pointless. Ribs and muscles protect the internal organs well. However, there are several places where a good strike can drop even a large, tough opponent. Generally speaking, blows that travel slightly upwards are more effective at sliding under the body's protection than downward strikes. The exception is a downward attack on the collar-bone.

- **The Collar-bone** is vulnerable to a downward blow. Breaking it will also disable the arm.
- **The Sternum** is directly over the heart and has large numbers of nerves running through it. A blow can cause intense pain.
- **The Solar Plexus** is just under the sternum and is the best spot to 'wind' an opponent. It can be hard to hit. The whole line around the torso at solar plexus height

contains targets that can be usefully struck – the liver, diaphragm and so forth – but the ribs offer good protection unless your strike is angled up from below.

- **The Kidneys** are a good target from the sides or from the front if you are close enough to throw a 'body hook' or roundhouse knee strike. Again, a slightly upward strike is more effective.

- **The Abdomen** is well protected by the abdominal muscles. A hard enough knee strike can knock the air out of an opponent and wind him, but this is not an ideal target.

- **The Groin** is another area that cannot be protected by piling on muscle in the gym. A blow to the genitals might not discommode an assailant, which can be an unpleasant surprise if you were banking on it. However, striking or grabbing at the groin will usually obtain a defensive response.

The Arms

Arms are not an ideal target for strikes unless you have a weapon that can break bones. However, they are often the nearest part of an assailant and do offer some useful targets.

- **The Upper Arm Muscles** can be struck with a fist or elbow in the hope of causing a 'dead arm'.

- **The Shoulder and Elbow Joints** can be attacked using a variety of arm-locking techniques either to cause pain or to break the joint.

- **The Wrist** can also be locked. However, it is hard to get a good grip on a hand or wrist, and most wrist locks are too fiddly for use in combat.

- **The Fingers** (including the thumb) can be grabbed and twisted to break them. This is only likely to work on someone who has hold of you.

The Legs

Legs can be attacked with kicks, knees or stamps. The front or side of the thigh can be given a 'dead leg' by driving a knee or roundhouse kick into it. Kicks lower down the leg can take the foot out from under the assailant and cause him to fall.

- **The Knee** is the most vulnerable part of the leg. Stamp-type kicks from front or side can disable the knee, taking the whole leg out of action.

- **The Shin and Ankle** can be kicked to cause considerable pain. Stamping on the ankles of a downed opponent will break them.

- **The Foot** is vulnerable to being stamped on, especially on the top of the instep. Alternatively, you can step on a foot to trap it and push the assailant over. If you keep his foot trapped as he falls, the ankle will break.

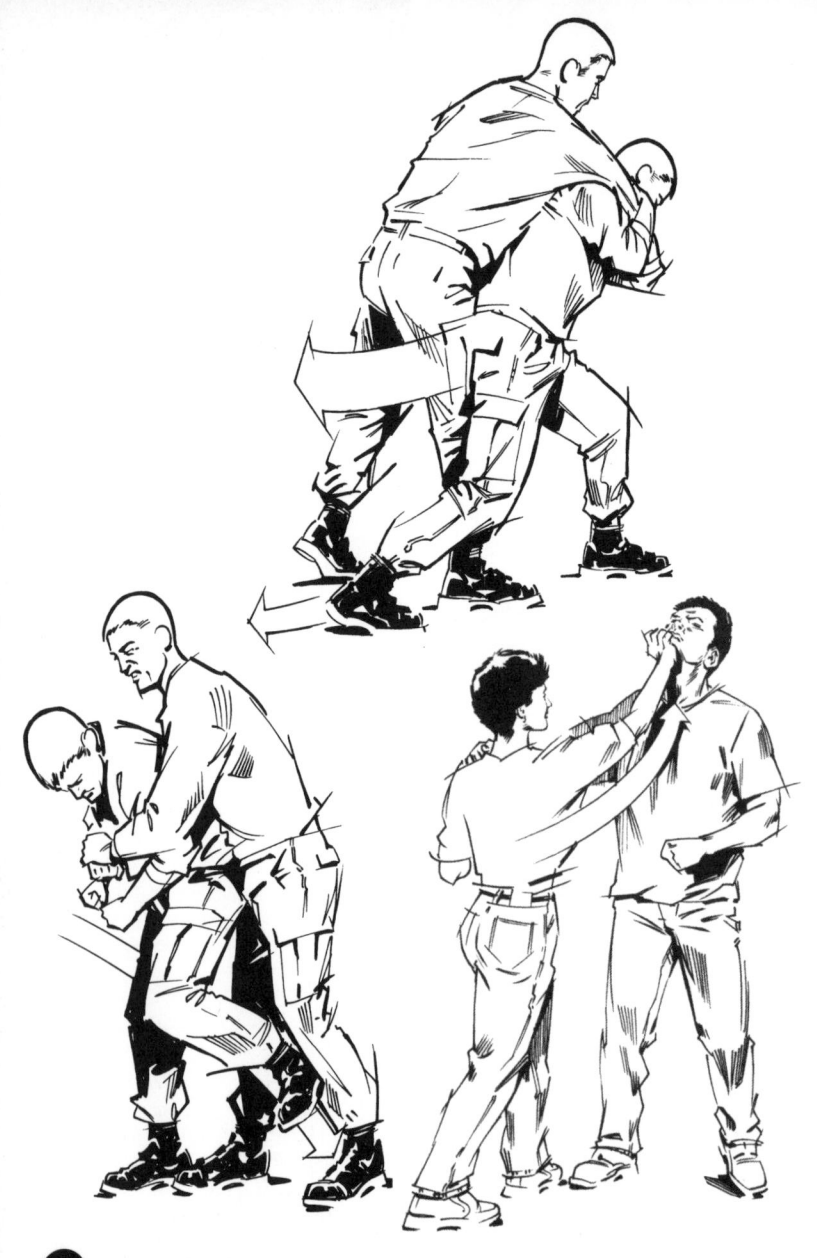

Any form of unarmed combat or self-defence training is best done under the supervision of a properly qualified instructor. Military instructors are experts in their field who can 'do' as well as teach, and this is a good guideline when looking for someone to teach you. Your life may depend on your unarmed combat skills, so it makes sense to find a teacher who understands real-world violence and who can perform what they show you. Talking a good fight is all very well but it would not be wise to trust your safety to unproven theories and big claims.

This section is not about specific techniques – the rest of the book deals with that – but about making your training as real as possible and preparing yourself to deal with what really happens in a fight. It also shows you how to test your skills under controlled but realistic conditions. As implied above, an instructor who cannot make his techniques work under this sort of fairly mild pressure-testing is probably not worth your time.

....

Left: There are essentially three aspects to unarmed combat training – defensive grappling to escape from a hold, offensive grappling intended to harm the opponent, and striking techniques.

5

Making your training as real as possible is the best preparation for real life fights.

Tools of the Trade

Unarmed Combat Training

TRAINING FOR REALITY

Anyone can perform what appear to be devastating techniques on a compliant partner in a class. The question is – will the same technique work on a wet pavement against an aggressive, possibly drunk, assailant who comes out of nowhere at 3.00 a.m. outside a nightclub?

TIPS:
REASONS FOR FAILURE

The key factors that can prevent you from successfully defending yourself are:

- Fear and adrenaline can debilitate anyone. Adrenaline is a natural reaction to the fear and stress of an impending fight, and can give you immense strength – but unless you know how to handle it, adrenaline can also exhaust you quickly and can actually inhibit you from acting when you need to. Good training incorporates some of the stress and pressure of a fight, so that you get used to the adrenaline and can think clearly under pressure.
- Uncertainty about the situation often prevents people acting until it is too late. Doubt about whether their actions will be successful can cause victims of assault to give in instead of fighting. Good training not only builds confidence in the techniques in use but also should involve some realistic 'scenario work' whereby the student can get used to how aggressors behave and learn to determine what is a real threat and what is simply a suspicious situation.
- Aggression is the main tool of the typical 'street' attacker. Many cannot actually fight that well, but rely on a barrage of threats and blows to overwhelm the victim. Good training includes specific techniques to deal with an extremely aggressive assailant, and also includes an element of 'stress inoculation' to prevent panic when faced with an apparently psychopathic individual.

Real fights never take place in a well-lit training area with mats on the floor, when you are well rested and prepared. Good training should involve at least some adverse situations so that the student learns to cope with whatever happens and fight on. There is a limit to how 'real' you can make training, but the more elements of real combat you can incorporate – at least to some degree – in your training, the better prepared you will be.

TACTICS

Good training includes use of tactics as well as techniques. Well-trained or experienced fighters play to their own strengths and try not to allow their opponents to do the same. For example, if you recognize that the attacker has little in his arsenal beyond big swinging blows, you might decide that grappling is a good choice because it will not allow him to use his strikes.

Good tactics also includes use of your surroundings and the situation. This is of paramount importance when dealing with a group. If you can move so that some of them get in each other's way or have to get past obstacles, you can buy time to deal with the others. You may also be able to manoeuvre so that you have a clear run out the door or to an object that you can use as a weapon.

> ### TIP: THE GOAL
>
> Your primary goal when confronted with aggression is to preserve your safety. If you have to fight to do so, then that is what you do. But do not let 'winning the fight' become your primary mission. Too many people have been badly hurt because they continued a fight when they had a chance to escape. Your goal is to preserve your safety, and every action should be directed towards that rather than incidental objectives like hurting the aggressor.

Taking the Offensive

Tactically, the most important thing that you can learn is how to take the offensive. You cannot win a fight by passively defending or running about dodging blows. It is sometimes possible to create an escape route, which can end the situation, but failing that you will have to take the fight to the opponent.

This may seem at odds with the philosophy of many martial arts – the ones that impose strict rules about not striking first. That is of no consequence; the reality of combat is that in order to win you have to harm the opponent. There is nothing unethical about striking first so long as it is justified. If you can see that someone intends to do you harm, then there is nothing to gain by waiting for him to start. He has already committed himself to hurting you, which is much the same as actually causing you harm – the only difference is that he has not yet achieved his aim.

The Offensive Mindset

An offensive mindset is extremely important to help you deal with fear. Military personnel know that it is much harder to cope with being shot at or shelled without being able to retaliate than when they are able to shoot back. The same applies in unarmed combat; fear saps your will to win while you wait for the assailant to make his move. By taking the offensive you are doing something positive. A blow that might have taken the fight right out of you will sometimes barely register if you are in the middle of launching an attack of your own.

Equally, an offensive mindset prevents the assailant from picking his shots. If you let him, he will accumulate all the advantages he

Air rage

Violence and aggression can erupt anywhere, but conflict is more likely in any place where people are frustrated and in close proximity to one another. 'Air rage' is particularly dangerous due to the close confines of an aircraft.

can get before committing himself. If he can erode your will by threats and intimidation, disorient you and establish dominance by shoving you or grabbing your clothing and ragging you about, then when he comes to actually hit you the fight will largely be over. Your chances are much better if you can at least force him to fight you without these advantages. And of course, the fact that you will not allow him to accrue his desired

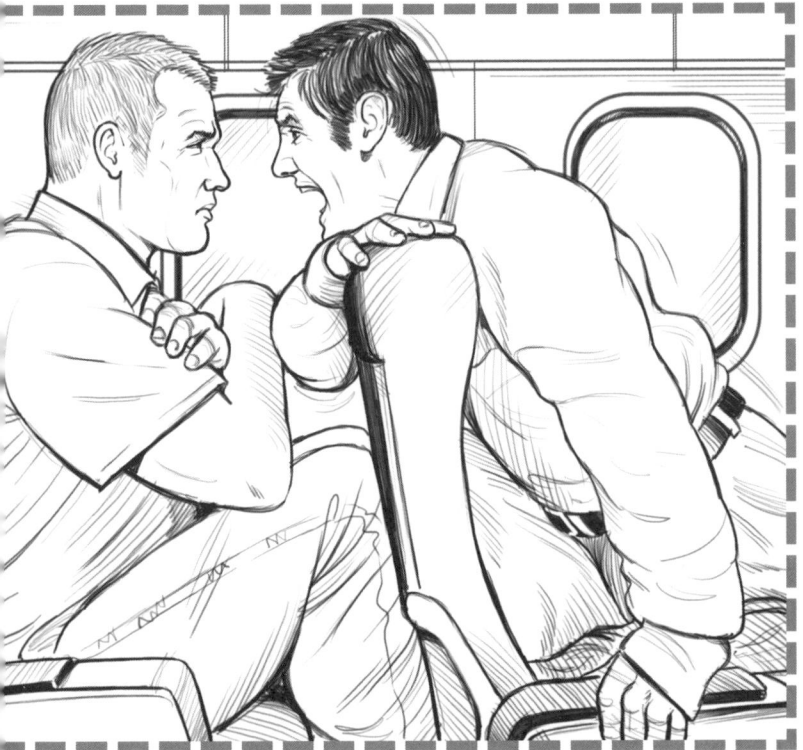

advantages might be enough to make him pick another, easier, target.

APPLICATION WORK

Once you have learned how to perform a given technique, you need to learn how to use it. Some techniques have absolutely zero chance of working under particular conditions – you need to know about this. Others are perfect for certain circumstances – you need to

learn how to set them up or to recognize the opportunity when it arises. You also need to try out different things to see what works for you and what does not; everyone is different and not everything works well for everyone.

All kinds of application drills are possible. For example, a student may have to face an instructor wearing boxing gloves who will wade in swinging like the typical 'outside a nightclub' attacker. Each student who participates is free to respond as they think appropriate. One student might choose to strike, another to grapple. This kind of drill allows students to try out different tactics and to make their mistakes in the training area rather than the real world.

Conventional Application Work

Most martial arts and combat sports use some form of application work which can be useful in relation to self-defence training.

- **Sparring** is normally associated with boxing or kickboxing techniques. Sparring is an opportunity to practise striking, defensive and evasive techniques. Less obviously, and just as important, sparring teaches the use of mobility and footwork, as well as learning to 'read' an opponent to see what they are about to do.
- **Rolling** is to grappling on the ground what sparring is to striking. Normally students are not permitted to strike and must grapple to a successful finish. This is normally signified by the opponent 'tapping out' to signify that they cannot escape from whatever technique has been applied. Students tend to spend a lot of time rolling around trying to get a dominant position – hence the name.

- **Randori** is a term borrowed from the martial art of Judo, for a contest where the combatants start standing and cannot strike one another. They fight for a takedown or throw and then seek a finish on the ground. Randori is one of the most physically demanding activities known to man, and builds both stamina and good, functional muscle.

Effective Application Work

All kinds of 'application work' can be hazardous, and indeed can be counterproductive. Once a student has developed some basic skills and has some confidence, they can start into application work, but the intensity needs to be built up gradually in order to avoid making the student lose confidence.

Varying intensity is a good idea even with experienced students. For example, lighter sparring is good for practising technique while heavier contact teaches students to deliver power and to take shots. Being hit hard encourages students to develop a good defence, but it is necessary to build up to this gradually to avoid becoming 'glove-shy'. This is counterproductive and must be avoided.

That said, there has to be some kind of challenge for application work to be anything more than a game. Non-contact sparring is of little use, but the degree of contact

Sparring

If someone has a good hold on you, it will not be possible to just pull it off. By inflicting pain, you can weaken the grab and make escape possible.

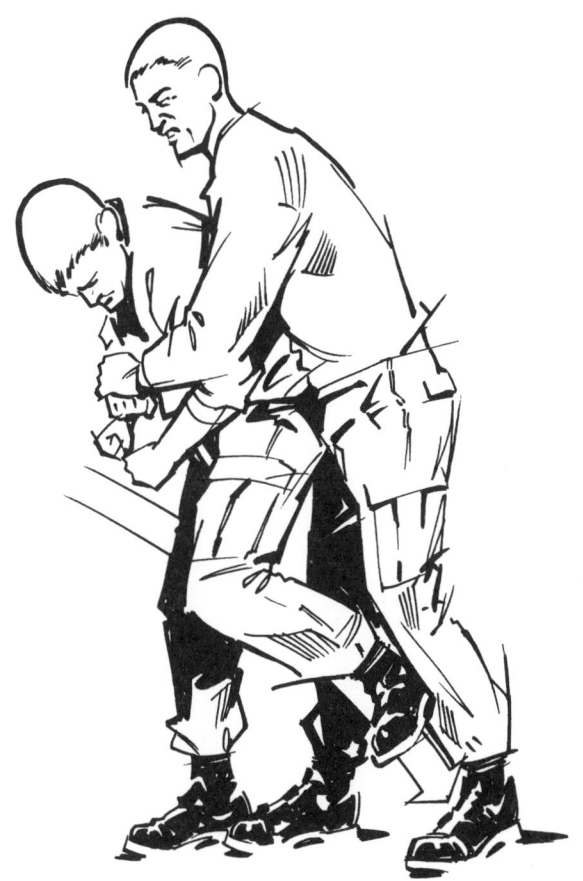

TIP:
TRY IT FOR YOURSELF

A lot of the time, techniques work really well when a partner 'feeds' you whatever attack you need in order to do the technique. But what about someone who just swings a punch at your head? Will it work then? This is an important question; your life could depend on it. It is one thing to hear an instructor say a technique will work, or to do it in the class with a compliant partner, and quite another to know for sure if it will work for real. Obviously, it is not practical (nor very wise) to go around picking fights in order to try out your skills. However, you can test out your skills under fairly realistic conditions.

Get a partner with boxing gloves on (16oz gloves are recommended for safety) and have them attack you with a real intent to hit. You can start quite light and work up to a full-on assault as you get more comfortable with the situation. If you can make your technique work on someone who is just swinging at you rather than feeding you a specific attack then it is valid. If not, either you cannot do it properly or it is not a useful technique.

can be varied from extremely light up to a full-on attempt to knock one another out depending on the circumstances. Realism in training should always be balanced against safety, and students should be offered challenges (and encouraged to meet them) rather than being pushed into something they are not ready for.

Pressure-Testing

Pressure-testing is essentially a very intense form of application work. As the name suggests, a student is put under stress and tested to the limit – but not beyond. Pressure-testing is designed to build the student's confidence, not to break the spirit.

Similar methods can be used to pressure-test as are used in

Body drop

This powerful throw is an effective counter to a grab from behind. Pull the opponent's arm forward as you take his lead leg out from under him by thrusting back with your hip and leg.

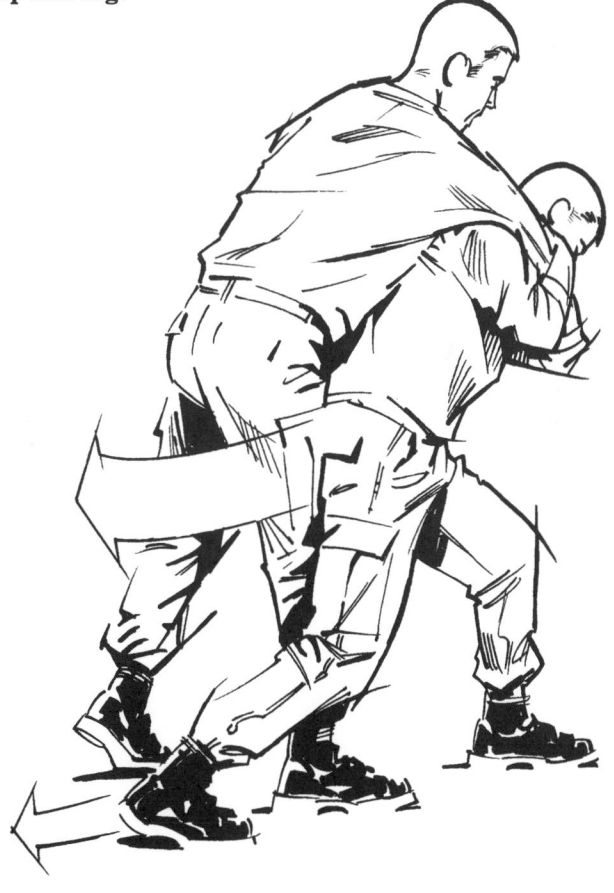

TIP:
**MAKE YOUR
MISTAKES IN
TRAINING**

Nobody likes to screw up,
but the more mistakes
you make in training, the
less chance there is that
you will get it wrong
when it counts. Push your
limits and seek out your
weak areas in training –
and fix the problem.
Embarrassment in the
class hurts less than a
beating in the street.

application work, only with greater intensity. For example, a student might have to go several one-minute rounds of groundfighting (rolling), with a fresh opponent coming in each time. He could then be required to spar a round with a fresh opponent when he is exhausted.

Alternatively, specific drills can be used. For example, a student might be confronted by several potential opponents, all of whom have boxing gloves on. They all grab and push, shouting and threatening the 'victim' to create stress, and then one of them launches an attack. The student must deal with the situation as best they can. This can be varied by having one or even several of the other aggressors join in. The resulting scramble goes on until the student achieves a dominant position, escapes, or the instructor calls a halt for safety reasons.

Benefits of Pressure-Testing

It is important to set a challenging but not impossible level of difficulty for any kind of drill. The aim, as already stated, is to test the student rather than defeat them. Disasters will happen, along with bizarre occurrences that make good 'war stories' for the pub later on, and the outcome should be talked through to show where the student made a good choice or a dubious one, to find out what went right and what really did not.

Quite apart from the ability to practise techniques under as close to real combat conditions as possible, pressure-testing enables the student to develop an almost instinctive understanding of what goes on in the chaos of a fight. Most importantly, to have been through the wringer and emerged victorious is a great feeling, which helps build self-confidence.

DEVELOPING AND USING SITUATIONAL AWARENESS

No amount of training or equipment is any use to a soldier who steps on a mine or is hit by an unsuspected sniper. Similarly, if an attack catches you completely unawares, you could be taken out of the fight before you have a chance to respond. Even if you are not knocked clean out, it is very hard to get back into a fight if you started out losing badly.

Habitual Awareness

The best way to avoid this happening is to develop habitual awareness of your surroundings. Special forces training teaches soldiers to constantly watch what is going on around them, and more importantly to make the right connections between the situation and what an enemy might do. A special forces patrol member will automatically note good points for an ambush or locations for a sniper. This may enable him to avoid the location altogether or to look more closely for an enemy.

If hostiles are spotted, it may be possible to turn the tables on them by sneaking up to ambush the ambushers, or the area might simply be bypassed. Even if the enemy cannot be avoided, awareness gives the special forces soldier an advantage in the vital first few seconds of an action. Instead of having to look for where fire might be coming from, the patrol will already have noted likely locations and can take cover or return fire quickly. Even if a sniper is well hidden, shooting up

his likely location will make it difficult for him to make a shot.

Awareness on the Street

By spotting potential trouble in the form of suspicious people and places where an attack is more likely, you can avoid many possible problems, or at least be mentally prepared to either de-escalate a situation and withdraw or fight your way out.

You can train yourself to automatically note potential hazards and to keep track of your surroundings. This helps formulate a gameplan quickly if you have to deal with a situation. For example, if you are in a room with one door, then there is only one likely direction a threat can come from – and only one easy route out.

One good way to learn this skill is to try to spot hazards around your home or workplace. For example, shoes left where family members could trip over them, objects close to the edge of a work surface, fragile ornaments located where toddlers can reach them … once you get into the habit of spotting hazards, all kinds of things become obvious. This can help prevent the occasional domestic disaster, in addition to any other benefits.

Using Awareness

Good driving instructors teach students to watch the road well ahead and deal with hazards early. A

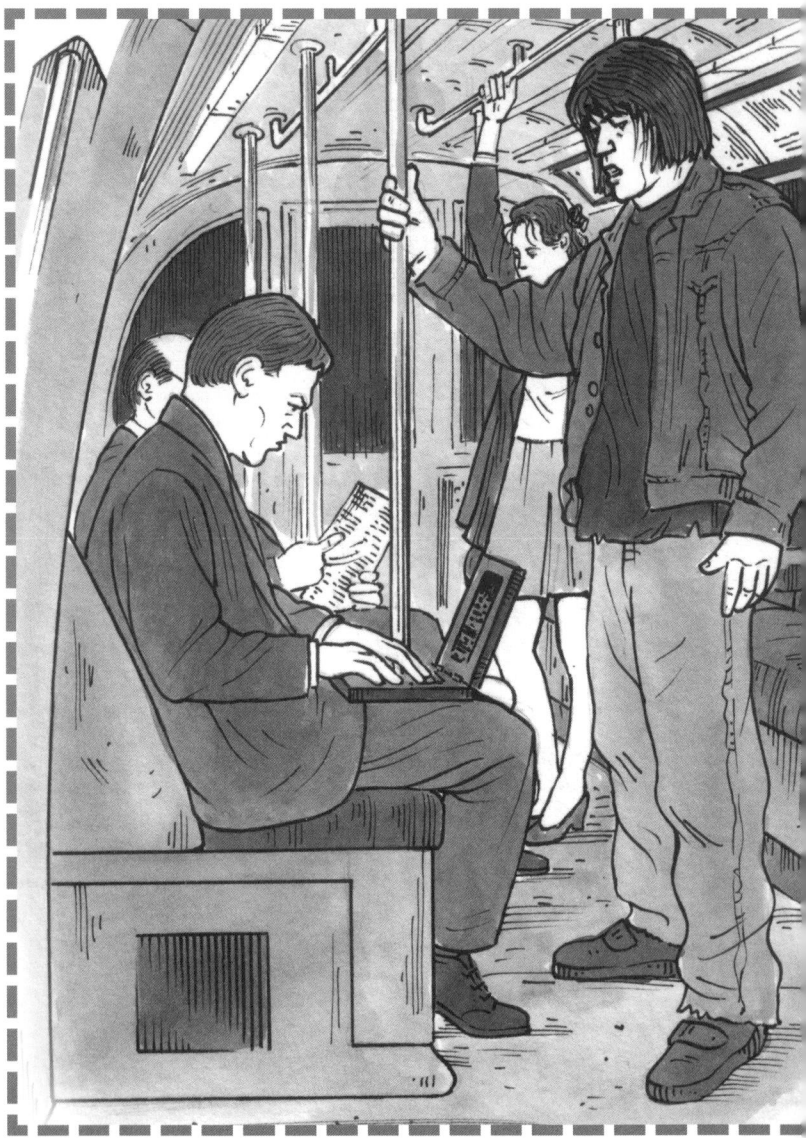

Situational awareness

Do not become so absorbed in whatever you are doing that you lose track of your surroundings. Not only does this make it impossible to deal with an attack, it also makes one more likely.

TIP: SIGNS OF AGGRESSION

- Flushed or very pale face.
- Jerky, violent movements.
- Contemptuous, angry or smirking expression.
- Speaking in very short sentence fragments or insults.
- Threats.
- Splayed hands.
- Very wide eyes or very small pupils.

timely lane change is a better solution to a motorway hazard than a tyre-smoking emergency stop, just as choosing not to walk past a gang on a street corner is better than battling them.

You can apply the same principles to self-protection. Watch out for poorly lit areas and for places where you have to pass close to a corner or to another area where an assailant could be concealed, and of course keep an eye out for people who just seem a bit suspicious. Ideally, you should avoid these people completely but if this is not possible then at least you can put some distance between you and them,

Avoiding dangerous areas

Trust your instincts. If you don't like the look of an area, leave or stay out. Complacently telling yourself 'it'll be all right' is a recipe for disaster.

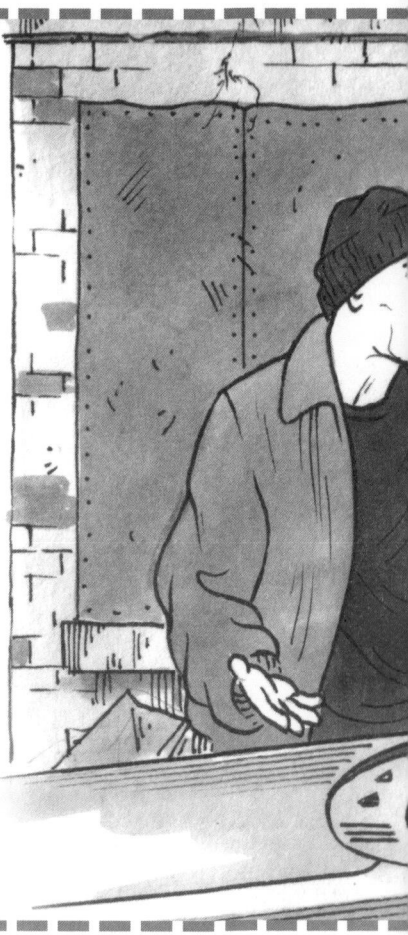

and be mentally prepared if they decide to approach you.

Of course, no amount of awareness is any use if you simply ignore your instincts, shrug and tell yourself it will be all right, and carry on regardless. You must be willing to act upon your observations in an appropriate manner. This can mean instant violence if necessary, or simply noting the threat and keeping an eye on it as you pass by.

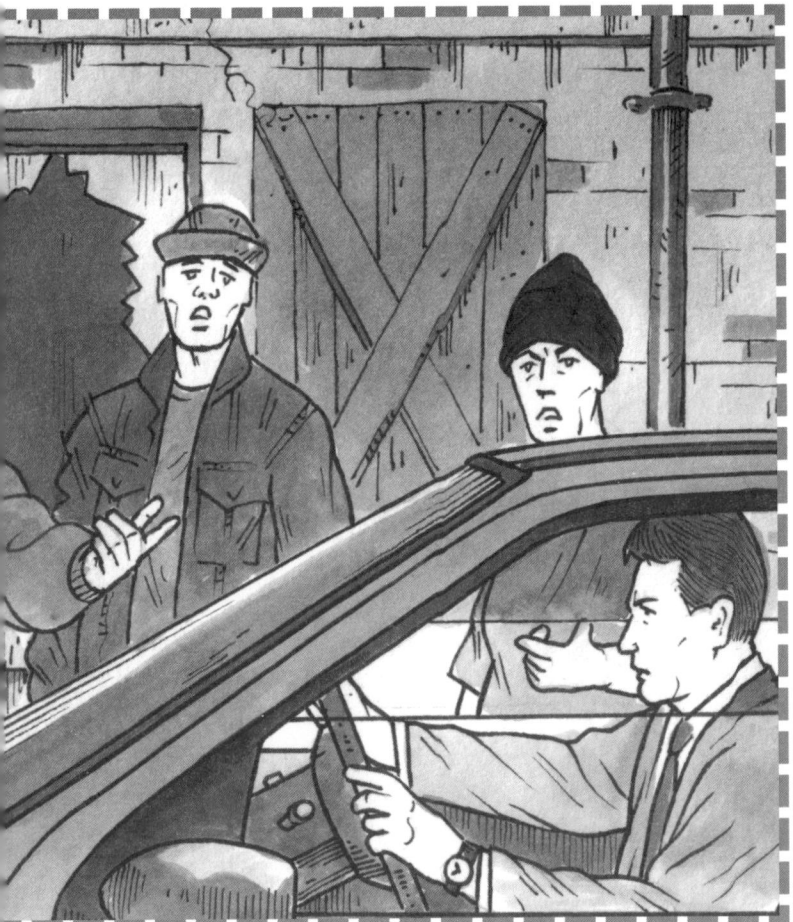

The Colour Code

We use a colour code to identify states of awareness and potential threats.

• **Code White** means you are completely oblivious to your surroundings, boogying down the street with your hood up and personal stereo blasting the greatest hits of 1972 in your ears … or whatever. Code White means you are not looking for

123

potential hazards and not in a mental state where you would even recognize a hazard, let alone act upon it. An attack against you will come as a complete surprise and will almost certainly succeed.

- **Code Yellow** indicates normal, habitual awareness. If a potential threat appears you will note it and decide what action needs to be taken, without being unnecessarily paranoid and nervous. Code Yellow indicates that there is no specific threat but you are aware enough that you would spot one if it appeared.

- **Code Orange** means that you have spotted a specific threat or opportunity for an aggressor but do not think that you are about to be imminently attacked. You might go to Code Orange when getting money from an ATM, because common sense suggests that this is a time when muggers might see an opportunity. Code Orange might also be triggered by someone approaching you in a manner that makes you suspicious. Code Orange indicates that you have recognized a hazard and are formulating a response in case it develops into an imminent threat.

- **Code Red** means that you are under attack or have reason to believe that you are about to be attacked. Code Red requires a physical response, which might be to flee, or to fight, or to dodge through a nearby doorway and bolt it behind you … the response must be appropriate to the goal of getting yourself out of the situation to safety. Thus Code Red probably means you are in a fight, but you must remember that winning the fight is just a means to an end – protecting yourself from harm is the real goal. If you are at Code Red then you must act to save yourself, fighting or doing whatever else offers you the best chance.

Making Use of the OODA Loop

'OODA' stands for Observation, Orientation, Decision, Action. If you have habitually observed your surroundings (Code Yellow), spotted a potential threat and evaluated it (Code Orange) and realized that you are about to be attacked (Code Red) then you will have already formulated the most basic of gameplans (probably something like 'hit him first') and are already at the Action stage. Your response will be quicker and more effective than if you had to figure out what just happened, realize you need to fight, orient yourself and the attacker, decide what to do, and do it.

TIP:
THE OODA LOOP

The 'OODA Loop' is a constant cycle that everyone goes through, no matter what they are doing.

- Observation – you see, hear, feel, smell and possibly taste what is going on around you.
- Orientation – you use the data from your senses to build up an image of where you are in relation to objects and people around you.
- Decision – you decide what to do next.
- Action – you act.

Since any action may change the circumstances around you, however slightly, the loop repeats before your next action. Usually, observation and orientation are constantly going on but they can be interrupted. If you are hit suddenly from the side and sent reeling away, you will have to reorient yourself, which requires observation of the new circumstances. This is a very quick process, but when under attack you have very little time. Thus if you can shortcut your initial response then your chances improve greatly.

The OODA Loop can work in your favour. If you hit the bad guy and then move, it will take him an instant to observe the new situation, orient himself, decide what to do and then start to do it. By that time, benefiting from an uninterrupted OODA Loop (you observed and oriented while you were changing position) you can be halfway through hitting him again.

Maintaining constant observation and orientation is a difficult business in a fight. The relevant skills are developed and honed in application work, as noted above. Thus the more sparring, randori, rolling or application drilling you have done, the better your in-fight awareness will be, and thus the better your chances of dealing with an assault.

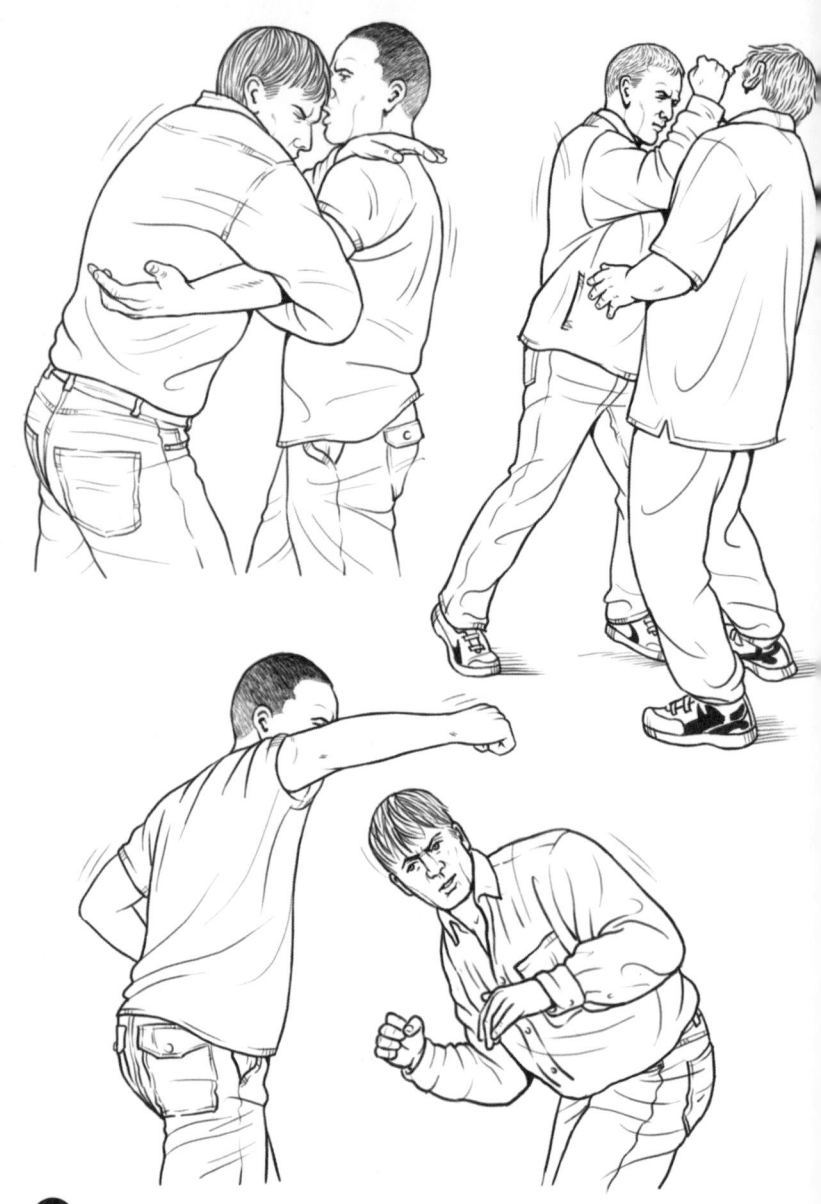

Occasionally, someone is described as being 'able to kill a man with their bare hands'. Truth is, everyone is capable of that if they know how. Compared to, say, a tiger or a shark, the human body's weapons are rather puny. However, they are entirely sufficient to cause severe harm to another human being. You can strike at another person with your hands, feet, knees, elbows and head, and can use your ability to grab and push or pull to good advantage too.

As noted already, even if you cannot do enough damage to subdue an attacker you may be able to make him give up attacking you, or switch his attention from hurting you to making you stop clawing at his eyes. An attacker whose easy victim turns out to be a screaming banshee intent on tearing his eyes out and biting chunks out of his flesh may well decide that you are more trouble than you are worth.

STRIKING WITH HANDS

Striking with the hands is perhaps the most obvious of your options.

....

Left: You can make use of your body's weapons in many ways, such as striking an opponent or applying pressure against his joints to disable them.

6

Your body has many weapons: fists, elbows, knees and feet are the obvious ones.

Tools of the Trade

Your Body's Weapons

Making a fist

Make a good, tight fist, tucking the thumb down the side against your fingers (A). Do not leave the thumb sticking out (B) or tuck it into the fist (C); both will result in a broken thumb.

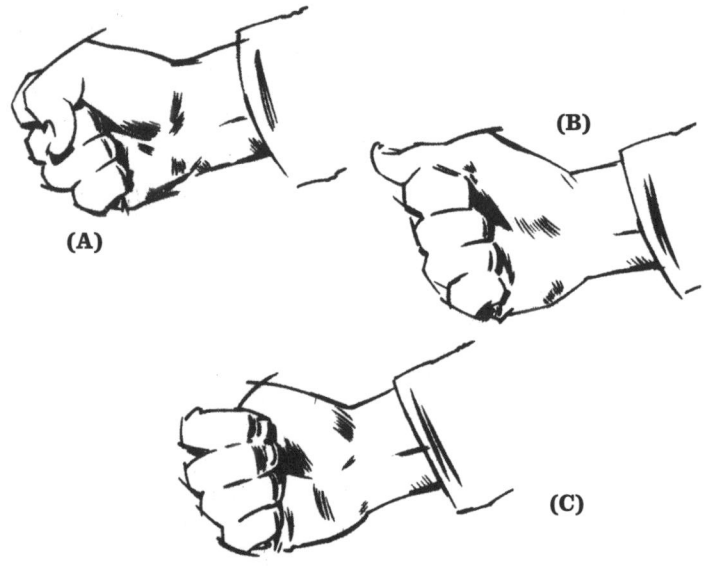

(A)

(B)

(C)

However, there are a number of possible ways to strike. The hand contains a great many small bones which can be broken by impact with a solid surface. Thus it is important to make a tight fist when striking, in order to support the hand and wrist.

Striking with the knuckles against the jaw is an excellent way of obtaining a knockout, but you need to connect cleanly to avoid damaging your hand. Fists are good weapons to use against softer tissue such as the solar plexus or kidneys.

Alternatively, a hammerfist is a good option, especially for downward blows. Make a tight fist and strike with the base of it.

Hammerfist

Striking with the base of the fist instead of the knuckles is very effective, especially against hard targets like the head. There is no risk of breaking your hand with a hammerfist.

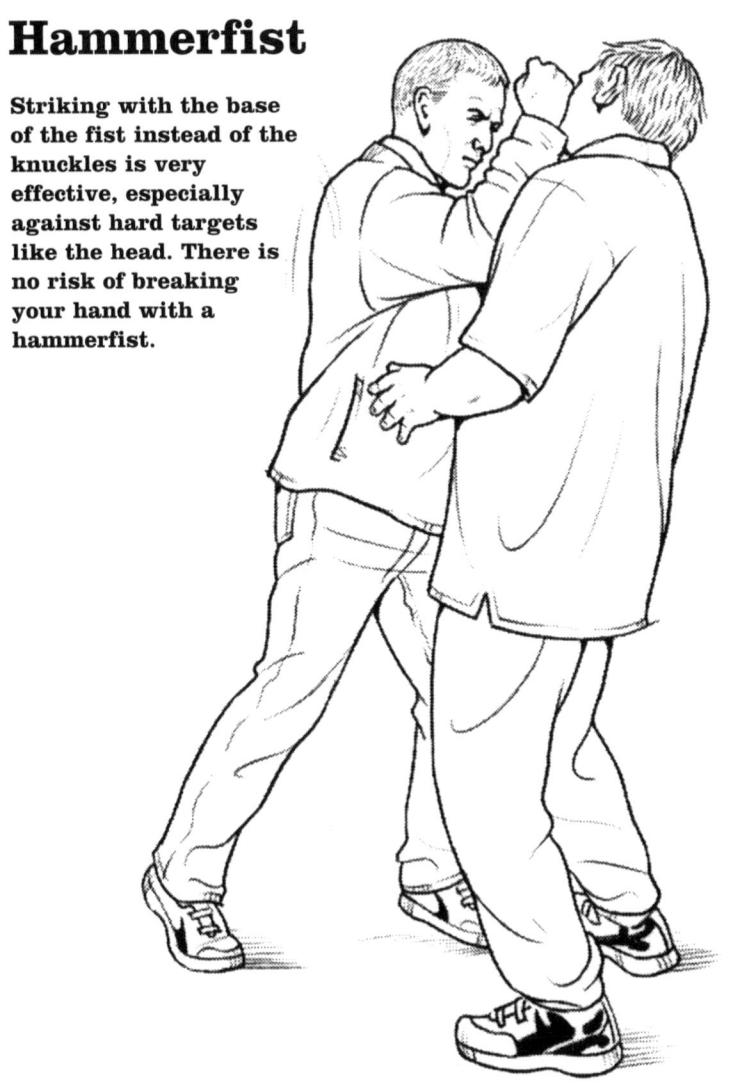

Palm strike

Striking with the base of the palm is another good way to protect your hands when hitting hard targets like the jaw. The mechanics of the strike are the same as for a straight punch.

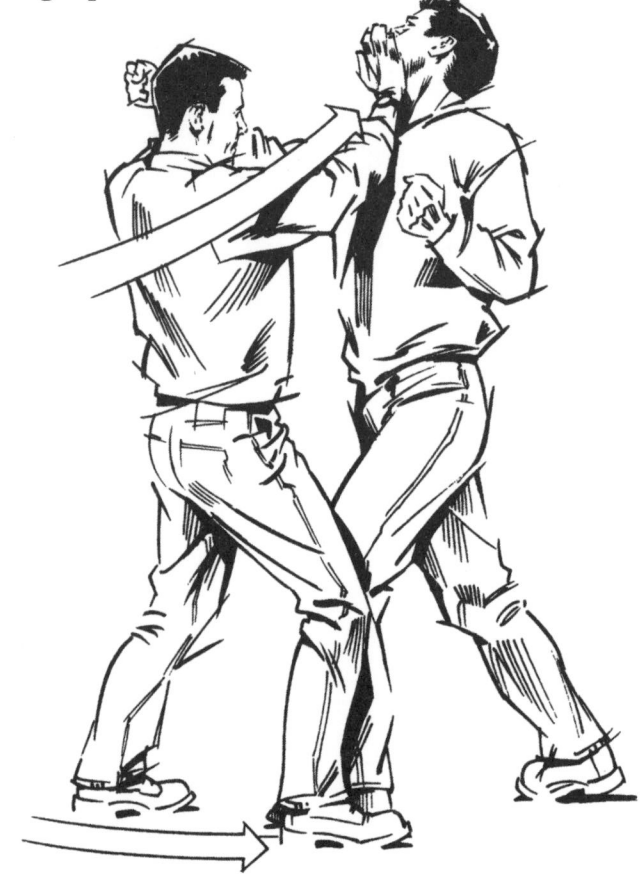

Edge-of-hand strikes

Edge-of-hand strikes are useful for soft targets like the neck, but are ineffective against hard or bony areas like the jaw or ribs.

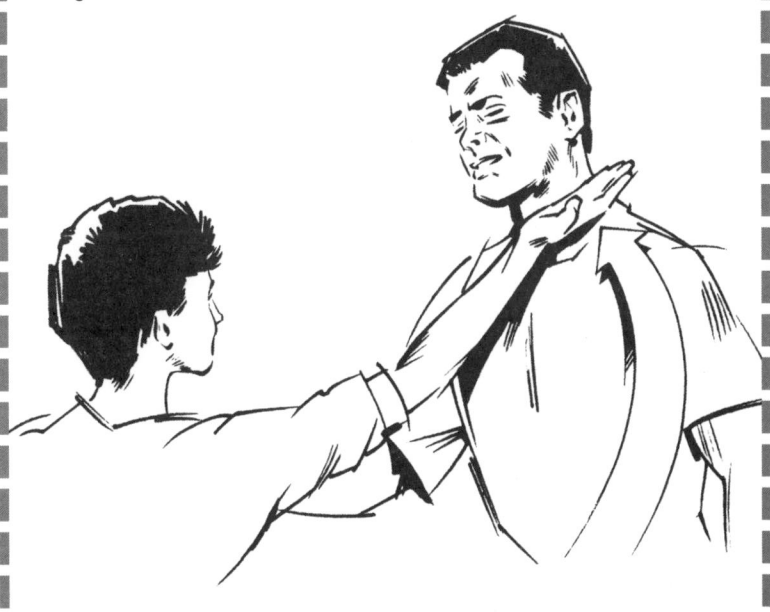

Other Hand and Arm Strikes

Striking with an open hand, using the palm, is good against bony targets such as the head. You use the same pushing or hooking action as a punch, and the natural padding of the base of your hand prevents damage. You can also strike with the edge of your hand.

Use the base of the hand rather than the fingers.

Your forearms and elbows can also be used to strike with, especially at close quarters. Elbows can be used for hooking (curved) strikes or straight ones. The bone in the elbow is very hard and will not be damaged easily by even the hardest strike.

131

Kick to the groin

Stabbing kicks with the toes are highly effective against soft body parts, especially if you are wearing hard shoes.

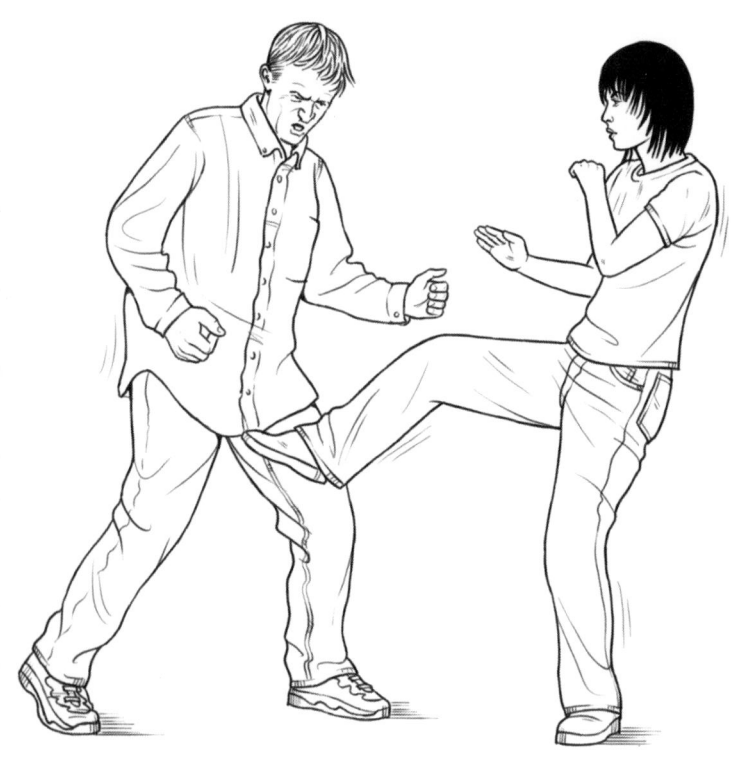

LEGS AND FEET

When you lift a foot up to kick, you lose at least 75 per cent of your balance. High kicks are an invitation to be knocked over, and should not be used. Some kicks are too complex or require too much space to be much use, so it is best to stick to the simplest of kicks and stomps.

Striking with the knee is instinctive and does not compromise your balance much, especially if you have a good grip on your opponent at the time. Knees are excellent close-quarters weapons.

If you want to strike with your foot, a simple stomping action is easy – strike with the heel first if you can. For more 'martial arts' type kicks there are various opinions on how to strike with your foot. However, most martial arts are performed barefoot and you are likely to be wearing shoes or boots, so a slightly different approach can be taken.

OTHER OPTIONS

A headbutt can be a powerful weapon, and need not be particularly precise. Drive a corner of your head (or any part of your skull above the eye line) into the target, ideally with a drop-step. Aim to hit below the eye line – otherwise you are simply banging two rocks together; the hardest will usually survive but both can end up cracked.

Even if you have no other options, you can bite and scratch. Using

TIPS: STRIKING WITH THE FOOT

- Top of foot (instep) can be used for a rising strike to the groin or the face of a bent-over opponent. The instep is sometimes used as the striking surface in a roundhouse kick.
- Shins are used (along with the instep) to strike with in a roundhouse kick.
- Ball of foot is used with many straight kicks. Some styles strike with the ball of the foot in a roundhouse kick, but this can be difficult with shoes on.
- Heel is used in stomps and thrust kicks (which are basically just sideways stomp kicks).
- Edge of foot is used in some martial arts styles but is not ideal for anyone wearing shoes.
- Toes can be used to 'stab' with if you are wearing hard shoes or boots.

Headbutt

There is nothing complex about a headbutt. Drive any part of your head above your eye line into the opponent, anywhere below his eye line. Cheekbones and nose are ideal targets.

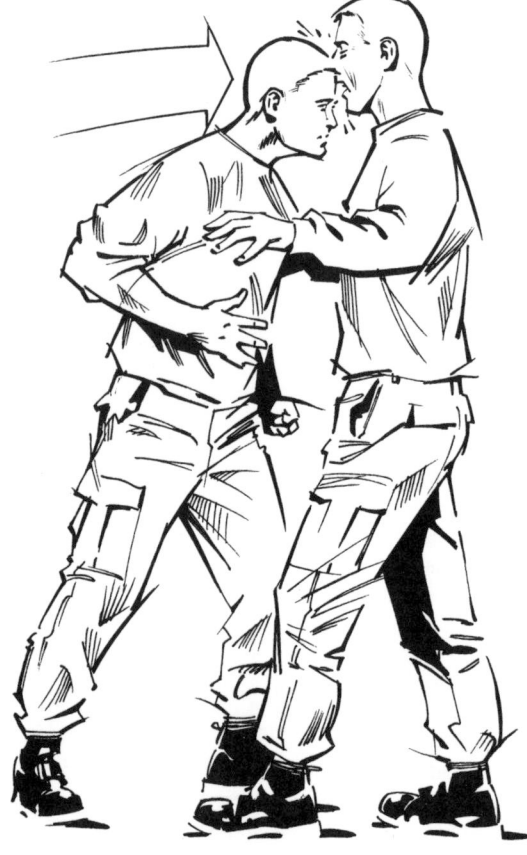

your nails as claws, your best target is the eyes and face, but any scratch is painful and collects DNA evidence which can be used to secure a conviction later. Biting also works surprisingly well. Rather than trying to bite through flesh, biting and ripping, or nipping a fairly small amount of flesh is highly effective.

Similarly, you can grab and rip at an opponent's flesh. Ears, noses and hair are fairly easy to get hold of, but you can also grab any fairly loose flesh such as cheeks or the sides below the ribs. Crunch up a handful of flesh and twist it to cause pain. None of this will seriously inconvenience an attacker of course, but it may be enough to make him give up, or to create an opportunity to do something more decisive.

DEFENCES

Ideally, you should defend yourself by not being attacked, i.e. avoid the aggressor or de-escalate the situation. Failing that, defend by taking the initiative and putting your opponent out of action before he can hurt you. However, once an attack is launched you must do something about it.

Pure defence is not a good idea. In other words, if you simply dodge or block an attack, your opponent can just throw another one. Even if you try to block-then-counter, he may be able to attack again. An ideal defence not only prevents you from being injured but also acts as the first part of your counterstroke. Some defences actually hurt the aggressor; others give you control of one of his limbs. The defence you choose to nullify his attack will naturally lead into your response.

Remember that you are vastly more likely to be attacked with a swinging punch or a grab-and-punch than almost anything else. Thus most defences deal with these eventualities.

Deflection

Against any fairly straight arm, e.g. a straight punch or jab, or a grab attempt, you can bat the attack aside. This is best combined with a sidestep to take you out of the line of the attack. Move to the outside and knock the strike inwards, turning the attacker's weapons (hands, feet, etc) away from you for an instant. Your countermove could be almost anything. A simple palm strike to the head works well.

Evasion

Simply dodging is not a great option. True, it can stop you from getting hit, but merely moving back out of reach just ensures that the attacker has to swing again. At some point you will have to close in and take the fight to the enemy.

A far better option is to evade and counter at the same time. The bob-

Deflect and strike

Against a straight punch or grab, move to the outside of the strike and deflect it inwards, then follow up with a palm shot to the chin. Pushing on the assailant's arm will prevent him turning to face you.

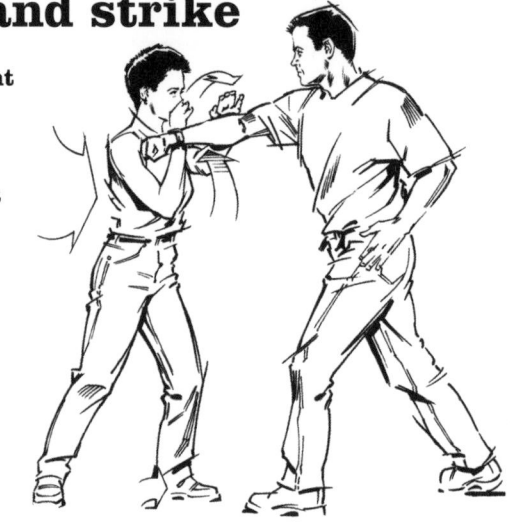

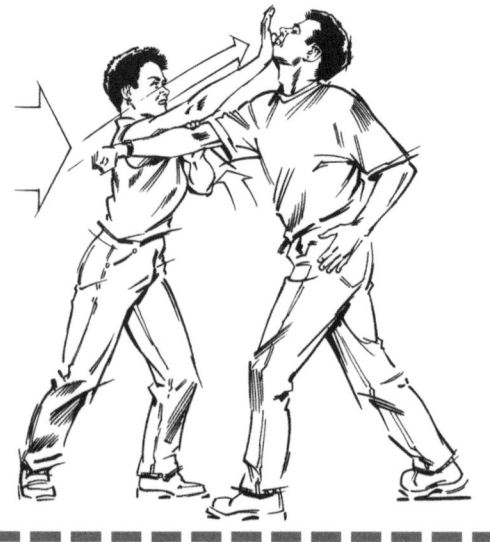

and-weave movement is used to dodge an opponent's blow whilst permitting a counterstrike. As he swings with his right hand, you duck under the blow by crouching slightly and bending your knees, moving to your left and 'bobbing' back up on the other side of the blow after it has gone past. Do not look at the ground as you bob; instead of

The bob

A favourite move for boxers, the 'bob' is a ducking movement in which you move towards the strike so that it passes over you more quickly. Ideally you can throw a body shot as you duck past the opponent's swing.

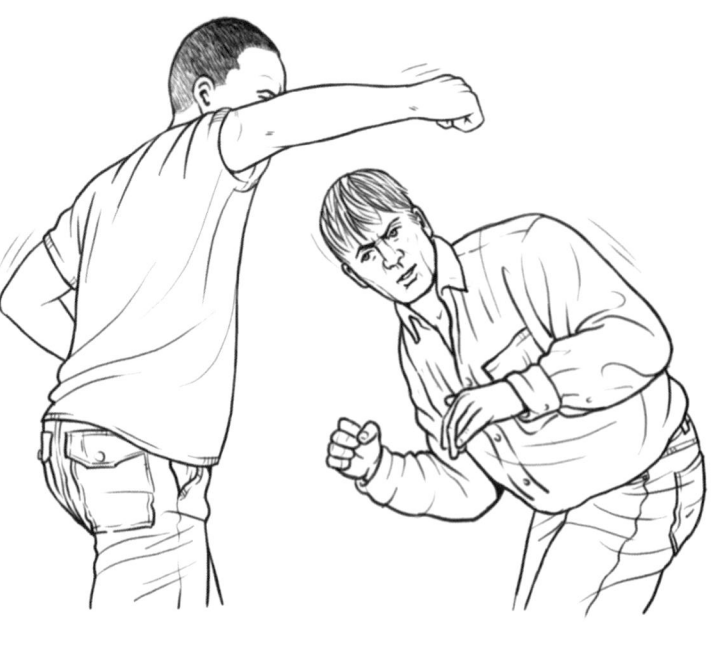

Smother block

As the assailant throws a hook punch, lunge forward and 'smother' it before it gets going. Drive one of your forearms into the crook of the elbow and the other into the assailant's shoulder.

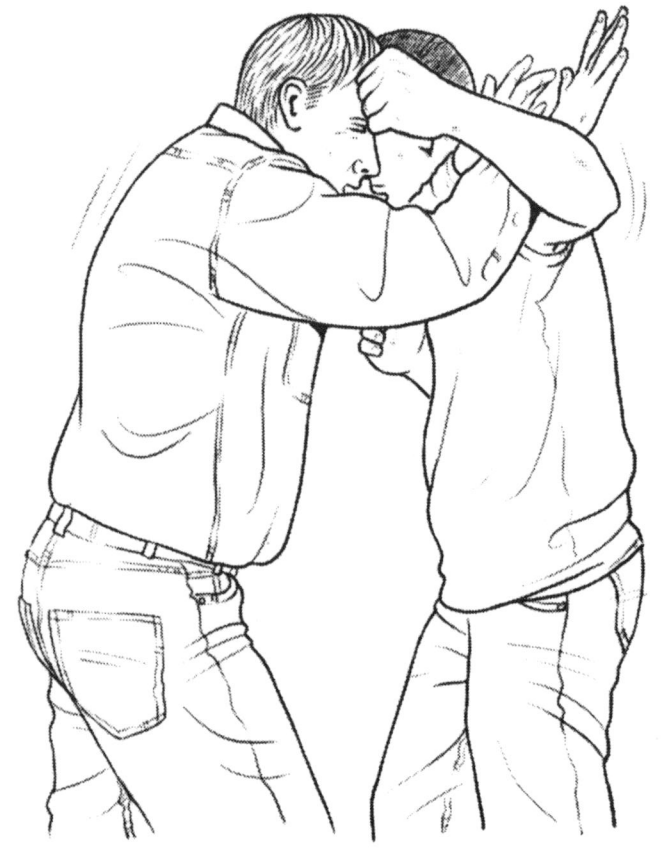

Arm wrap

Follow up a smother block by looping your arm over the opponent's and back under, behind his elbow. Your other arm grips his shoulder to immobilize the arm. There are many possible follow-ups from here. Knee strikes and headbutts are simple and effective.

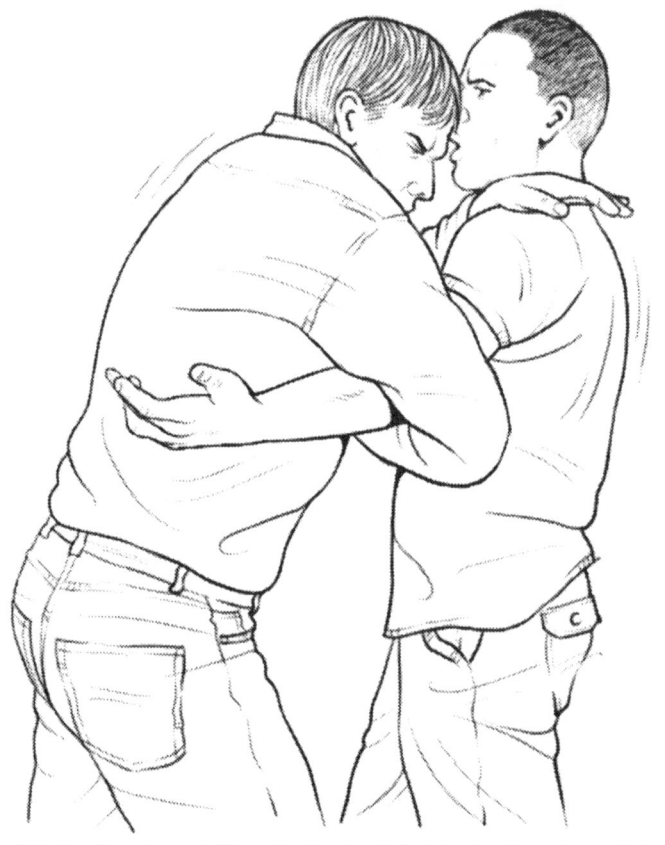

Cover block and arm wrap

If the opponent's swing is already on its way then it is too late to 'smother' it. Cover your head and move forward, inside the strike. As it glances off your covering arm, wrap the arm to control the opponent while you launch a countermove.

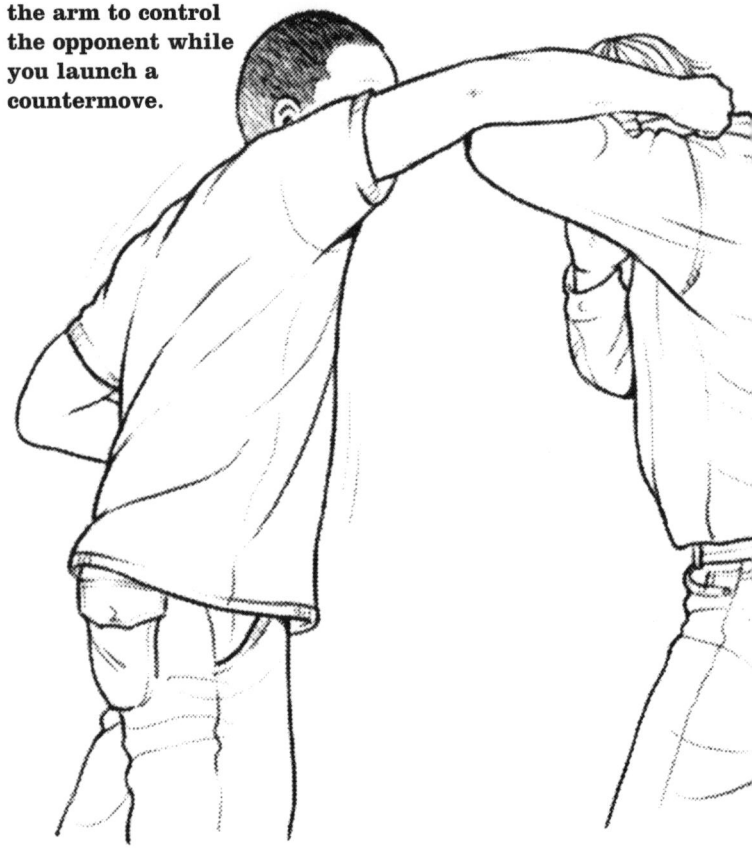

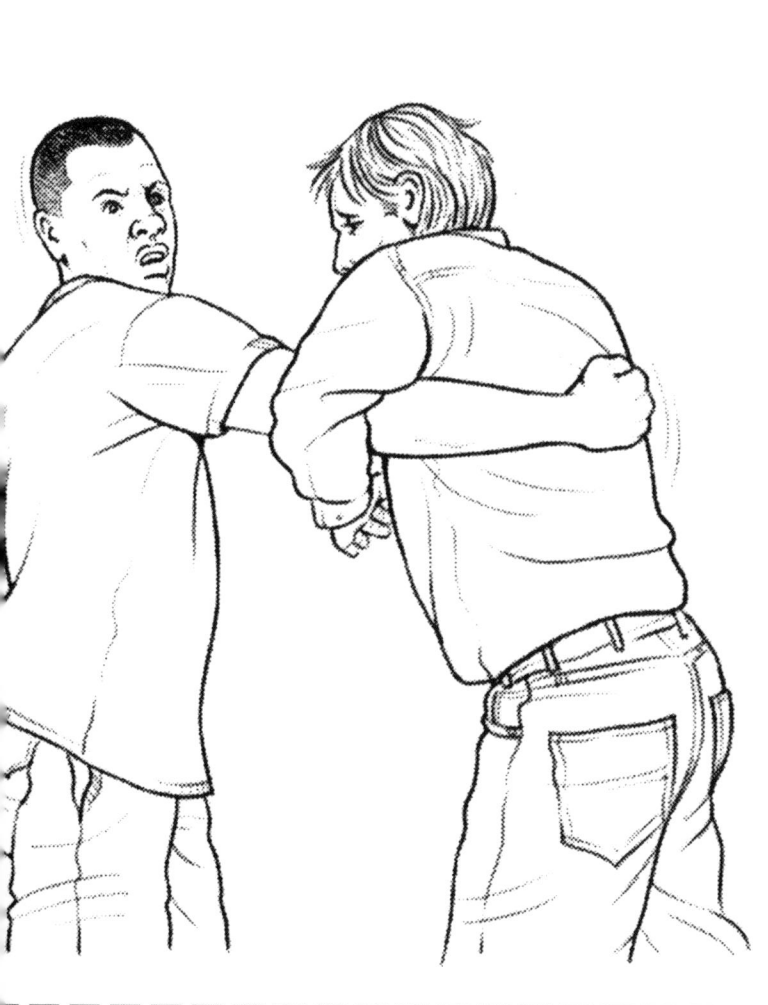

ducking, you dip down and keep looking forwards. You may counterstrike as you bob up, or 'weave' back into a position directly in front of the opponent.

Smother Block

You can 'smother' a hooked strike before it really gets moving. As your opponent 'chambers' his punch (i.e. draws it back to strike), lunge forward with your arms up protecting your head. Drive one forearm (near your elbow, or ideally your elbow itself) into his biceps or the crook of his arm. The other smashes into his shoulder. This can stagger the opponent backwards, and if you hit elbows-first it can cause stunning pain.

From this position there are several possibilities including takedowns and grappling. The simplest option is to use your outside arm (your left if you stopped a right hook) to trap the assailant's arm by wrapping it and holding it against your body, then delivering a knee strike.

Cover Block

If the attack is already on its way, a different response is necessary. A straight shot can be knocked aside with a single arm, but this is inadvisable against a committed hooking attack. Instead, protect yourself by raising your arm and curling your hand around the back of your head. Move forward, inside the path of the hook and drop your weight a little to avoid being knocked off balance.

The blow will strike your arm and skid around the back of your head. This is unpleasant but it will mitigate the blow while putting you in a position to win the fight. As soon as you feel the impact, wrap your arm around the attacker's. You have just gained control of his main weapon, his right arm. Meanwhile yours is still free to strike him in the face with palm and elbow shots. Chances are he will try to pull his arm free before doing anything else. This gives you what amounts to a free shot. You can follow up your first blows with knees, headbutts and possibly a takedown.

Defending a Knee Strike

If you are grabbed by an assailant, a knee strike is a likely follow-up. If you are upright, a knee strike can be 'jammed' by forcing your own leg or knee against that of the assailant. This prevents the strike from being launched. If you are bent over, perhaps having been pulled down, then you must protect yourself from a knee to the body or face. Putting your hands or forearms down works well enough, but you can get a better result by pointing your elbows down and allowing the opponent to strike them with the flesh of his thigh, just above the knee.

Knee defence

A knee strike can be 'jammed' with hands or forearms. This is a purely defensive movement of course; you will need to counterattack as soon as possible.

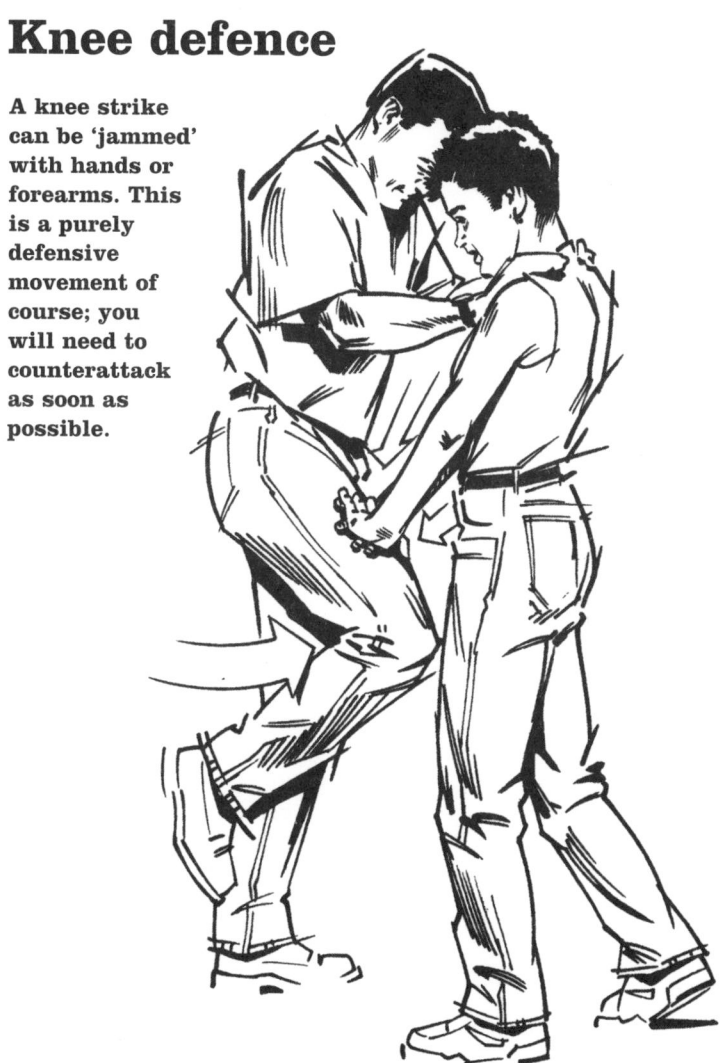

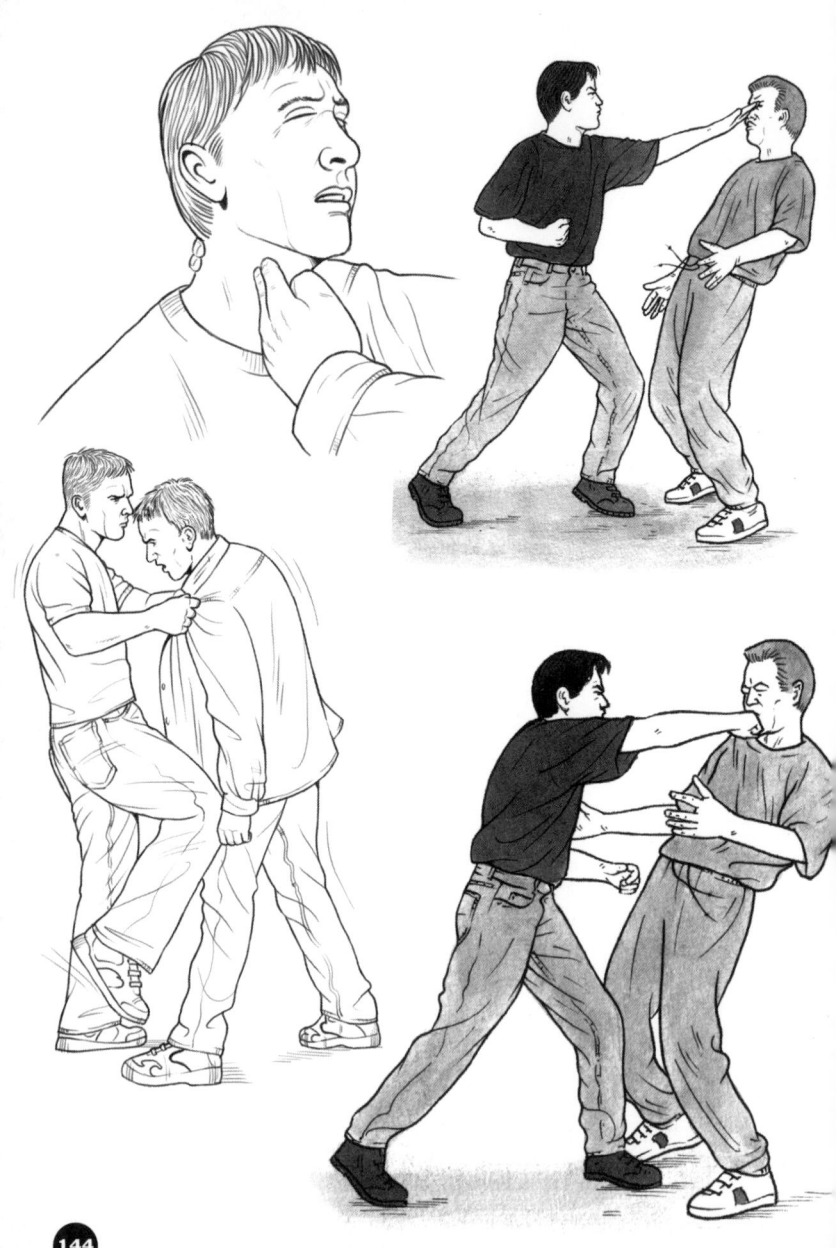

A s already noted, strikes are the main tools of unarmed combat. Even while grappling, you should be attacking with knees, elbows and anything else you can strike with, in order to keep the opponent on the defensive and to wear him down.

The basic rule for striking is 'hard weapon to soft target; soft weapon to hard target'. That is to say, hard weapons like clenched fists are best used against soft body parts like the solar plexus or kidneys. When striking bone, say the jaw, palm strikes are better as they reduce the chance of injury to your hand. However, it is more important to hit something with something than to hesitate while you try to decide upon the best weapon for the job.

STRAIGHT STRIKES
Straight strikes go straight from your shoulder to the target rather than moving in a curve. They are delivered with a pushing action. Note that it takes considerable training to become effective with the weak (lead) hand. For this reason it is rare to see people involved in a street fight throwing neat jabs at one another. Instead they will often use their lead

. . . .

Left: The method used should match the target; as a general rule your legs are used to attack low targets and your arms against higher ones.

7

There are many effective ways to strike an opponent.

Tools of the Trade
Striking and Grappling Methods

Knee to thigh

A knee to the thigh will probably not end a fight, but it hurts a lot and will make an opportunity to do something more decisive.

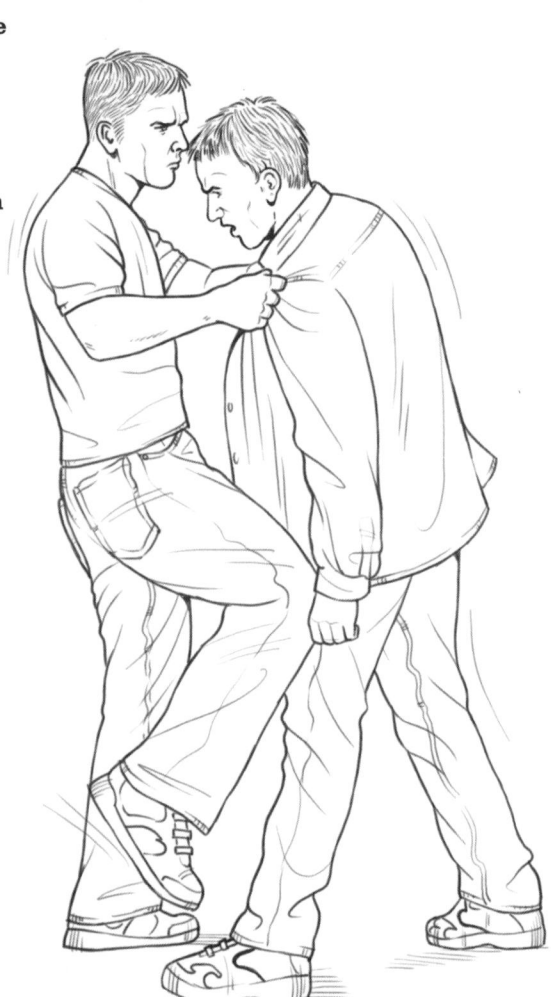

hand to grab with, pulling the opponent onto a strong-hand blow.

This approach is entirely valid – until you have trained up your lead hand into a useful combat asset, do not try to hit with it. Stick to grabs and eye jabs unless you can be sure of getting a useful result with a lead-hand blow.

Eye Jab

This works especially well off the 'fence' position as your lead hand will be close to the assailant's face when you launch the strike. Spread your fingers slightly and bend them a little so that if you hit the forehead you do not break your own fingers. Then simply push your hand forward and upwards, towards the assailant's eyes. Aiming a bit low and skidding up the cheek into the eye sockets works better than going in too high.

Note that it is virtually impossible to destroy an eyeball this way; the most you are likely to achieve is to make the assailant double up in pain or flinch away, so be prepared to follow up with a suitable finishing technique.

Lead-Hand Punch (Jab)

A lead-hand punch follows almost exactly the same path as an eye jab, but targets the nose or jaw instead. Drive your hand hard forward and push with your back foot, putting some weight behind the punch. Contact can be made with a fist or a

> ## TIP: DELIVERING FORCE
>
> In order to deliver maximum force on a strike, you should aim to hit through the target. That way your blow is still accelerating as it goes into the target area, rather than slowing down.
> - You should never reach full extension of your arm before hitting a target with a punch, or have to lean.
> - Learning your distance is an important part of training. It can be done on focus pads or a punchbag, or in sparring.

palm. A lead-hand shot (sometimes called a jab) is highly unlikely to drop an opponent but can create an opportunity for a more powerful follow-up shot.

Cross

The 'straight right', 'right cross' or just 'cross' is a staple move of boxers everywhere, and rightly so. It comes from the rear hand (the right if you are in an orthodox left-lead

Eye jab

An eye jab is unlikely to cause permanent harm but will stop an opponent long enough for you to escape or do something more effective. An upward movement is best; hit just below the eyes and skid up rather than striking the forehead.

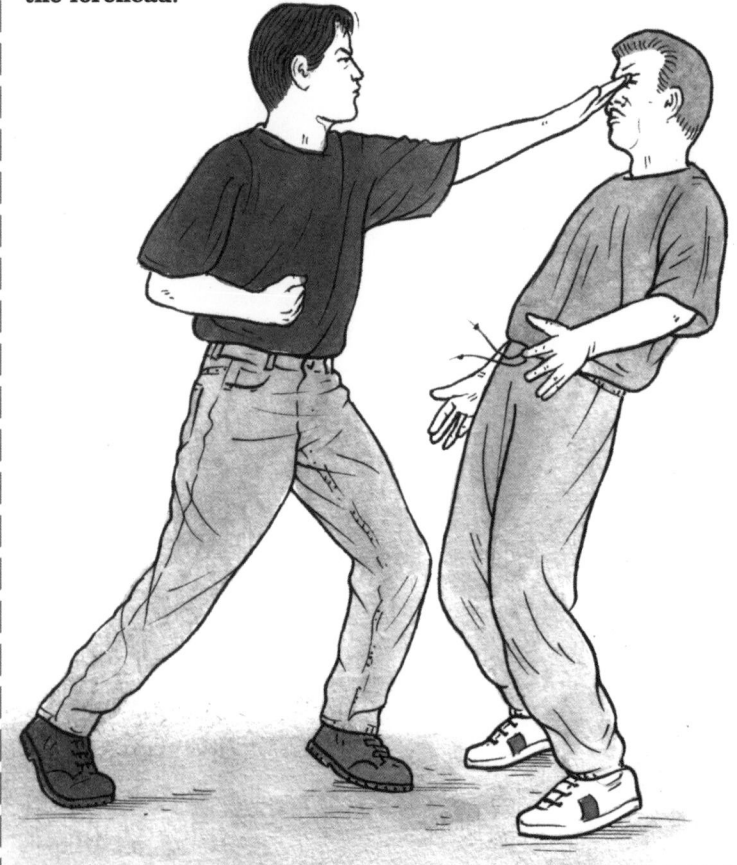

Straight left

It takes a lot of training to be able to throw an effective lead-hand shot, but it is worth it. A fast, hard left will interrupt whatever the assailant is doing and set him up for a more powerful right to follow.

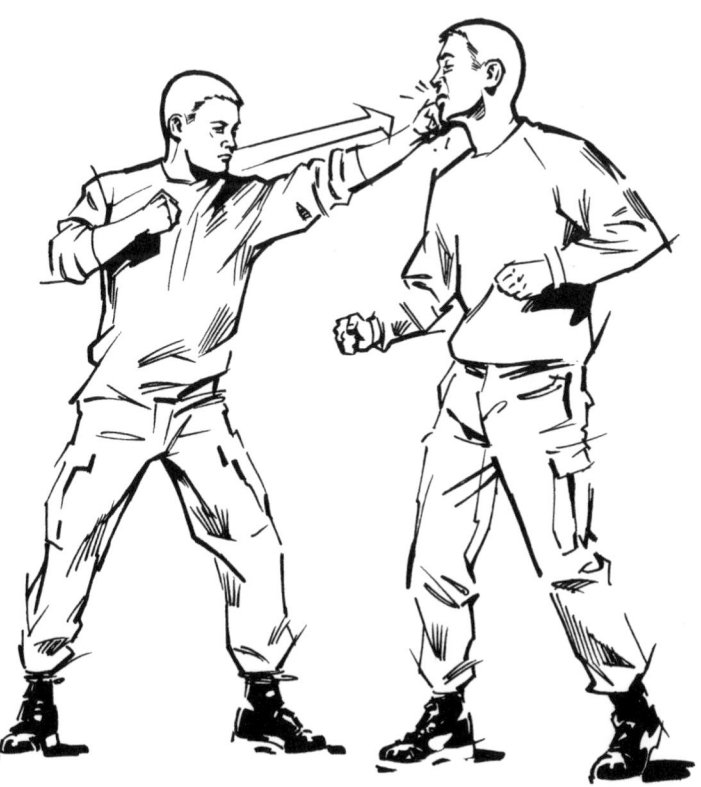

stance) which is driven hard and straight towards the nose and jaw. Contact can again be made with palm or fist.

The cross is a powerful blow, and it is important to get your weight behind it, driving with your back foot and bringing your right hip forward. However, this is not a hooked shot – it goes in a straight line, not a curve.

Against someone taller than you, you might have to angle the cross upwards. This can be a good thing, as a palm shot under the jaw is an excellent knockout tool. This is the reason it was among the very small number of extremely potent techniques taught to World War II commandos.

Throat Strikes

Striking the throat can be lethal, so is used only as a last resort in civilian self-defence. Military systems, on the other hand, are designed to kill and so make extensive use of these strikes. The two main variants are the web hand and the straight-fingered strike. Both are delivered with a hard, straight pushing action.

The web-hand strike uses the 'L' shape between thumb and forefinger as a striking surface. This is driven hard into the front of the throat. With some care, it is possible to strike just hard enough to make the opponent cough and choke a bit, then grab his larynx and squeeze hard enough to get his full attention. This is a useful deterrent technique if you do not simply want to knock him out, but all throat strikes and chokes must be done with great care.

The other common throat strike is to make a spear out of your stiff fingers and ram it into the throat, just

---

TIP:
END THE SITUATION

Remember that your goal is to preserve your safety. Simply getting an aggressor to let go of you does not end the situation.

- Be prepared to do enough to guarantee your safety or facilitate your escape. Many people have been hurt because they took half-measures then allowed the assailant to have another go at them.
- But remember that your goal is to end the situation and preserve your safety, not to punish the attacker. Do what you need to and remove yourself from the threat, do not hang around to get a few extra blows in if you do not need to.

Striking first

Your best chance to end the situation on your terms is to hit first and hit hard. Once you do deliver a blow, you must keep going until the threat is nullified. Do not hit and then stand back to see what happens next – you will not like what does!

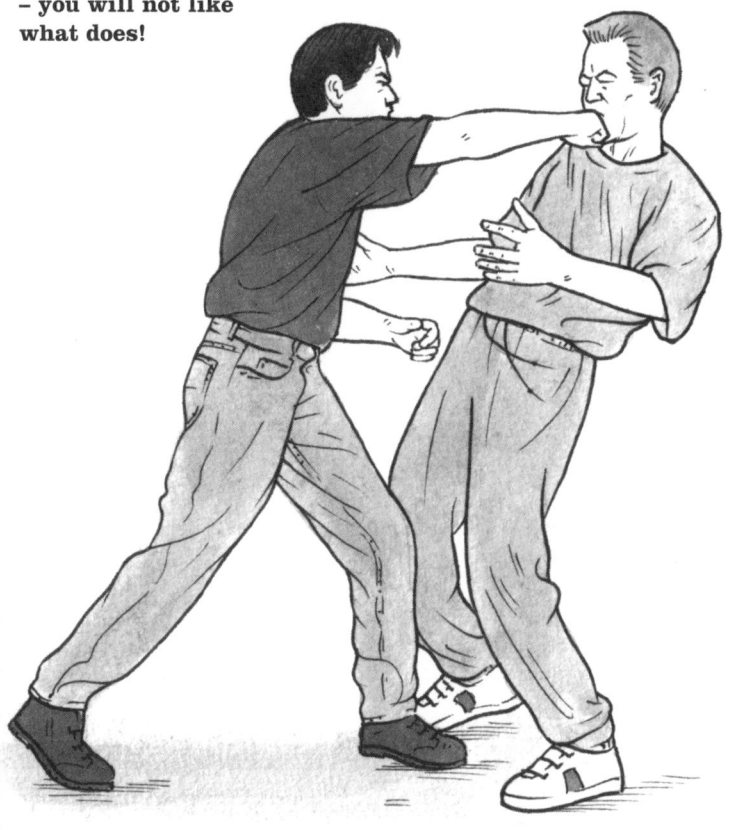

Throat strikes

Throat strikes can kill, so should be used only in the face of a very serious threat. Strike the larynx with the web of the hand between thumb and fingers, or jab stiff fingers into the softer parts of the neck between the larynx and carotid arteries.

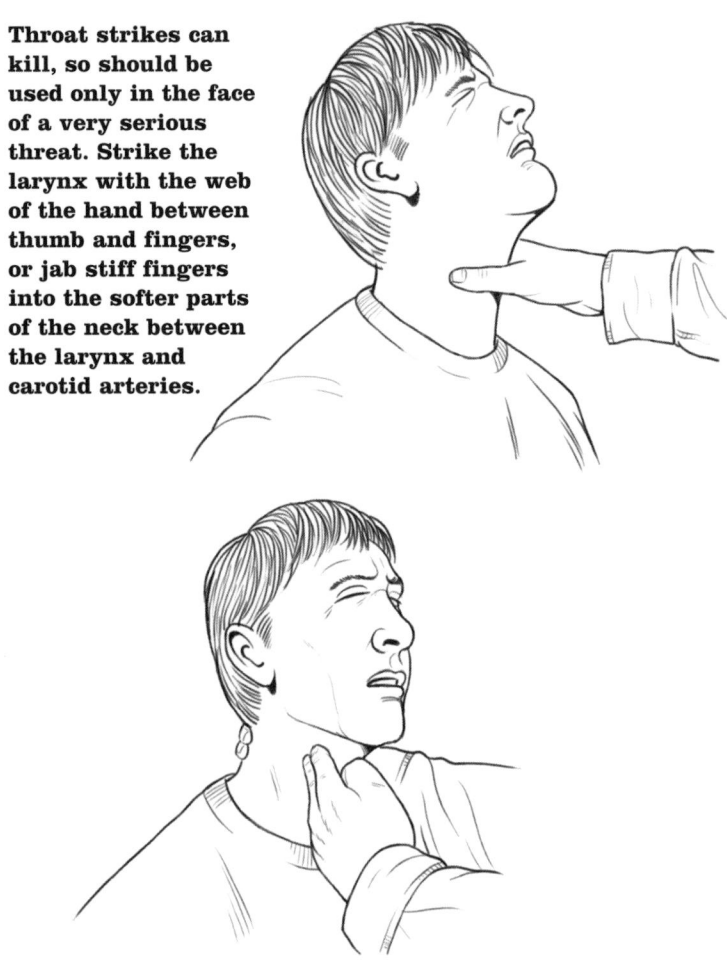

Disciplined hook

A skilled fighter will also throw hooked punches, but these will be tight and follow a smaller arc. A hook is a much more effective punch – keep your own hooks tight and well disciplined for the best effect.

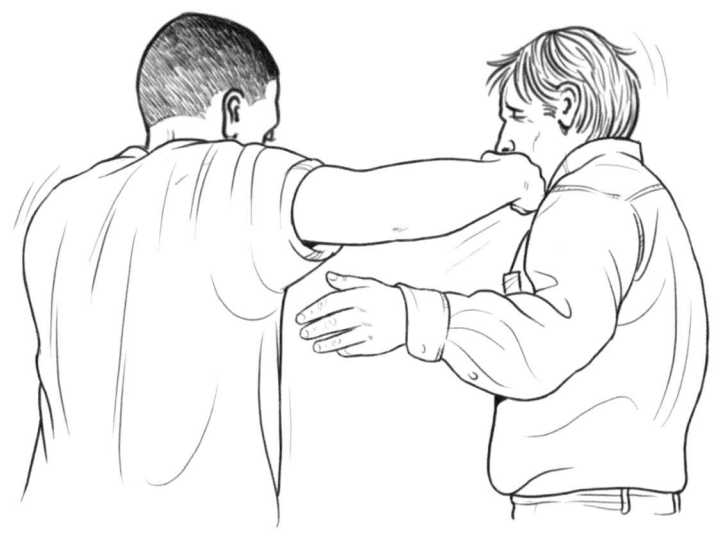

to the side of the larynx and angled inwards. This can kill, so it should be saved as a last resort.

HOOKED STRIKES

Hooked strikes travel in a curve and can generate great power. They are also useful for getting around an opponent's guard. The usual target

for hooks is the side of the jaw, though body hooks to the kidneys are effective from in close.

Hooked punches to the head are the most common attack in unarmed combat. Most untrained people throw wild 'haymakers' that are very easy to see coming and deal with if you know how. This does not mean

Haymaker

Most people throw wild, hooking 'haymaker' punches which are very powerful but easy to spot. If you see someone 'chamber' a fist like this then you know what is coming – a big swing at your head.

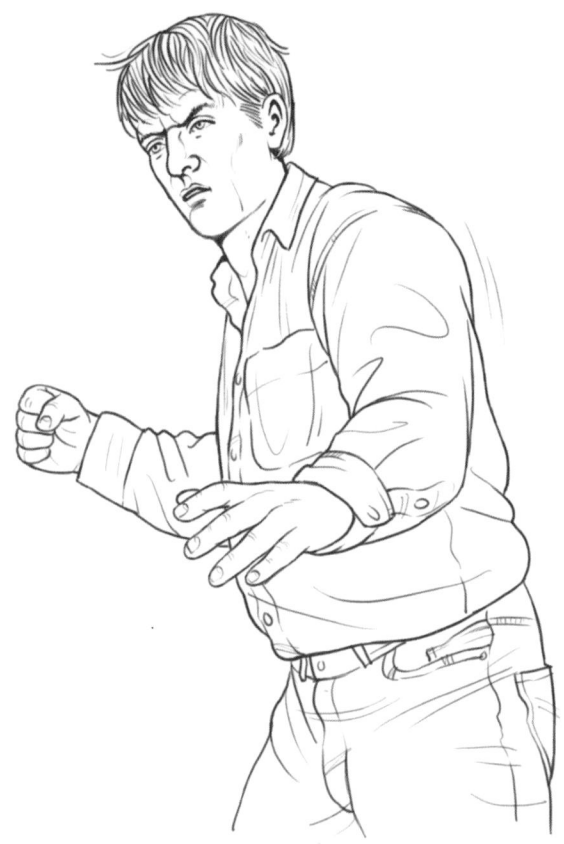

Uppercut

The uppercut is a very effective knockout blow. Drive your fist up under the chin like a piston. For added power, crouch slightly and straighten your legs as you strike, driving your whole bodyweight upwards into the target.

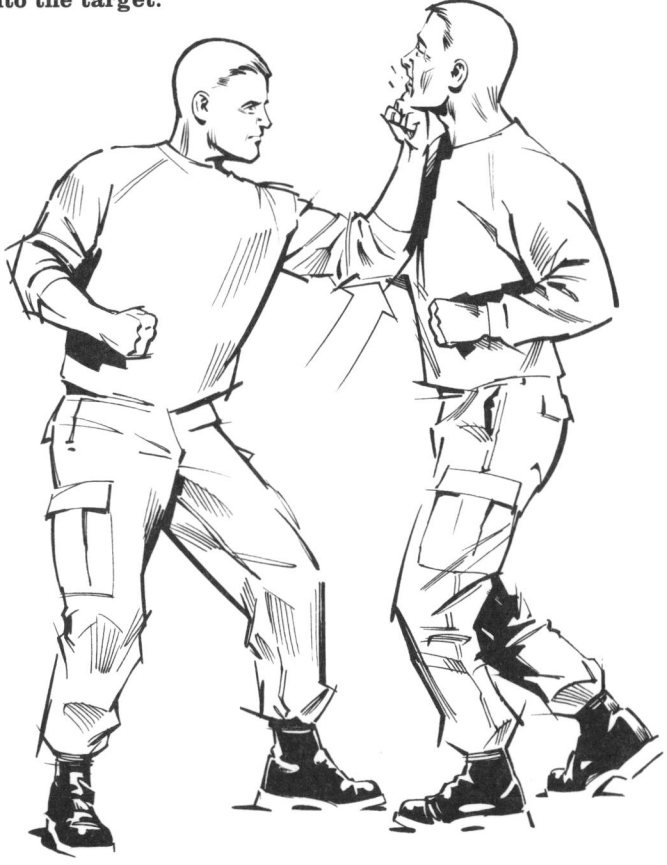

they will not hurt you badly if they land though.

A disciplined hook follows a much tighter arc and is harder to see coming. Contact can be made with a fist or an open hand, again using the palm to deliver force.

Body Shots and Uppercuts

The uppercut is one of the best knockout shots possible, but it is tricky to execute. Begin with your forearm parallel to the ground and swing straight upwards under the opponent's chin. Straighten your legs as you make contact to increase the impact and to lift his head up and back. Contact is made with a fist.

From the same starting position, you can instead drive your fist forwards into the solar plexus. Like the uppercut, this is a close-in strike. In both cases, unless you can perform the strike well, it is not worth throwing at all.

ELBOW STRIKES

Elbows are excellent close-quarters striking tools. There is no part of the human body that will damage an elbow hitting it, so there is no need to worry about breaking your elbow.

Rising Elbow

From close-in keep your arm bent and bring the elbow up in a sharp arc under the opponent's chin. Imagine you are trying to reach straight back over your shoulder.

Downward Elbow

Again, keep your arm bent so that the elbow becomes a point. Drive it downwards into the back of an opponent bent over in front of you. The same strike can also be used to finish off an opponent in groundfighting.

Thrusting Elbow

An elbow can be driven straight backwards into someone who has hold of you from behind, or can be thrust out to the side. This is best accompanied by a step towards the opponent, putting your bodyweight behind the strike. This is one of the few times when hitting an opponent in the chest is worthwhile – a pointed elbow with your weight behind it will bring almost anyone to a momentary halt.

Hooked Elbow

A hooked elbow strike follows much the same path as a hooked punch, but a shorter arc. Since the elbow is close to your body there is little 'give' in the strike, resulting in incredible power delivered to the opponent. Hooked elbows can be driven into the head or ribcage.

KICKS AND KNEES

A good kick can end a fight very quickly – and so can a bad one, but not in a way you like. Military personnel use kicks and stomps to finish off downed opponents. This is fine in a military context but should

Rising elbow strike

An alternative to the uppercut, a rising elbow is thrown as if you were reaching back to scratch your shoulder blade. If the opponent is not knocked out, you can bring the elbow back down into the face, collar-bone or pectorals.

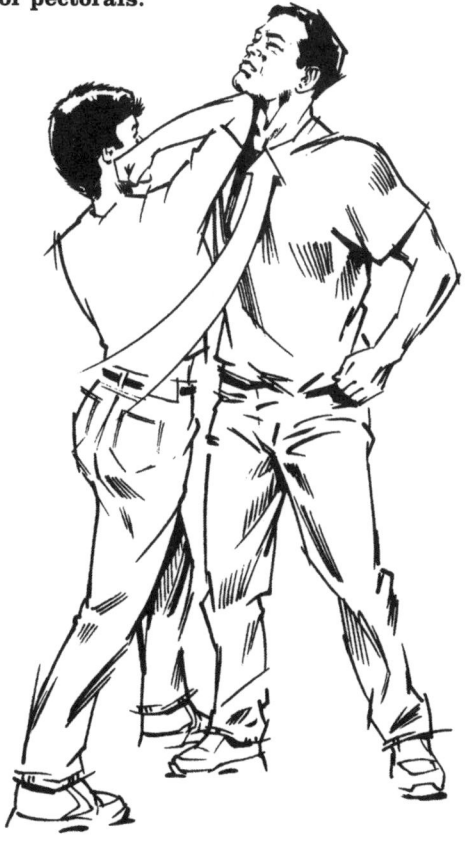

Downward elbow strike

This is an excellent 'finishing' technique against an opponent whose head is down for whatever reason. A 'stab kick' to the groin with your toes will put his head in position for a dropping elbow to the back of the head, or behind the ear.

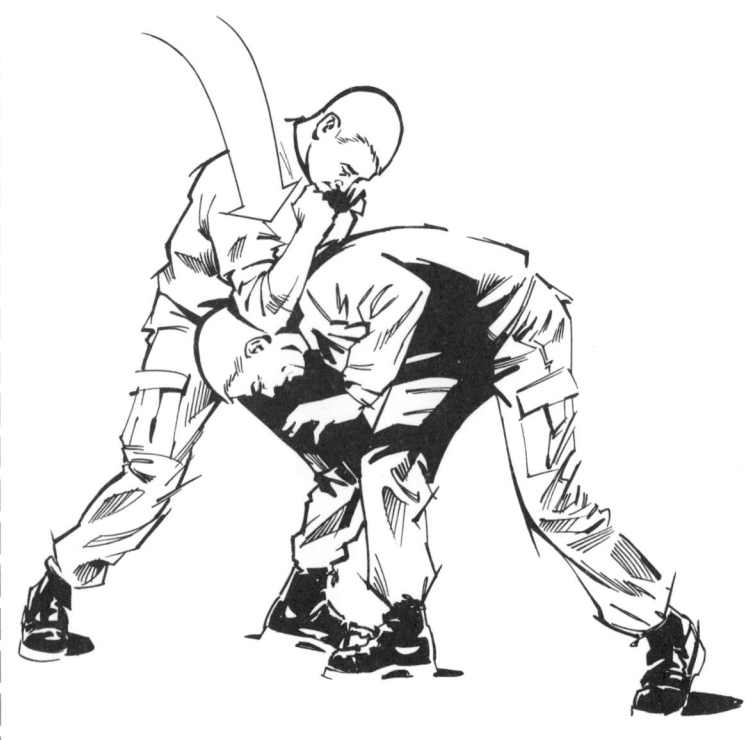

be viewed with caution for self-defence applications. If the assailant is getting up to attack you again, then you are probably justified in kicking him as he does so, but stomping a helpless individual on the ground – however much the person deserves it – can land you in serious legal trouble.

Stomp

The simplest and most effective way to finish off a downed opponent is to stomp on him with your heel. This is simply a matter of straightening your leg and driving the heel downwards into the target. You can also stomp on ankles to stop a pursuit or on a hand that is reaching for a weapon.

Groin Kick

Attacking the groin is not the sure-fire fight-ender that some people think. Men become skilled at protecting their groin at an early age, and in any case even a straight shot to the testicles will not always stop a determined assailant.

That said, a groin kick can produce very effective results. Simply swing your leg up and contact with the instep or, if you are wearing hard shoes, use your toes. The same kick can be used to the face of an opponent who is bent forwards – perhaps as the result of your groin kick. A groin kick of this sort should be fast and can be delivered with the front foot.

Shin Kick

The shins have large numbers of nerve endings close to the surface and are thus a very painful place to receive a kick. Use the inner side of your foot and strike with a sweeping action fairly low down on the shin. The combination of pain and impact may drive the opponent's foot back, compromising his balance. If you are wearing hard shoes, you can impact with the toes instead.

Front Kick

This basic kick can be delivered to the legs or abdomen of an opponent. It is launched off the back foot, never the front, and can be combined with a step forward for added power. The kick is not swung; instead you should lift the knee to 'chamber' the kick then drive your foot forward in an arc. The kick itself is delivered as if stomping on a vertical surface in front of you. Contact is normally made with the ball of the foot, but the heel can also be used.

Roundhouse Kick

This curved kick is extremely powerful. It is best delivered to the leg, ideally just above the knee or halfway up the thigh, or under the ribs. Contact is made with the instep and shin, and there is no attempt to pull the kick back after impact – allow it to drive right through the target. This can buckle a leg even if the kick does not put it out of action.

Foot stomp

If you need to stomp on someone, use your heel. Stomping on the head can kill. However, stomps are useful to disable an opponent's ankles or to neutralize a hand that is holding a weapon.

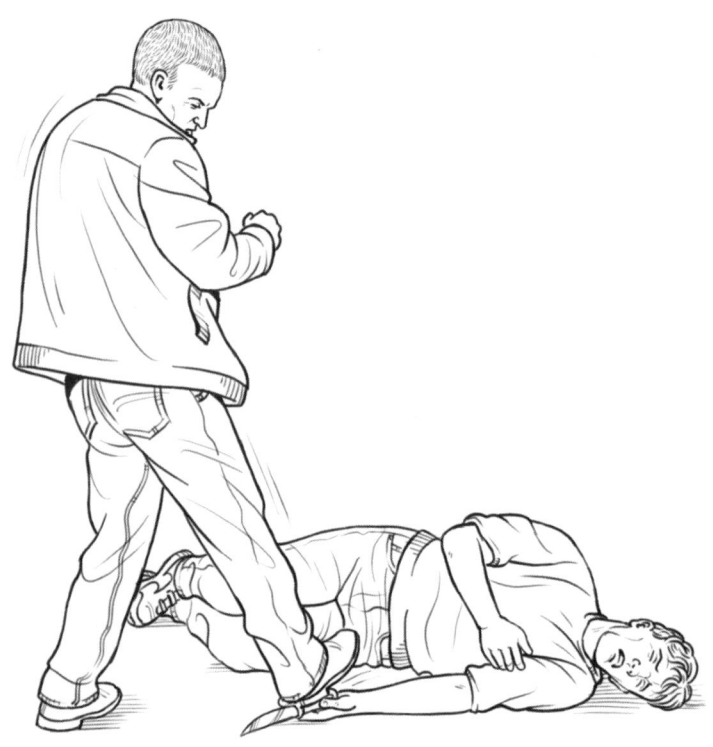

Groin kick

A good kick to the groin with the toes or instep, if timed right, can stop an opponent. However, groin kicks are not the all-powerful fight-enders that some martial arts systems believe. It is easy to miss and hit a leg or the abdomen, so do not gamble everything on a single kick. Be prepared to have to continue fighting.

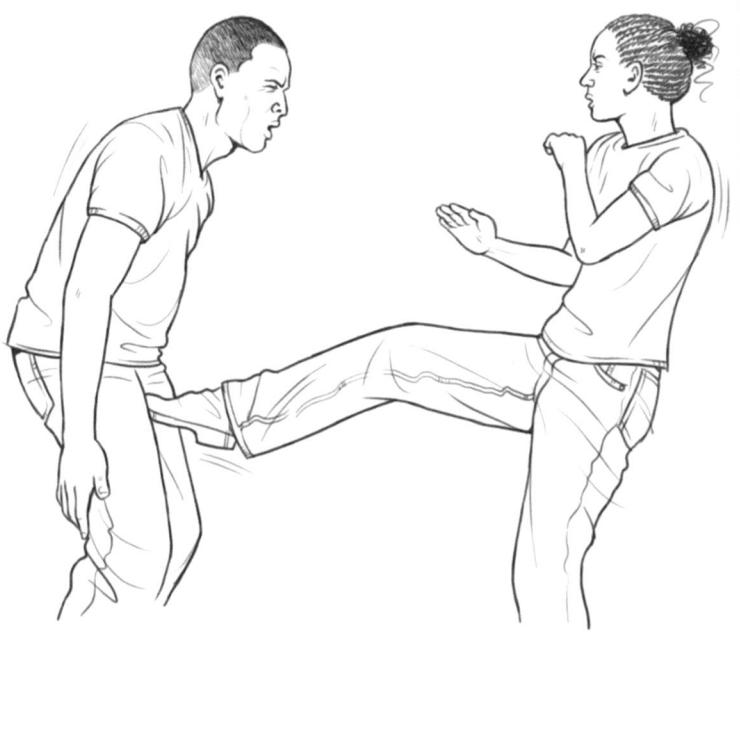

Side kick

A side kick is essentially a stomp but launched sideways. Straighten your leg fast and drive your heel into the target for maximum impact. Ideally you want to crumple the opponent, rather than push him away.

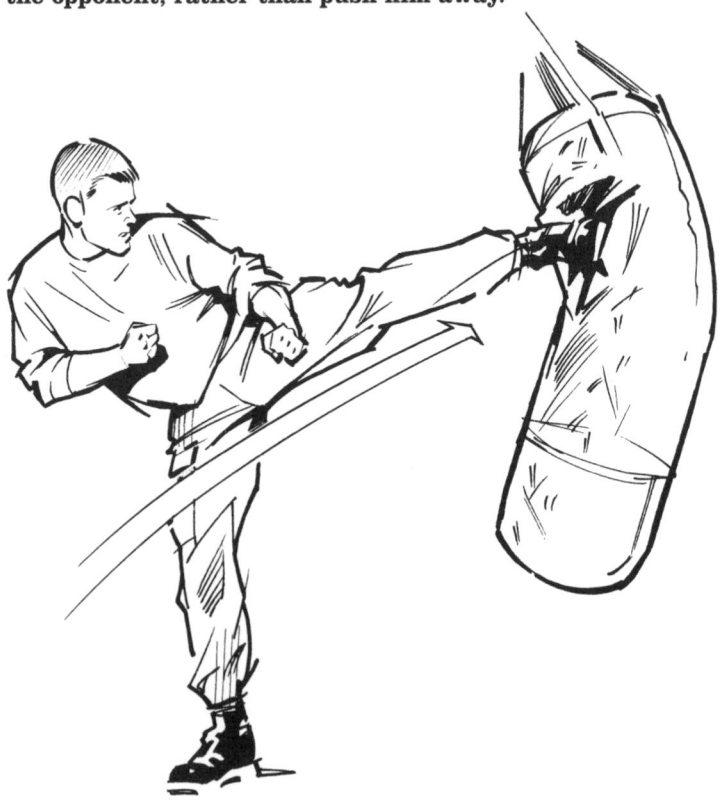

Shin kick

A 'sweeping' kick with the side of your shoe not only causes intense pain but it can take the opponent's leg out from under him. Shin kicks do not compromise your balance as much as higher kicks.

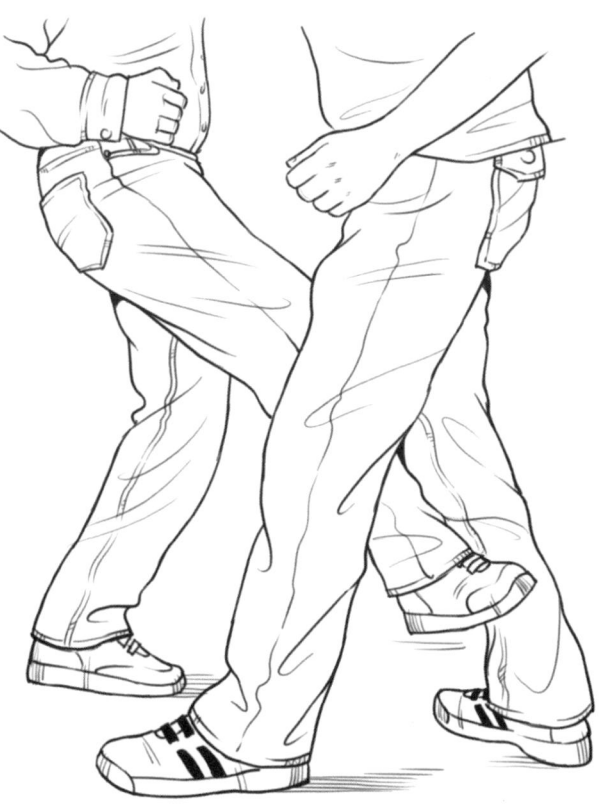

Roundhouse kick

This extremely powerful kick is delivered with the shin and instep. It is important to turn the foot you are standing on to point in the direction of the kick, and to raise your knee to the height you want to kick at. Straightening the leg as you twist into the kick delivers incredible force.

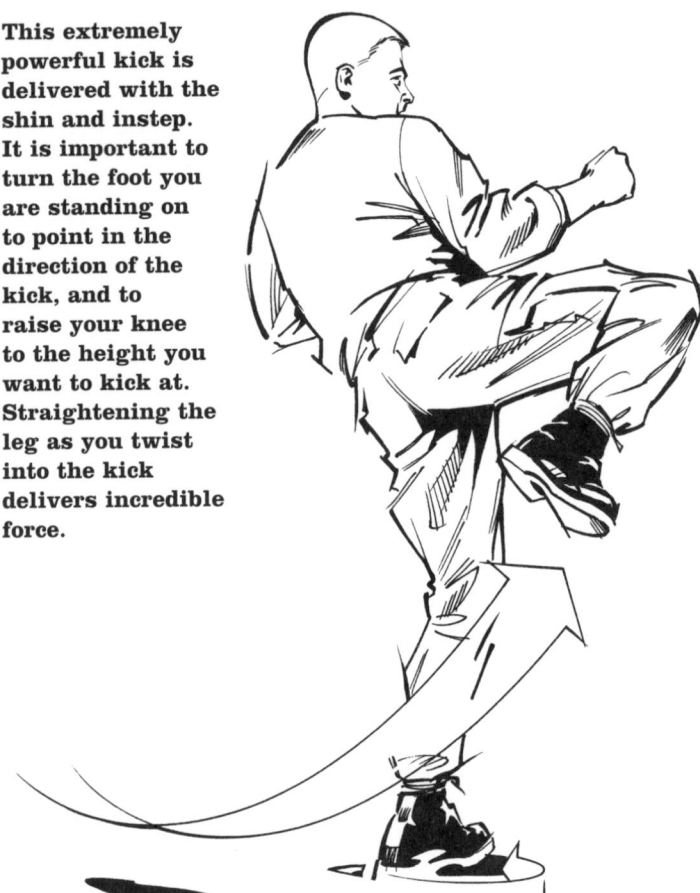

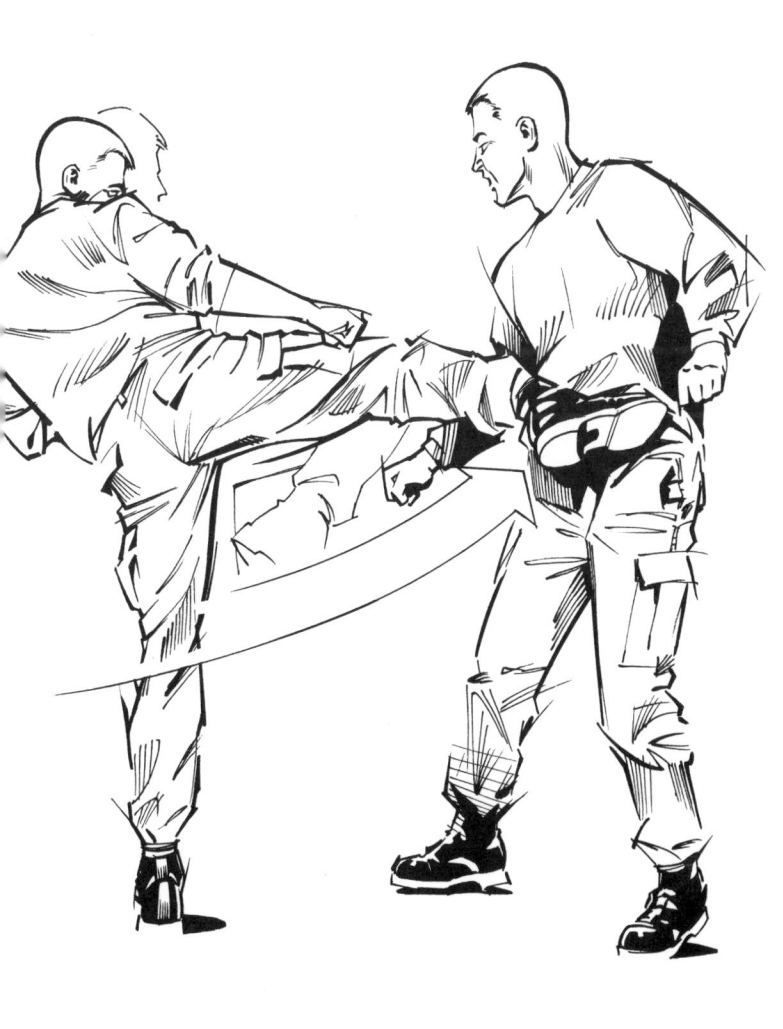

Side kick mechanics

'Chamber' the kick by raising your knee to the height of the impact point, then straighten your leg into the target. You may have to lean your body away from the kick to prevent your kicking leg from dropping.

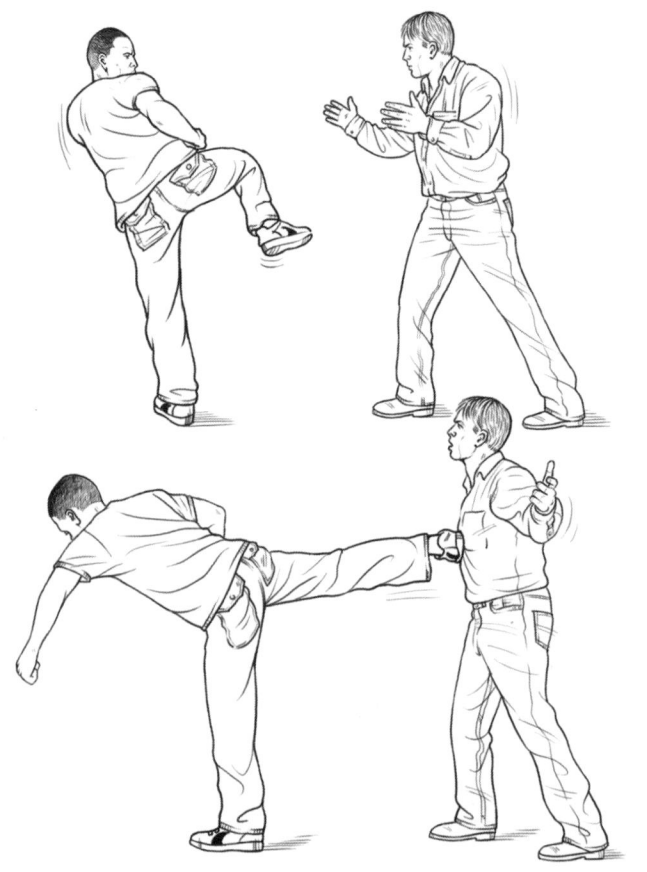

A roundhouse kick is launched from the trailing foot. Turn the toes of the lead foot outward (in the direction the kick is going to travel), lift the kicking leg to aim the kick and then straighten it while pivoting into the target.

Side Thrust Kick

A side kick of this sort will normally push an opponent away from you if directed at the torso. If directed at the legs, it is likely to break the leg or knee instead. To deliver a side kick, turn side-on to the target, lift the kicking leg by bringing your knee straight up, then thrust or stomp out sideways at the target.

A side thrust kick can also be used from the ground, directed at an opponent's legs or groin.

Knee Strikes

Knees can be considered grappling tools as much as striking weapons. Military and law enforcement personnel are taught to use a knee to the thigh as a 'distraction' while trying to restrain a struggling captive or suspect.

A straight knee is simply driven up or forwards into the opponent's legs or body. This works best if you can pull him onto the strike. A roundhouse knee travels out and back in, in an arc that strikes the side of the thigh or under the ribs. In both cases, use your back leg to strike with.

Knee Drop

The 'knee drop' is a finishing technique used against a downed but still combative opponent. Place your foot next to the target's torso or head and allow the knee to bend, dropping your weight straight down onto the opponent. Done lightly, this can be used as a hold-down, or by dropping your full weight you can crack ribs and put the assailant out of the fight. If necessary, after knee-dropping onto an opponent, you can keep your weight on him and deliver more strikes or a choke with your hands.

THROWS AND TAKEDOWNS

An enemy who is on the ground is a far lesser threat than one who is standing up. In a military context, downed opponents are often finished off with a soldier's boots, but this is not always desirable in self-defence. If an opponent hits the ground hard enough, he can be taken out of the fight. A hard fall can result in winding, and an awkward one can break bones.

Care must be taken when training in throws and takedowns. It is strongly advisable to join a Ju-Jitsu, Judo or Mixed Martial Arts class if you wish to learn to use throws. They require a fair amount of practice to be useful, and should be trained only under qualified supervision. Particular care must be

Straight and roundhouse knee strikes

As a general rule you should not try to knee someone unless you have hold of them. A straight strike is launched by simply raising your knee into the target. A roundhouse knee follows a similar path to a roundhouse kick, curving into the target from the side.

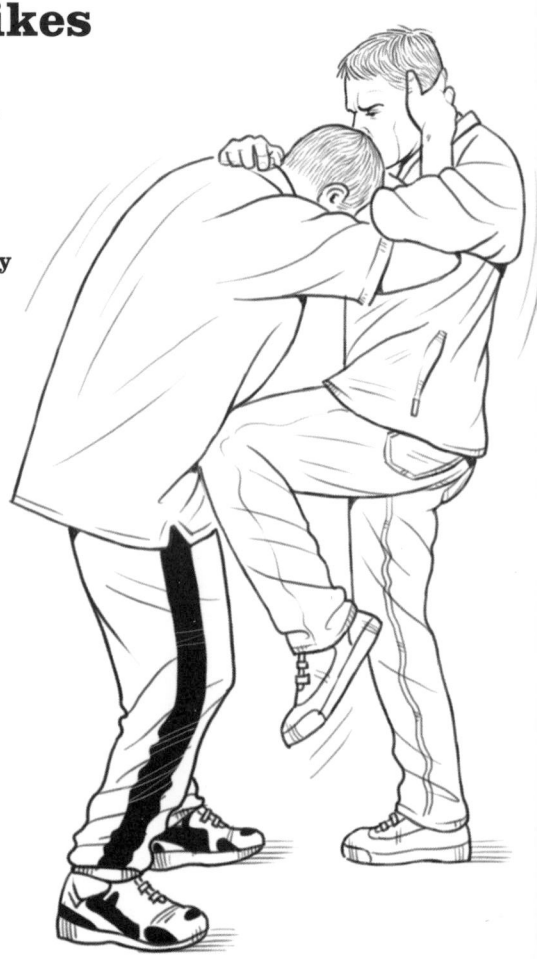

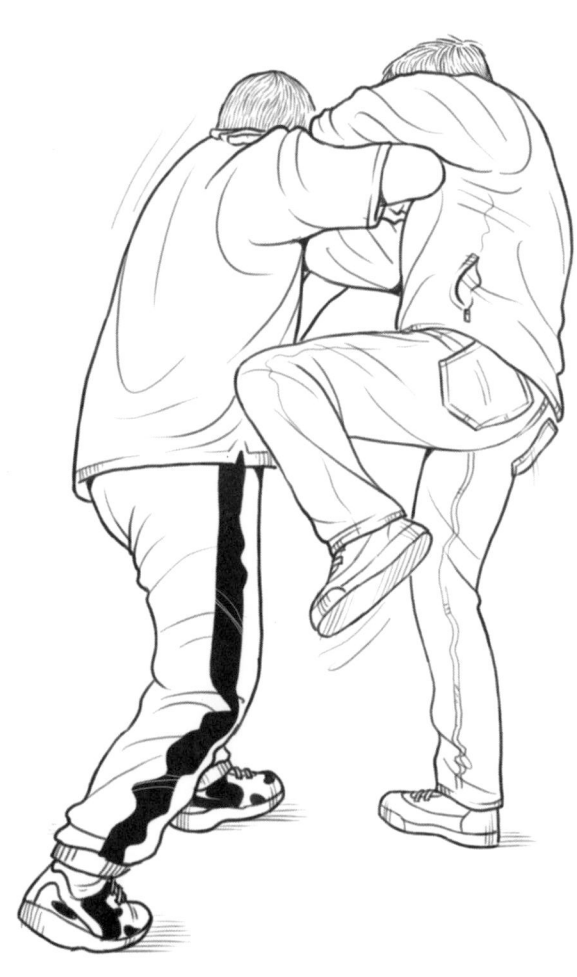

Outer reap takedown

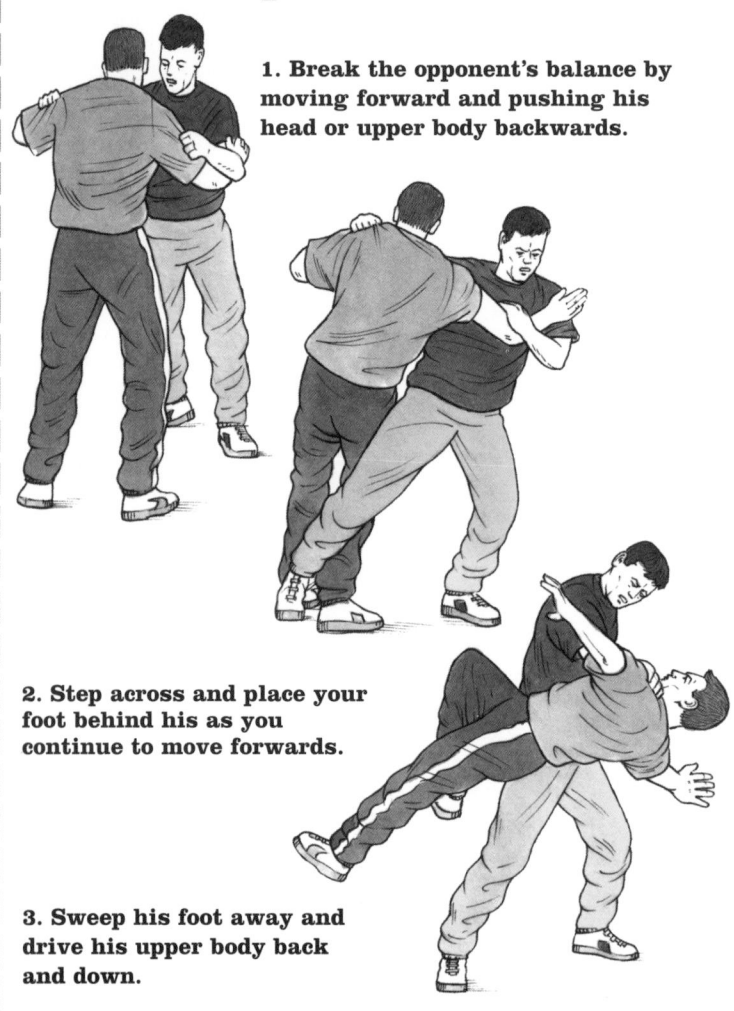

1. Break the opponent's balance by moving forward and pushing his head or upper body backwards.

2. Step across and place your foot behind his as you continue to move forwards.

3. Sweep his foot away and drive his upper body back and down.

taken to avoid hard contact between a student's head and the ground.

Outer Reap Takedown
This takedown dumps the assailant hard on his back. It is most often performed after 'smothering' a hooked punch. Move past the assailant, bringing your foot round behind his. At the same time break his balance by pushing his head back. Now sweep your leg back, taking his foot out from under him, and drive him back and down as hard as you can.

Inner Reap
Similar to an outer reap, but this time you are square-on, almost chest to chest. Tip the assailant's head back to break his balance and step through, hooking one of his feet away with yours as you shove him back. If he has a good grip in you, he may drag you down with him which is not ideal, but at least you will land on top where you have a significant advantage.

Sideways Reap
This takedown only works if it is performed suddenly and fast. Pull the opponent violently sideways, twisting him so that the shoulder nearest the direction you want him to fall comes forward and the other one goes back. At the same time kick or sweep his foot away, causing him to spin out of control and fall on his back in front of you.

Haul and Turn
Grab your opponent around the back of the neck with both hands and haul him forward and down so that he bends forward. Keep your elbows down so that he cannot escape. Now step back and drag him with you, pulling down on the back of his head. Pivot to the side and out of his way as he falls. This will cause the opponent to land on his back where you were just standing. The key is to bend him forward far enough that his balance is destroyed – a groin kick or body blow will help achieve this.

Single Leg Takedown
'Shoot' in under the opponent's guard, grabbing his ankle or behind the knee with one hand while you drive the other elbow into his hip joint on the same side as the leg you grabbed. Pull his leg up and towards you while driving his hip back with your elbow. He will fall on his back.

Double Leg Takedown
Once again 'shoot' in under the opponent's guard and grab him around the backs of his knees. Drive your shoulder into his hip or groin and pull his legs up and towards you. For added force, straighten your legs and pull his legs upwards as if you were trying to put his knees in your trouser pockets. This will result in a

Leg sweep principles

All 'sweeping' takedowns use the same basic principles. Move the opponent's upper body one way and sweep his foot away in the other direction. The aim is to create two forces moving in opposite directions, thereby turning the opponent over.

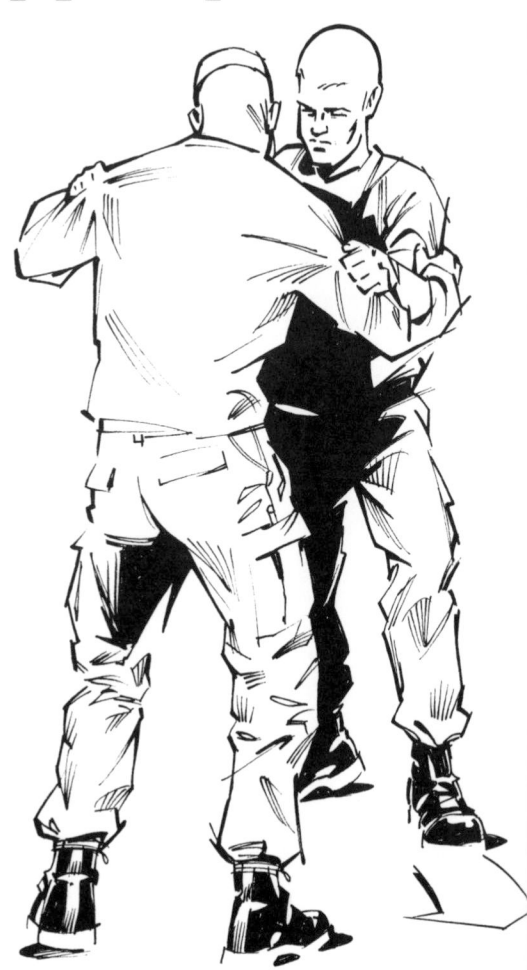

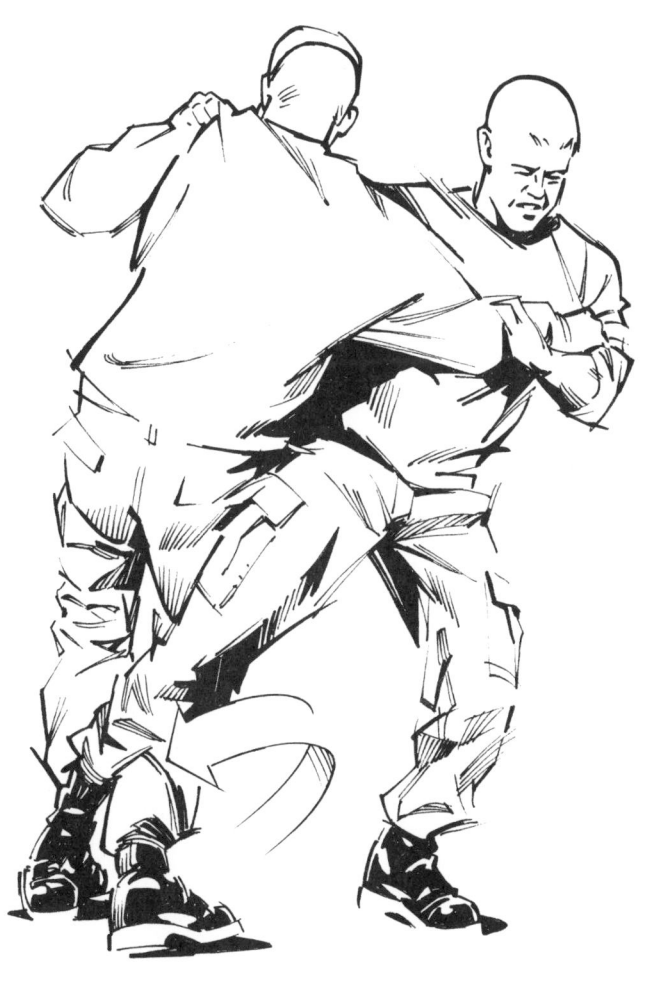

Sideways reap

Grab the opponent's arms or upper body and pull or push him off balance. The aim is to get him to elongate his stance front-to-back, making him vulnerable to a sideways movement. Pull violently to the side and kick or sweep his lead foot out from under him. The higher you can get his foot, and the more violently you pull him sideways, the harder he will fall.

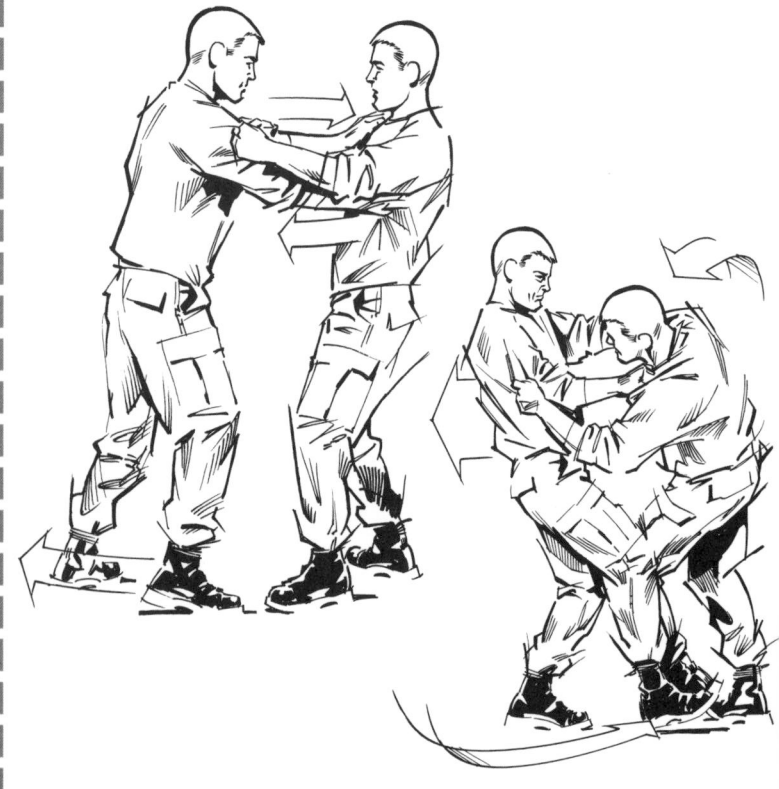

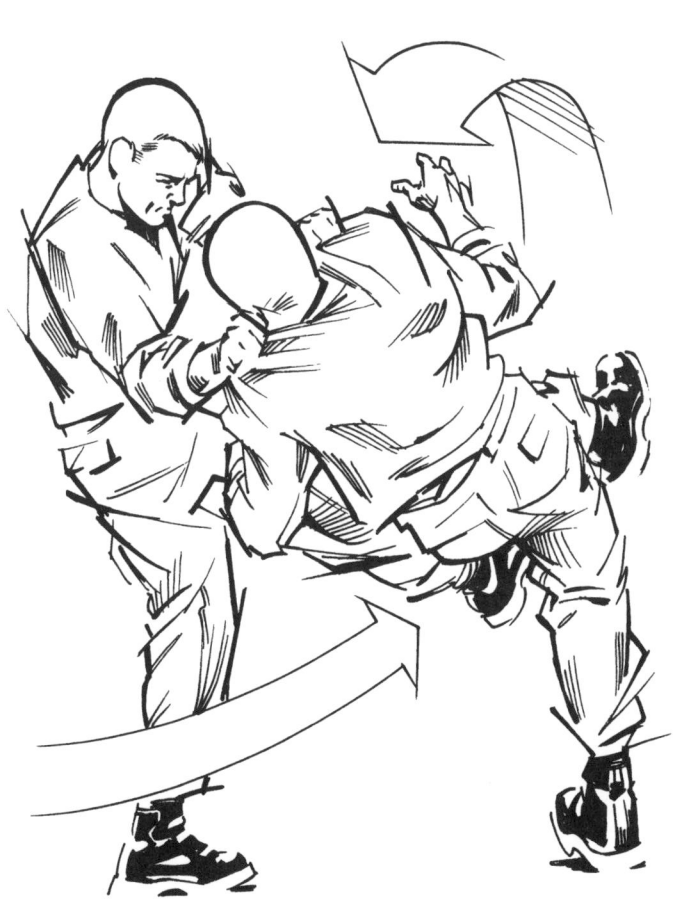

Double leg takedown

'Shoot' in below your opponent's hands and grab him around the backs of his knees, pulling upwards vigorously. At the same time push him backwards with your shoulder to dump him hard on his back.

Shoulder throw

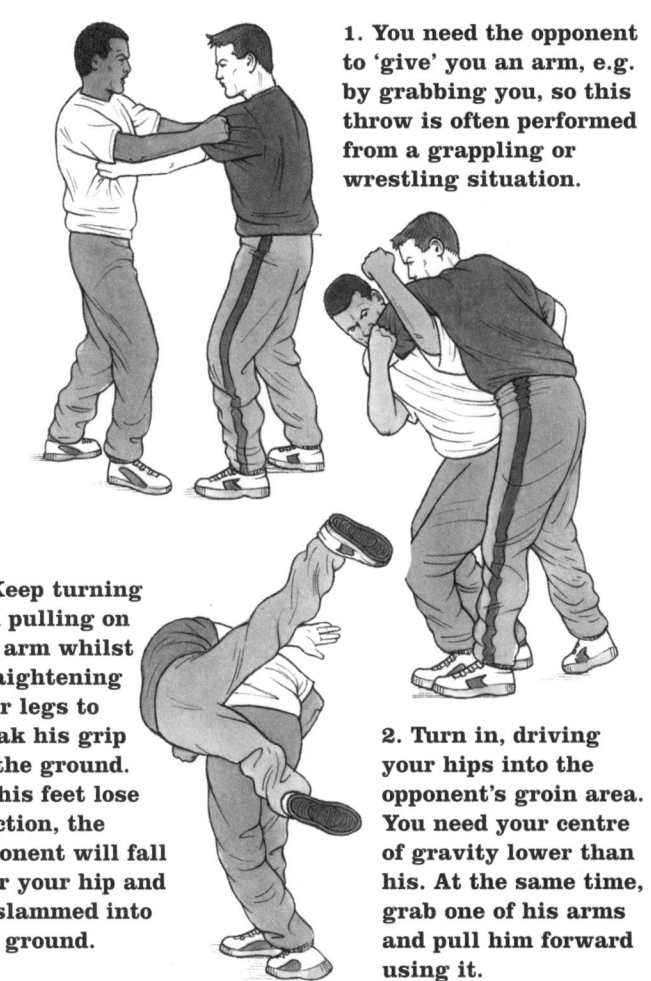

1. You need the opponent to 'give' you an arm, e.g. by grabbing you, so this throw is often performed from a grappling or wrestling situation.

3. Keep turning and pulling on the arm whilst straightening your legs to break his grip on the ground. As his feet lose traction, the opponent will fall over your hip and be slammed into the ground.

2. Turn in, driving your hips into the opponent's groin area. You need your centre of gravity lower than his. At the same time, grab one of his arms and pull him forward using it.

much harder takedown. The easiest finish, if one is needed, is a knee drop on the groin.

Shoulder Throw

Drag your opponent towards you so that his balance is broken. Turn in

place and keep hold with one arm, using it to pull with. Bring your other arm through and wrap it over the opponent's arm. Keep turning in the direction you are already moving and bend forward, straightening your legs. As you do this haul the

TIP: THROWS AND TAKEDOWNS

The difference between a throw and a takedown is that in a throw you have to carry the weight of the opponent, however briefly. Some techniques that are traditionally called throws are actually takedowns.

Some takedowns and all throws are designed to slam the opponent into the ground and damage him. Some takedowns are designed to make him fall so that his weight breaks a locked joint, while others are simply ways of getting an opponent to the ground and do not cause much damage. Generally speaking, the easier a technique is to perform, the less damage it does.

Rear takedow

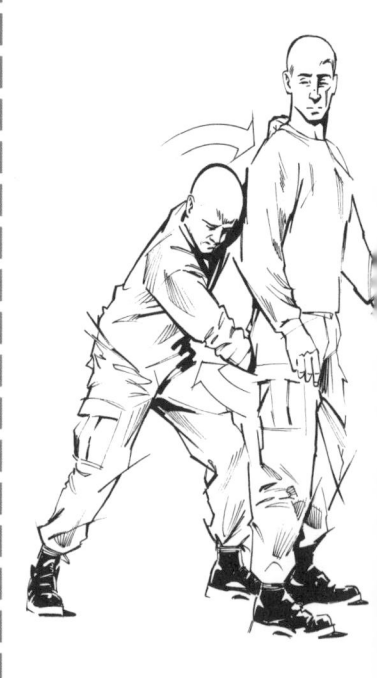

opponent over your shoulder. He will land on his back in front of you.

Rear Takedowns

Grab the opponent by the shoulders and pull him sharply backwards. At the same time, push or kick one of his legs forwards with your foot. Step back whilst still pulling and allow him to fall on his back in front of you.

Or grab the opponent's groin and yank back while gripping his collar and shoving forwards. The aim is to slam him face-first into the ground.

Grab the opponent by the collar and groin (or belt), pulling back on his groin whilst lifting and pushing forward at the collar. Let go of the collar as he falls but keep pulling up at the waist or groin to increase the impact of his head on the ground.

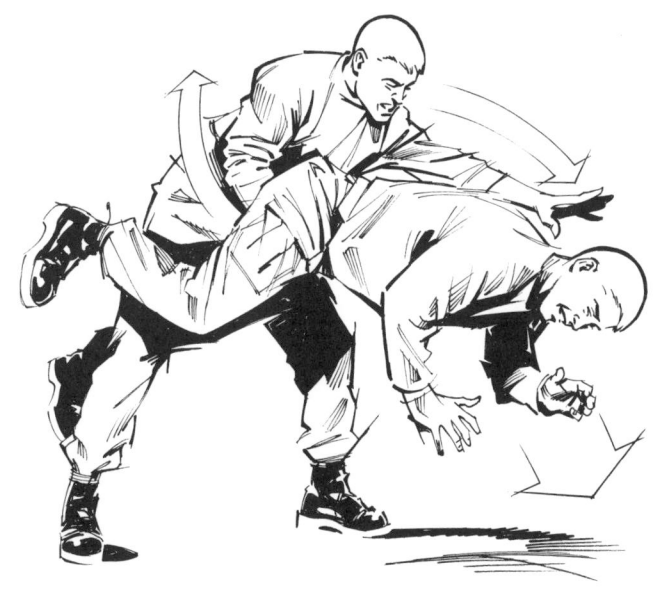

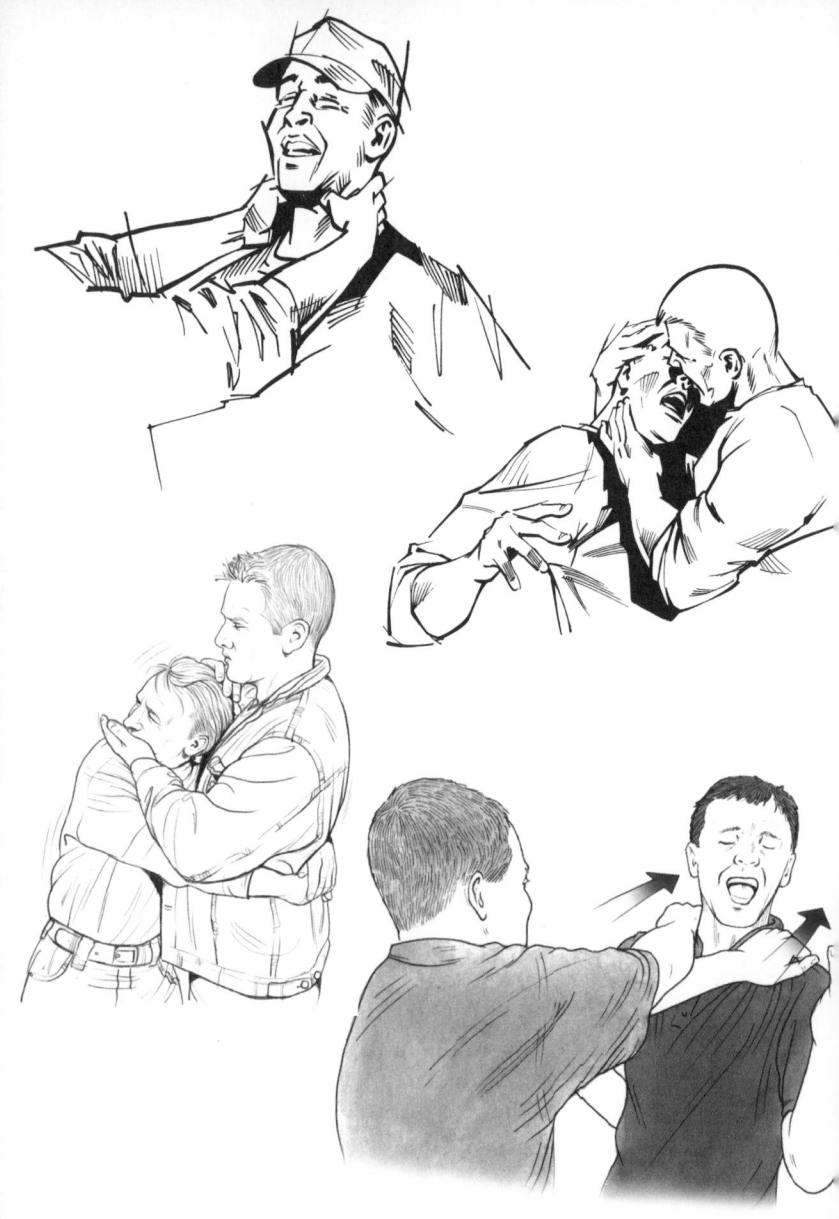

J oint-locking techniques were not invented as a way to cause an opponent to 'tap out' in a contest; they were designed to cause damage. An enemy soldier whose arm is broken cannot use his weapon effectively and is thus neutralized. Of course, a lesser degree of force can be used in training or when the situation merits it.

In military combat systems, joint locks are primarily used for arrest and restraint, which may be necessary when involved in peacekeeping duties. However, in a combat operation, troops may need to take out their opponents and move on to the objective. Thus locking techniques can be used to injure an opponent or put him where the soldier wants him. For example, a special forces soldier might use an arm-locking technique to turn an armed opponent around and put him in a position to be killed or disarmed.

USING JOINT LOCKS IN COMBAT

It is not generally a good idea to fiddle about looking for a tricky joint lock in the middle of a fight. If you are presented with the opportunity for one, take it for all it is worth, but do not become over-technical when your life is in danger.

. . . .

Left: Joint locks and chokes are most effective from a position of control.

8

Sometimes it is best to get an opponent under control rather than striking him or hurling him to the ground.

Tools of the Trade
Locks, Controls and Chokes

Thus the locks presented in this section should be considered as options in a lower-threat situation, while aggressive joint destructions can be used to disable an attacker if the opportunity arises. However, if you are in serious danger then stick to simple techniques, which normally means strikes.

WRIST LOCKS

The biggest problem with wrist locks is that it is very hard to catch hold of a wrist in the middle of a chaotic fight. Ironically, wrist techniques are often easier to use on someone who has a weapon as this provides some leverage.

Wrist grabs

Most people are right-handed, so the 'main event' comes from the right hand. If someone grabs you with the weak hand, they are almost certainly about to hit you. If the grab is with the strong hand, as here, then the intent is usually to gain dominance rather than an immediate attack.

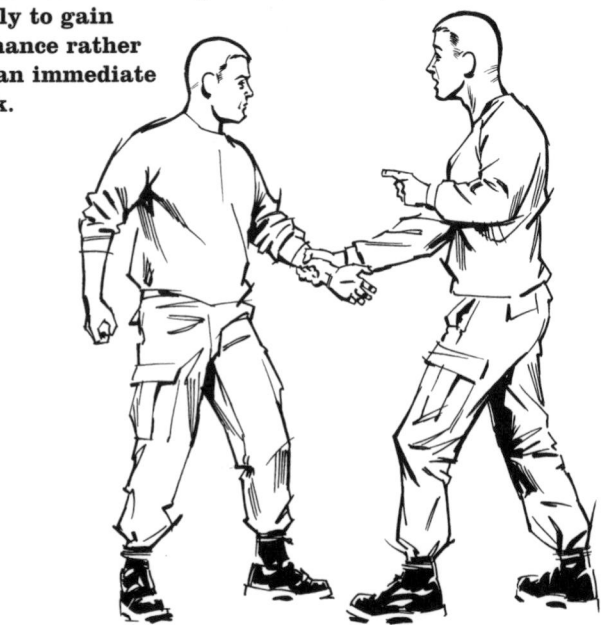

Many civilian martial arts teach wrist locks as a counter to an opponent who has grabbed your clothing or limbs. This is valid in theory, but combat experience shows that once someone has achieved a good grip it is very hard to peel it off and apply a lock. Rather than fighting for a wrist lock, you may be better off striking the assailant, who has just taken one or both of his hands out of action by grabbing your lapels.

The simple rule for wrist techniques is: if you find yourself in possession of an opponent's hand or wrist, use a wrist technique. But do not go looking for one – just hit him instead.

Outward Wrist Lock

Grab the opponent's hand with your opposite hand (e.g. his right with your left) and place your thumb on the back of his hand. Rotate your hand outwards until his arm cannot go any further. Additional pressure will cause pain or damage and may force him to twist around. Some martial arts teach this as a 'wrist throw' but it is not really a throw; the martial artist throws himself into a flip to get out of the lock. An untrained opponent or someone caught by surprise will not be quick enough and can end up with a fractured forearm if you apply enough pressure.

If you need more force, use your other hand as well, with both thumbs on the back of the opponent's hand. Alternatively, grab his elbow with your other hand and wrench it inwards (i.e. to your right if you have hold of his right hand) as you turn your left hand outwards. This is not really a wrist technique any more – it tears the shoulder joint – but it is extremely effective.

Wrist Crush

Grab the assailant's hand with your same-side hand (e.g. right to right) with your thumb digging into the pad between his thumb and first finger. Your fingers go around his. Now turn your hand over so that your thumb is pointing at your face, and rotate it vertically to try to point it at the opponent's face instead. Dig your little finger into the point where his wrist joins his hand and use this as a point to pivot around. If you need extra leverage use your other hand as well.

This causes intense pain and usually forces the opponent down, where he can be kicked or kneed easily. It can also be used as a pain-compliance technique to get someone under control.

Wrist Fold

Grip the opponent's hand around the widest part, where the fingers meet the hand, and 'fold' his wrist as far as it will go. With your other hand, grip his elbow and ram your hands together. This will tear tendons and ligaments in the wrist and make it useless. Alternatively, ram his elbow back against something hard such as a wall. This works particularly well as a finish against a downed opponent.

Joint locks

Top:
To apply a wrist lock, grip the opponent's hand with your thumb on the back. Try to rotate your hand by pushing your thumb forward, twisting the opponent's wrist. For added force, pull his elbow in the opposite direction.

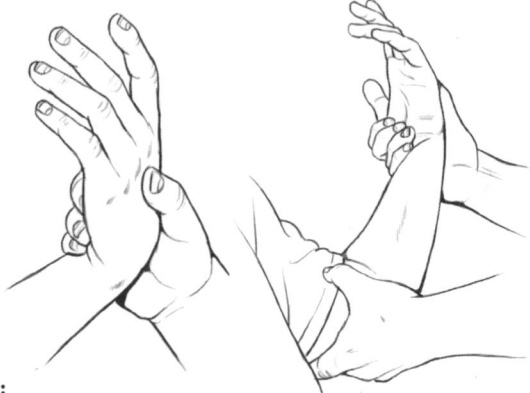

Bottom:
To apply a wrist crush, grip the opponent's hand so that your little fingers are at the very base of his hand. Rotate your hand, again by pushing the thumb forwards. Your little fingers act as a fulcrum to rotate around. The harder you twist, the more it hurts.

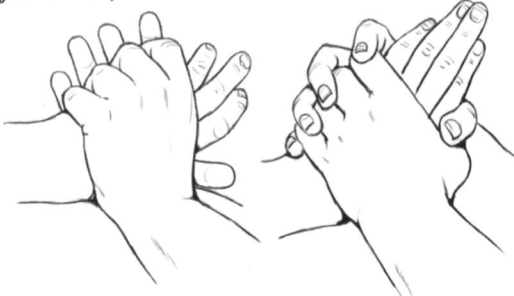

This basic wrist fold is used as the foundation of several more complex wrist locks, but these are too complex to deal with here and should in any case be taught by a properly qualified instructor.

ARM AND SHOULDER LOCKS

As with wrist locks, arm and shoulder locks can be used to restrain or control an opponent, but were originally invented as ways to disable enemy soldiers by breaking their limbs. Care must be taken when training arm locks. In particular, if your partner starts to stumble or fall, let him go. Sudden weight on a locked joint can cause irreparable damage. Of course, in a military context, locking a joint then dropping the opponent's weight on it is a highly effective combat technique.

Arm Bar

There are many variations on the arm bar, or 'straight arm lock'. In all cases the arm is pulled out straight from the body and something – usually a part of your body – is used as a fulcrum just behind the elbow. Pushing the elbow against its normal range of movement while pulling on the wrist places great strain on the joint and can tear it apart.

There are also many uses of the arm bar; we will see several of them in the next chapter. For now, it is sufficient to learn the basic arm bar. Applying more pressure on a straight

TIP: CONTROL AND RESTRAINT

'Control and restraint' methods should only be tried with opponents who are relatively low-threat or when backup is readily available. Tying yourself up by putting an arm lock on someone while his friends pound on you is not a great idea. As a rule 'C&R' is the province of security and law enforcement personnel rather than people who have to defend themselves from a serious attack.

arm lock will tear the joint. Another variation can be used to break an arm quickly. Simply grab the opponent's arm and yank it to you. At the same time push your chest forward to use as a fulcrum.

Shoulder Arm Lock

Many martial arts teach this as a 'finishing' move, but it is not really. It can immobilize someone and cause them pain, but that may not be enough to end a fight. However, this

Shoulder arm lock

Wrap the opponent's arm by looping your 'outside' arm around it, with your forearm behind his elbow. Your 'inside' arm grips his shoulder. Grab your 'inside' arm with your 'outside' hand to fix the lock in place.

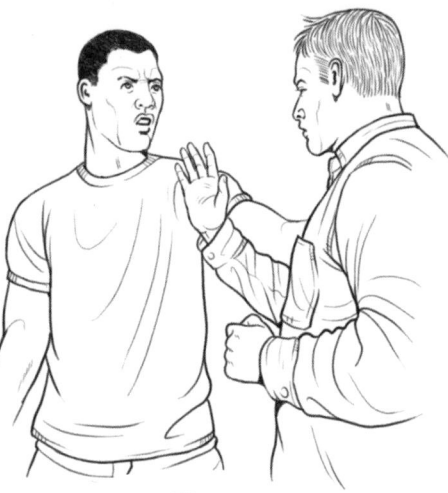

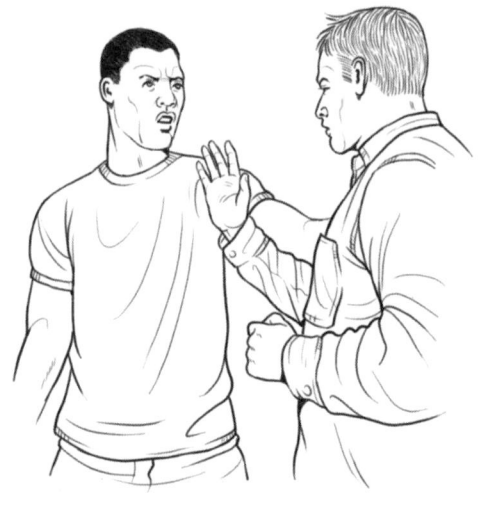

lock is useful to get the opponent's arm (usually his right) under control so that you can do whatever you have in mind. This is very important if he is holding a weapon. Once you have established the locking position, it is a simple matter to follow up with knee strikes or a takedown.

To perform the lock, wrap or 'snake' your arm around that of the opponent. This is particularly easy from a cover block as described above. The important thing is to get your forearm behind the opponent's elbow. This prevents him pulling his arm out and applies pressure to the elbow joint. Your other hand extends forward to grab his shoulder, and your wrapping hand grabs the straight forearm to anchor the lock. If you now straighten your arms, this will cause pain in the opponent's elbow joint.

Alternatively, just wrap the arm and grab his throat instead. This is not an arm lock as such but it is a useful control and restraint technique.

CONTROLS

Some techniques do not cause any real harm to the opponent but are useful to get him under control. This can mean putting him where you can do him most damage, or simply protecting yourself. For example, if you are fighting a good puncher, it makes sense to get in close and tie up his striking arms.

This may not win you the fight but it reduces the chances of losing while you seek a victory.

The Clinch

All manner of clinches are used in combat sports and martial arts. The term simply means getting in close and grabbing the opponent. The most basic clinch is to grab around the head. This can be done one- or two-handed, or with one hand round the head and one grabbing an arm or striking.

Go in fairly low and cup your hand or hands around the back of the neck and head, using the bulge of the skull to prevent your hands sliding off. Pull the opponent down and towards you, ideally dragging his head onto your shoulder. The obvious follow-up from here is to pull him onto knee strikes.

It is also possible to clinch around the body. Ideally you want your arms under his (wrestlers call this 'underhooks') and round his back, pulling yourself tightly into the opponent. Tuck your head in to protect it. This may look like a weak position but it is possible to set up a range of takedowns from here. The body clinch is a good defensive position if you have been hit – it protects you while you recover your wits and places you for a counterattack once you are ready.

From a body clinch, you can drop hammerfists into the opponent's thigh muscle or kidney area whilst keeping hold with the other hand. Biting and headbutting are also options from this position.

Head Controls

Grabbing an opponent's head is a highly effective way to get them under control. Where the head goes, the body follows. Thus if you pull the head in close to you, you can bend an opponent forwards and off balance. Pushing it backwards bends the opponent backwards ready for a takedown. Alternatively, the head can be twisted which forces the body to turn with it. This can be used to effect a release from a bear hug or similar grabbing attack. 'Headlocks' are another effective control and are instinctive to most people. The key is to bring the opponent's head down and lock it against your body.

SHUTDOWN TECHNIQUES

'Shutdown techniques' is a catch-all term for a number of techniques that can be used to 'shut down' an opponent and change his mindset from aggressive to defensive. Shutdown techniques are unlikely to be decisive but can give you a chance to take the offensive with something more effective, or can at least take some of the pressure off.

In general, you should take any opportunity you can to cause shock and pain to the opponent. This means relatively weak knee strikes,

blows and headbutts should still be delivered if you cannot land anything harder. Obviously there is no substitute for fight-winning blows, but that does not mean that it is not worth throwing, say, a relatively weak elbow strike when in close.

The most effective shutdown techniques target the face. Stick your fingers or thumb in an eye socket, or grab and rip at ears, lips, cheeks and anything else you can get hold of. Simply raking your hand across someone's nose and eyes can make him flinch away and allow you to gain an advantage. You can also drive your thumbs into the nerve centres just under and in front of the ears, or anywhere on the throat and neck.

Shutdown techniques of this sort are a bit undignified and not at all in keeping with a 'gentlemanly' ethos of a clean fight. But so what? It is necessary get the job done anyhow you can, and while a neat knockout is elegant, an opponent mauled into submission is still a win. Be willing to fight as dirty as you possibly can if your survival is at stake.

CHOKES AND STRANGLES

Correctly speaking, a 'choke' cuts off the air supply (like the choke in a car) and a 'strangle' cuts off blood supply to the brain. Most choke or strangle techniques end up being a bit of both. Of all the possible combat

Control the head

Where the head goes, the body follows. Twisting the head can turn an opponent round and break a grab, while a simple headlock can be used to get someone under control quickly.

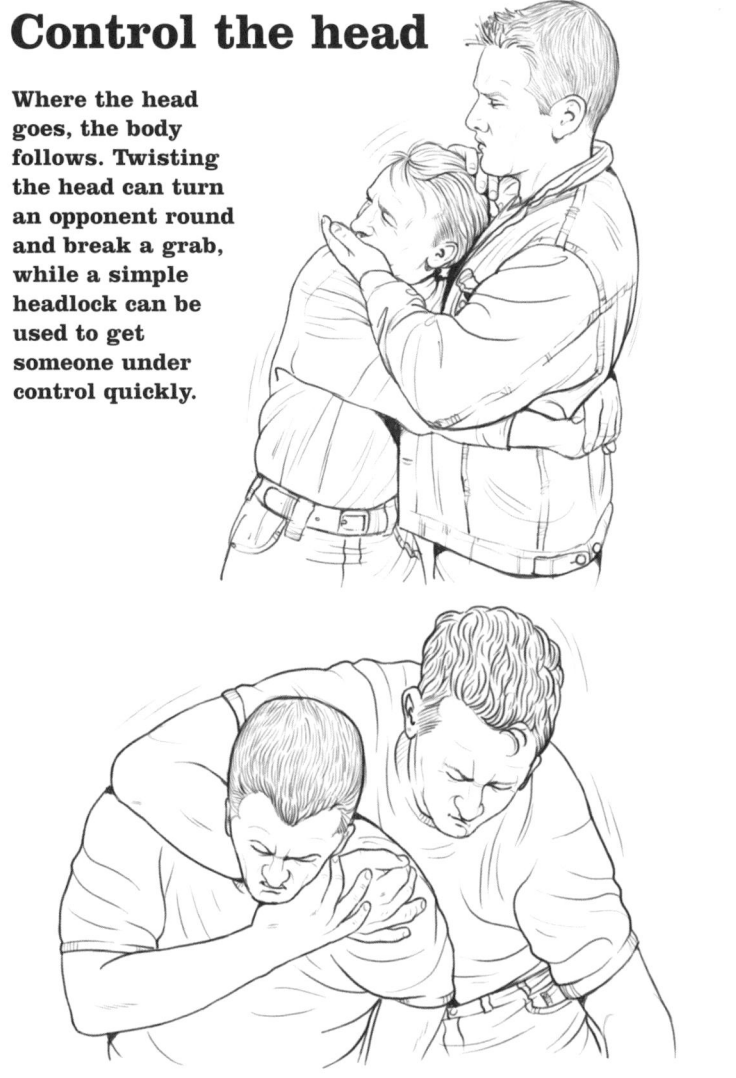

Strike and grab

Striking and grappling can be combined to defeat a close-quarters attack. Break the grip and stun the opponent with strikes, then grab and twist the head to get him under control – and on the ground.

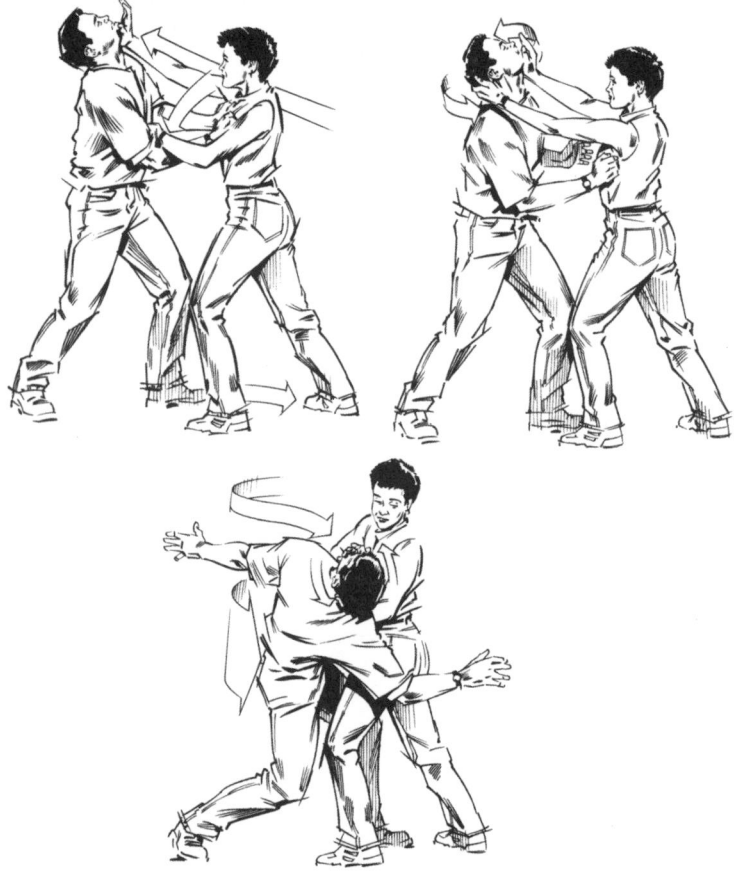

Attack the head

The head can be attacked in many ways. At close quarters it is effective to bite, rake fingers across the eyes or poke them into the eye sockets, or to squeeze the throat. These painful techniques can 'shut down' an attacker and force him onto the defensive.

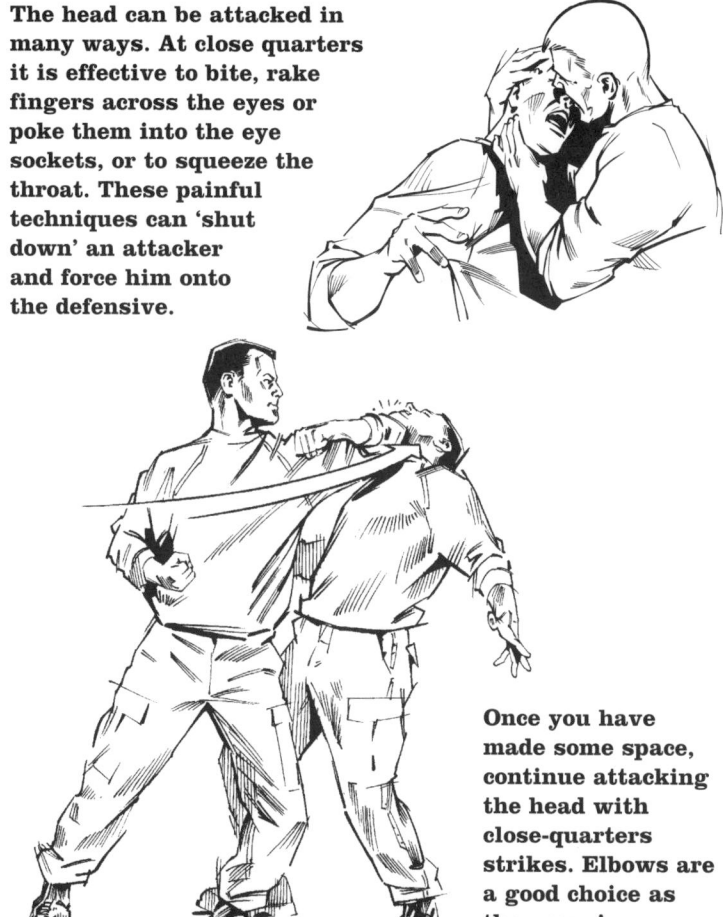

Once you have made some space, continue attacking the head with close-quarters strikes. Elbows are a good choice as they require very little space to use.

techniques, these are the ones that require the most care in training and should only be learned from a qualified instructor.

Chokes and strangles give different results. A choke can take some time to subdue an opponent, and having your windpipe constricted is one of the most terrifying things that can happen to you. As a result, if you start to choke someone they will usually go berserk trying to escape. Chokes can be useful in getting control of someone, frightening them and then loosening the hold a little. The added advantage is that if you have a good grip on head and neck, the rest of the body tends to follow.

Strangles are more insidious. If a strangle is properly applied, it will usually cause unconsciousness in a few seconds, typically 5–10 but sometimes less. If the strangle is kept on for even a few seconds after unconsciousness occurs, the victim will usually die. Thus strangles are extremely dangerous – and conversely, anyone trying to strangle you must be treated as a potentially lethal threat.

Rear Naked Choke and 'Sleeper Hold'

The most basic choke is performed by putting your forearm across the opponent's throat and pulling back towards you. Lock the choke in by placing your hand in the crook of your opposite elbow and bending that arm, placing the hand on the back of the opponent's head. Push his head forward with your hand as you pull back with your forearm.

A version of this choke can be performed with just one arm, leaving the other free. This version is used mainly to control someone as it is hard to apply sufficient pressure to choke the opponent with just one arm. However, someone in this position makes an excellent human shield against his friends. It is important, whether using one or both hands, to bend the opponent backwards towards you, breaking his balance and making it difficult to escape from your hold.

A 'sleeper hold' is a strangle rather than a choke, but it is applied much the same way, but you need to reach further through so that the front of the opponent's throat rests in the crook of your elbow. Squeeze his neck between your biceps and forearm, placing pressure on both carotid arteries (at the side of the neck). If applied hard and fast, this technique can cause unconsciousness in seconds and death soon after, so must be trained only under qualified supervision.

Two-Handed Strangle

A classic in movies, strangles of this sort are rare in reality, except in domestic violence situations. It is mentioned here mainly as it tends to be used by untrained opponents. The strangle is performed by squeezing the opponent's neck between your hands, with the thumbs on the front of the throat. This is not a very effective combat technique as it is useful mainly against much weaker opponents or someone who is already more or less helpless due to other techniques. The same strangle can also be applied from behind, but it is even less useful from that position.

Bar Choke

A basic bar choke can be applied from many angles. Place your forearm across the opponent's throat and push back. Obviously, he can escape by moving backwards so this must be prevented somehow. One way is to push him against a wall or

Rear naked choke

The choke is applied by a forearm across the throat, locked in by your other arm. Put your hand into the crook of your elbow, then place the other hand on the back of the opponent's head. Push his head forward and down for a powerful choke.

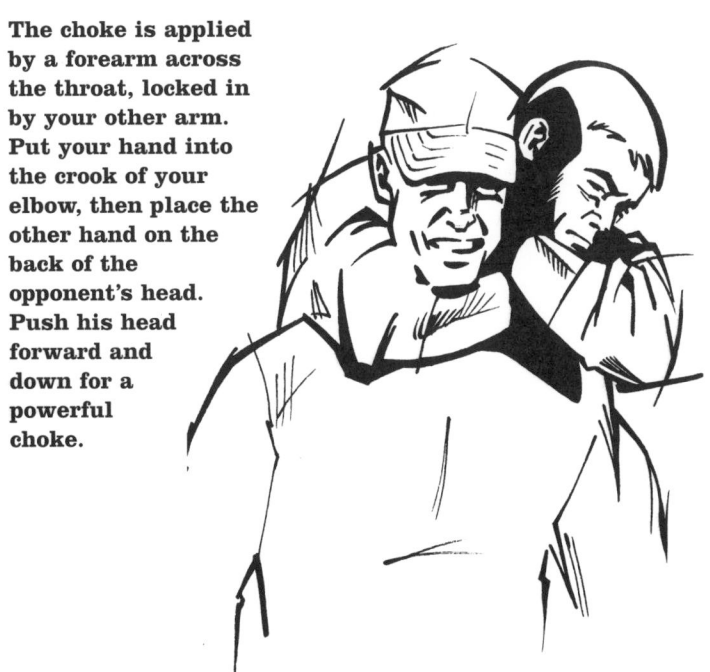

Bar choke

This easy choke only works when the opponent is pinned against something, such as the ground or a wall. Your forearm is used as a bar across the throat to squash the windpipe.

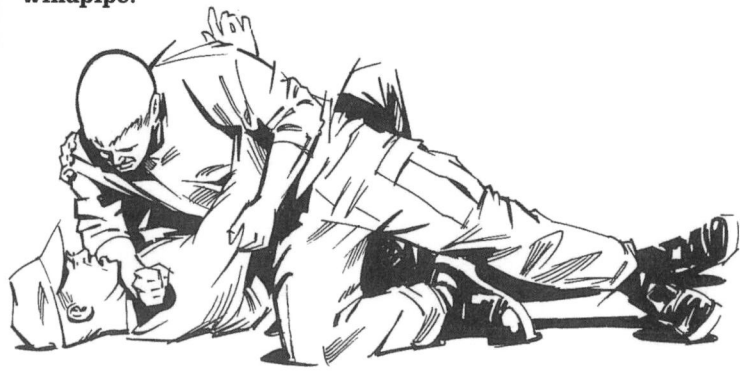

to apply the choke on the ground, pushing down on his windpipe. Alternatively, it is possible to grab the lapel of a jacket and pull down with the other hand, locking the choke in with his own clothing.

Clothing Chokes

In addition to the clothing-assisted bar choke noted above, clothing can be used to choke an opponent in other ways. A 'scissors' choke is performed by reaching both hands deep into the collar and grabbing hold, then pulling the opponent down and forwards while moving your elbows outwards. The effect is like a pair of scissors with your hands as the blades. A variant on this choke is to use one hand in the collar and to pull down on the opposite lapel with the other.

If you are behind your opponent, however, reach over the opponent's shoulder and grab his lapel on the opposite side, dragging it up and over his shoulder. This will pull his clothing across the throat and apply a choke. It does not work well with flimsy or stretchy clothing however.

Lapel choke

A lapel choke can be applied with any reasonably robust clothing. Pull one lapel across the throat and pull the other down hard to tighten the choke. Alternatively, slide your hand inside the opponent's collar and grip, using your arm instead of his jacket across his throat. The pull down on the other lapel remains the same.

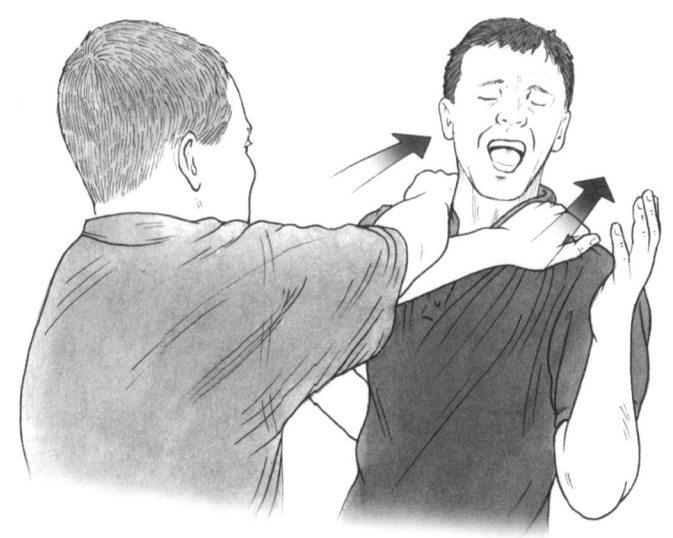

Guillotine Choke

To apply a guillotine choke, you need to bring the opponent's head down. A groin or solar plexus strike will assist with this. Loop your arm over his head and pull it down to just above your hip, pushing your arm under his chin from the outside inwards. Lock this arm in with your other arm and pull upwards. Ideally you want to push his head down while you pull his throat upwards. One advantage of a guillotine choke is that even if you do not quite get it, you still have a headlock and can deliver some knee strikes.

Headlock/guillotine choke

This position can be used to simply control an opponent, or to choke him. Pull up with your arm under the throat while pushing his head down by dropping your shoulder.

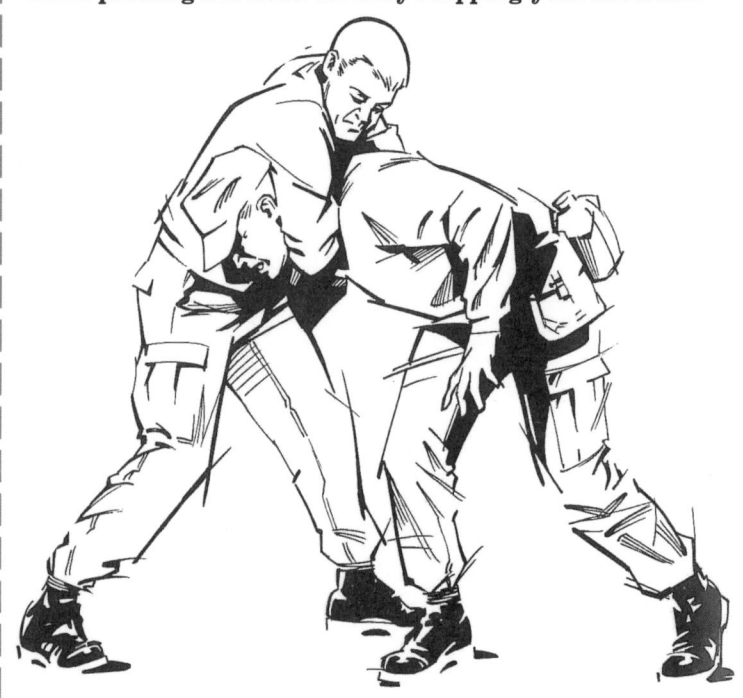

Throat Grabs

It is possible to apply a choke simply by grabbing the opponent around the larynx with a 'C-grip' and squeezing. Push in and up, and try to bring fingers and thumb together behind the larynx. The intensity of the choke can be varied depending on the result you want – a fairly light choke can obtain compliance from someone you are trying to restrain, harder chokes can be used to

Throat grab

An effective strangle can be applied by gripping the back of the neck with the fingers of one or both hands and digging the thumb(s) into the carotid arteries. This cuts off blood to the brain.

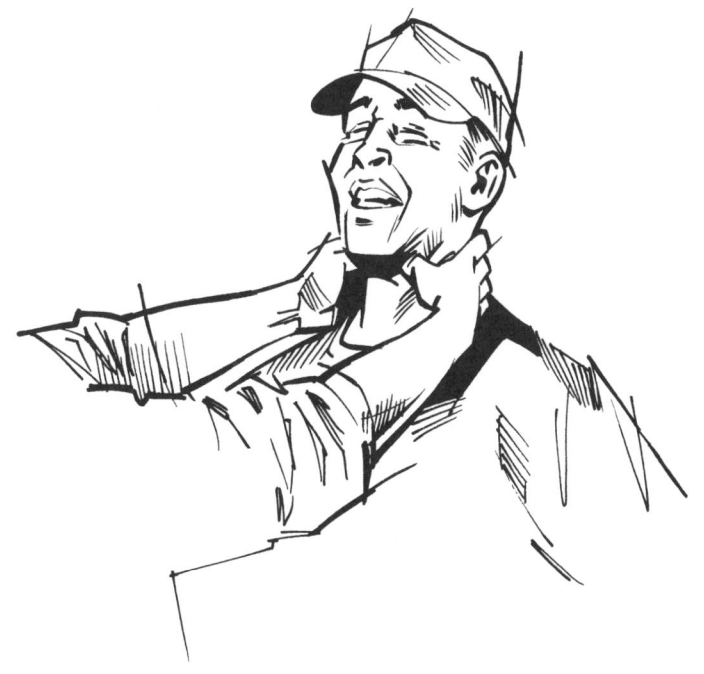

subdue someone who is trying to harm you.

A similar choke can be applied by gripping around the neck. Your fingers go around the back of the neck and the thumb digs in to one side or other of the larynx. You can use one or both hands. It is relatively easy to pull out of this choke, so it is best performed on someone you have hold of with your other hand or have pushed up against a wall.

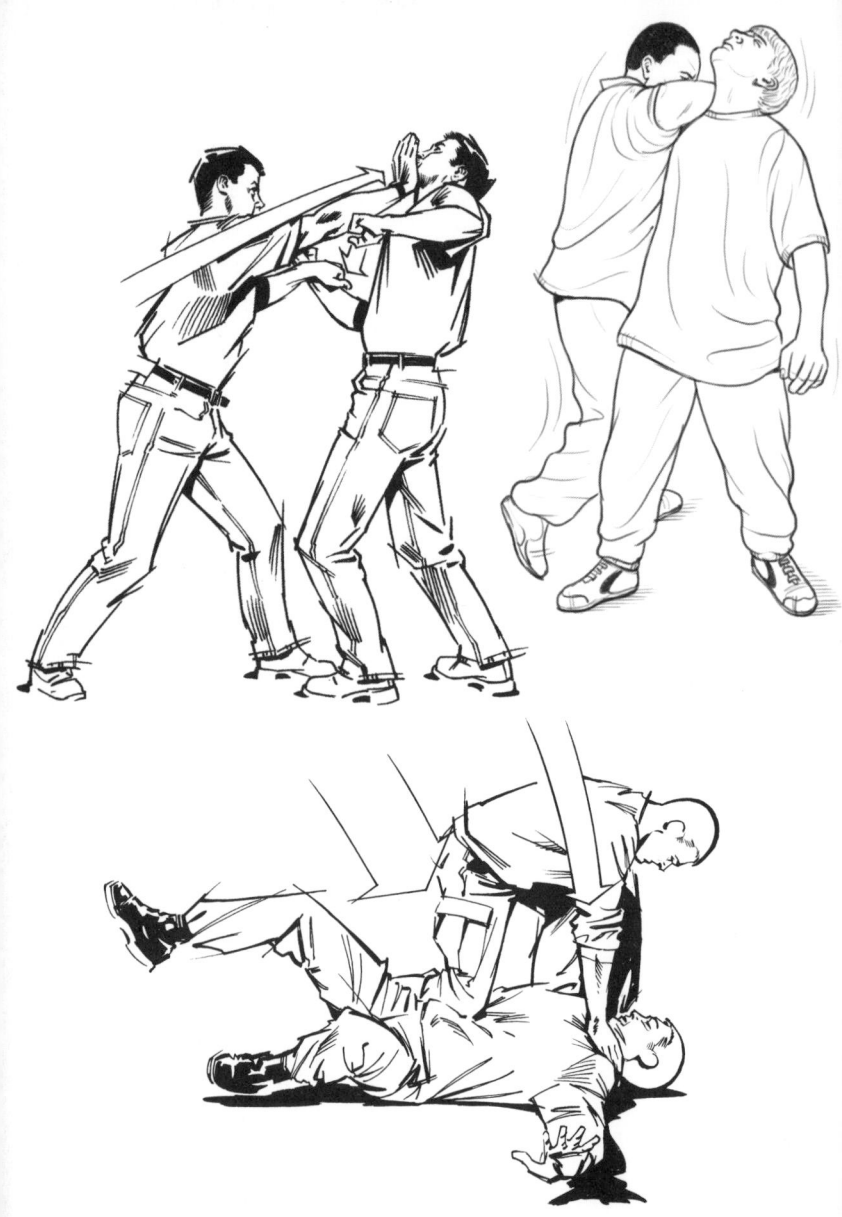

Once combat starts, you fight with what you have. Your preparation is done, your skills and fitness are at whatever level you have reached. There is no time to wish you had spent more hours in the gym or learned some extra techniques. If you lack skill, fitness, strength or any other factor, you will have to make up for it with something else. The mental aspect is of paramount importance – guts and determination can cover many other deficiencies.

Many people subscribe to the idea that 'violence solves nothing'. In fact, a great many problems can be solved with violence, provided you use enough and in the right way. However, using violent means will often create new problems. For example, it may be a simple matter to eliminate a sentry, but once he is missed the enemy will be alerted – the sentry problem is solved but now there is an active search underway. This is a different and possibly more serious problem.

Thus if possible it is best to deal with threats by non-violent means. However, sometimes there is no alternative but to use force. If you have tried and failed or been given

....

Left: Weapons, combat skills and physical prowess are all useless unless they are intelligently applied.

9

Good tactics can get you through a situation that would have been impossible had you just bulled in head-on.

In Action

Tactics

no opportunity to avoid trouble, de-escalate the situation or deter the assailant, then you must accept that the attack is going to happen and deal with it head-on. If this creates new problems, you can handle them as they arise.

Remember that your goal is always to bring the situation to an end on your own terms, and act accordingly. That might mean escaping or disabling the opponent. It might mean bundling him out through a door and locking it behind him, or applying a painful restraint and

outlining the consequences of continuing his attack. Decide what you need to do and then do it without hesitation or second-guessing yourself.

COMBAT PRINCIPLES

Many martial arts treat unarmed combat as something resembling a tennis match. One player serves, the other hits the ball back, and it goes back and forth until someone makes a mistake. This is fine in a sporting context but for life-or-death combat a different approach is needed.

TIP:
GETTING IT RIGHT

One of the author's students got it exactly right when a stranger barged into her house and began behaving aggressively. She ran to her room, locked the door and leant on it while calling the police. More importantly, she made a decision.

Her gameplan was, 'If he stays on that side of the door I wait for the police. If he's willing to kick through it to get to me, I hit him with the heaviest object in the room' – which she duly located and readied.

This was exactly the right thing to do. She removed herself from danger and summoned help. She also prepared a backup plan in case things got worse, rightly realizing that someone willing to smash through her door rather than just taking property that was easily accessible was probably after her personally. This was a very serious threat requiring an all-out response.

Rather than taking turns to attack and defend, military combat systems are all about demolishing the opposition as fast and efficiently as possible. If the opponent manages to launch an attack, you must deal with it, but the principle is to nullify the attack while making one of your own or at least putting yourself in a position to defeat the opponent.

Seeing it Coming
In order to deal with an attack, you have to see it coming. Obviously, this means looking at your opponent. Do not stare at one part of his body such as his hands, eyes or feet. Let your eyes rest roughly on the base of the throat and upper chest region, and allow your peripheral vision to take in a picture of what he is doing. This

Focus point

Allow your gaze to rest on the base of the collar-bone and take in the 'big picture' rather than fixing your gaze on any one part of the opponent.

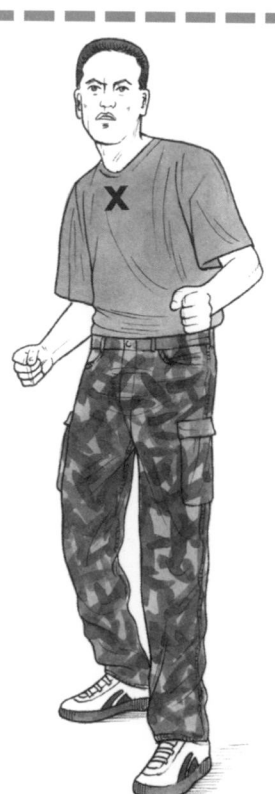

Returning to the tennis analogy, imagine a world-class tennis player throws up a ball to serve it at you. You are not going to win on his terms, are you? So how about you smash a ball of your own over the net while he is serving, and follow it with several more until you have won?

Or maybe you could just run over and beat him senseless with your racquet. Who said you have to play the same game as the attacker? If he is strong in one area, attack his weaknesses and do not let him play to his strengths.

way you will be aware of his movements without becoming fixated on any one part of his body.

Offensive Defence

Supposing the assailant throws a swinging right hook. You have several effective options, which include but are not limited to:

- Stop it cold by 'beating him to the punch', perhaps with a fast lead-hand shot or eye jab.
- Raise your elbow into the path of the punch and let him break his own hand by striking it instead of your head.
- Smother the attack as you move in for a takedown.
- Duck under the assailant's swing and punch him in the solar plexus as you do so.

None of these is really a 100 per cent defensive response. Instead, you are defeating the attack while making one of your own, which could be considered an offensive–defensive response. Once you have dealt with the attack and gained the initiative by landing one of your own, continue your attacks until you have nullified the threat.

The Steamroller Principle

Ideally, you will never allow the opponent to get into the fight. Even if he makes the first move, you gain the initiative with your offensive–defensive response and then retain it by constant aggressive actions. Everything you do keeps him off balance mentally and physically; if you cannot land fight-ending blows then you must launch a series of smaller but painful strikes. You can

Finishing techniques

If the opponent is down but still a threat to you, it will be necessary to put him fully out of the fight. Knee drops are an excellent finish, and against a very dangerous opponent a throat strike is an effective option.

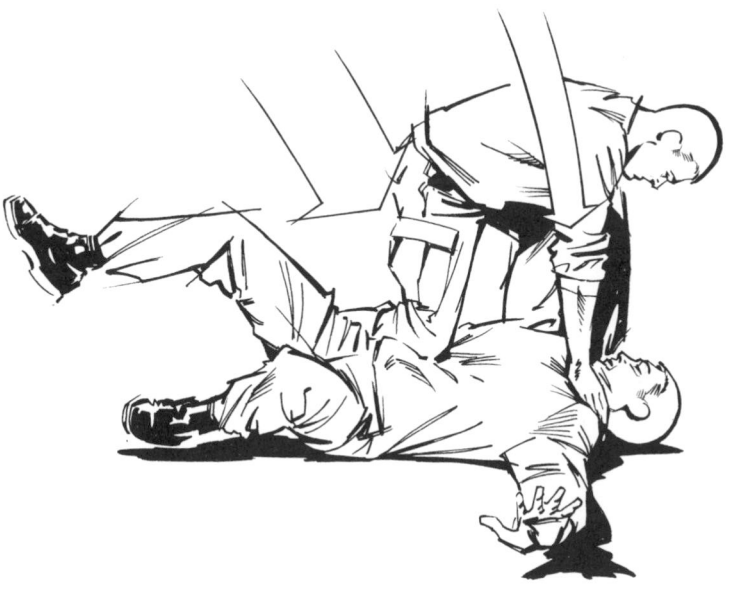

grab him and pull or push, kick him in the shins, bite, grab and rip, dump him on the ground with a takedown … and you must keep at it until he is out of the fight.

Obviously, you have to stop when the opponent is not a threat to you, but until then you must 'steamroller' him with constant attacks. If you let him regain his composure he might be able to turn the tables, and where you are willing to stop when it is over, you cannot guarantee that an assailant will have any mercy.

Taking the Initiative

Sometimes it is vital to gain control of a situation early on. The fence, coupled with an appropriate verbal gambit, can be used to change the course of a confrontation. So can a pre-emptive strike if you realize you are about to be attacked.

If you are facing a dangerous opponent or a group, getting the initiative is essential. This means either acting before they do or interrupting their actions with an offensive–defensive response to regain the initiative.

'Pincer' attacks are common, where one assailant confronts the victim while the other launches an attack from the side or rear. This can sometimes be prevented by movement and assertive behaviour ('Hey, where are you going? Stay where I can see you!') but if the attackers are determined, your best chance is to take the initiative by attacking one of them before they are ready. This will help even the odds and at least prevents them picking their time and manner of attack.

Change Tactics where Appropriate

Many people fixate on one kind of attack, throwing the same punch over and over whether it is the best option or not. Be willing to switch tactics, using close-quarters strikes and grappling to counter a puncher or blows to keep a grappler

at bay. Try to remember that you have many options. Often, once grappling starts people forget that they can strike, and end up struggling for a takedown or joint lock when they could knee, elbow or shin-kick more effectively.

If you keep your head you can disorientate your opponent by varying your attacks. Throw a couple of strikes then grab him, pull him in and knee, then dump him on the ground with a takedown. Or pull him off balance and kick him as he tries to regain his equilibrium. People are good at adapting to circumstances but if you keep changing the rules your opponent will never catch up and the fight becomes much easier.

SET-PIECE ATTACKS

If you succeed in gaining and keeping the initiative, you will be able to launch a set-piece attack designed to rapidly destroy the opponent. It is worth drilling a few such sequences on the heavy bag or with a partner. However, be prepared to adapt to changing circumstances. An opponent might stagger away after being hit, or fall over and spoil your planned combination. If this happens, adapt and carry on with something more appropriate rather than trying to finish a set-piece that will not work, or stopping in the middle of a fight because things have not gone to plan.

Take the initiative

If you are outnumbered, you have to attack or you will be overwhelmed. Attack intelligently; this blow actually takes two opponents out of the fight for a moment, leaving just one to be dealt with.

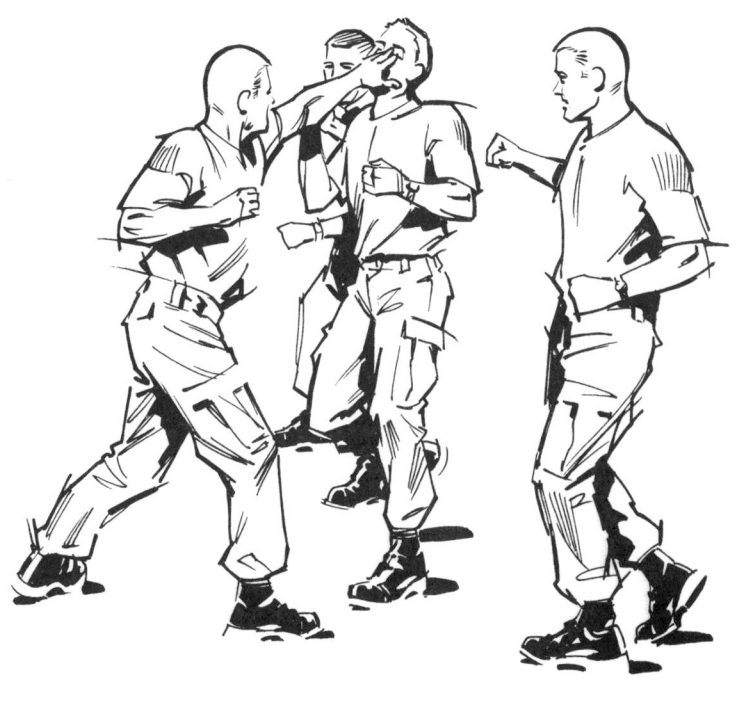

Set-Piece 1: Pre-Empt off the Fence
Confronted with an aggressive person, you have put up the 'fence' and tried to de-escalate the situation. No good ... you realize he is about to launch his attack. Pre-empt his attack with a right

Avoiding a 'pincer' attack

A common trick is for one assailant to get your attention and another to move behind you. Avoid this by moving so that both remain in your field of vision.

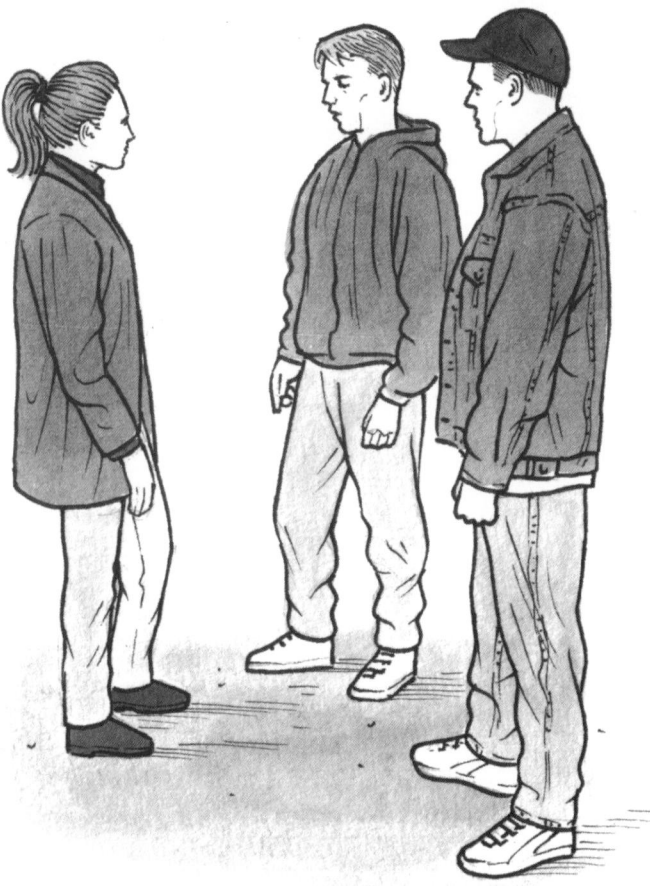

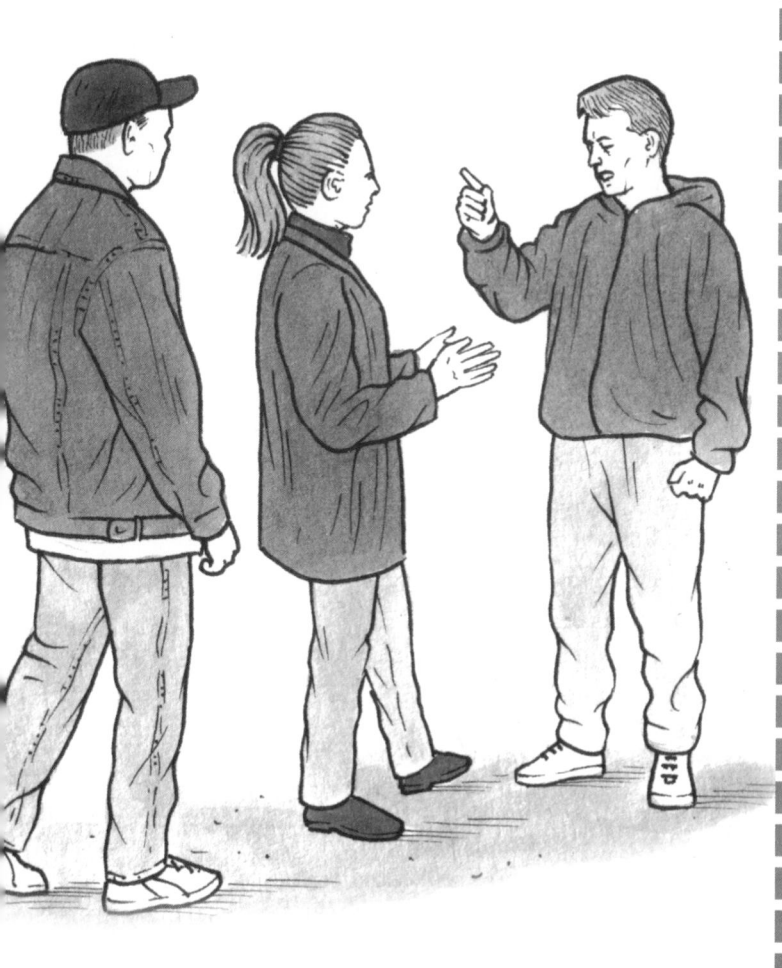

TIP:
SOMETIMES YOU GET MORE THAN YOU EXPECTED

During a training drill, the author was knocked out by a 'setup' strike launched by a student. He ended up sitting semi-conscious on the floor looking up at a disappointed student, who said, 'Aw, I wanted to do a takedown!' Comical, but there is a point here. The 'setup' strike worked better than expected and it took the student a moment to realize that he had won. He had quite rightly operated on the assumption that the strike might or might not work, and was mentally primed for the next step. This is wise; if you are 100 per cent sure something will work and it does not, panic can set in. However, sometimes a technique works unexpectedly well. As always, be prepared to change your plan.

cross or straight palm strike. This may result in a knockout or you may have to follow up with additional blows.

Hooked strike and takedown

This set-piece exploits the shock of the initial blow and the sideways movement it induces to set up a rotating takedown. The opponent can be finished once he is on the ground.

Set-Piece 2: Hooked Strike and Takedown

Again, you realize that the bad guy is about to 'go'. Throw a cupped-hand blow from your fence position, striking with the base of your palm along his jaw close to the ear. This might drop him but you cannot afford to take chances. Grab

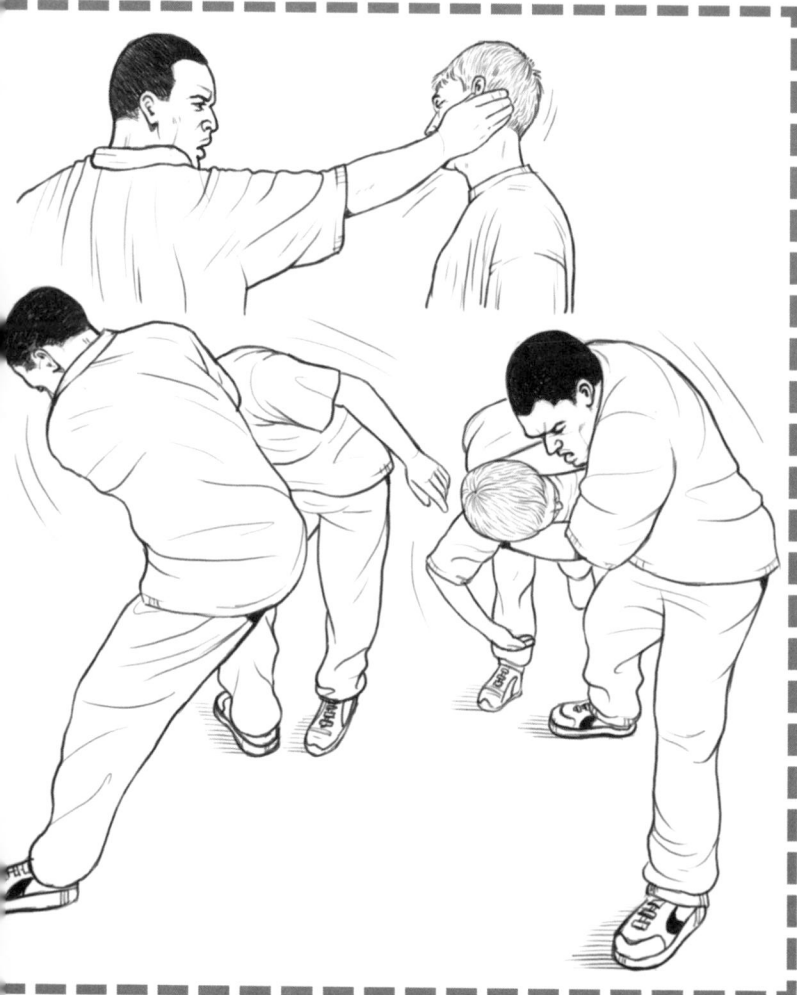

his head and pull him forward, launching a kick to his right shin with your right foot. This pushes his foot back and opens him up for a takedown. Pull his head forwards and down, pivoting back and out of the way. He should land on his back or side in front of you and can be finished off with a knee drop.

Eye jab–palm smash–elbow– knee

This is a 'steamroller' of blows. It is not pretty but it is certainly effective if you want to end the fight quickly. Create an opening with the eye jab and then keep on hitting until the threat is nullified.

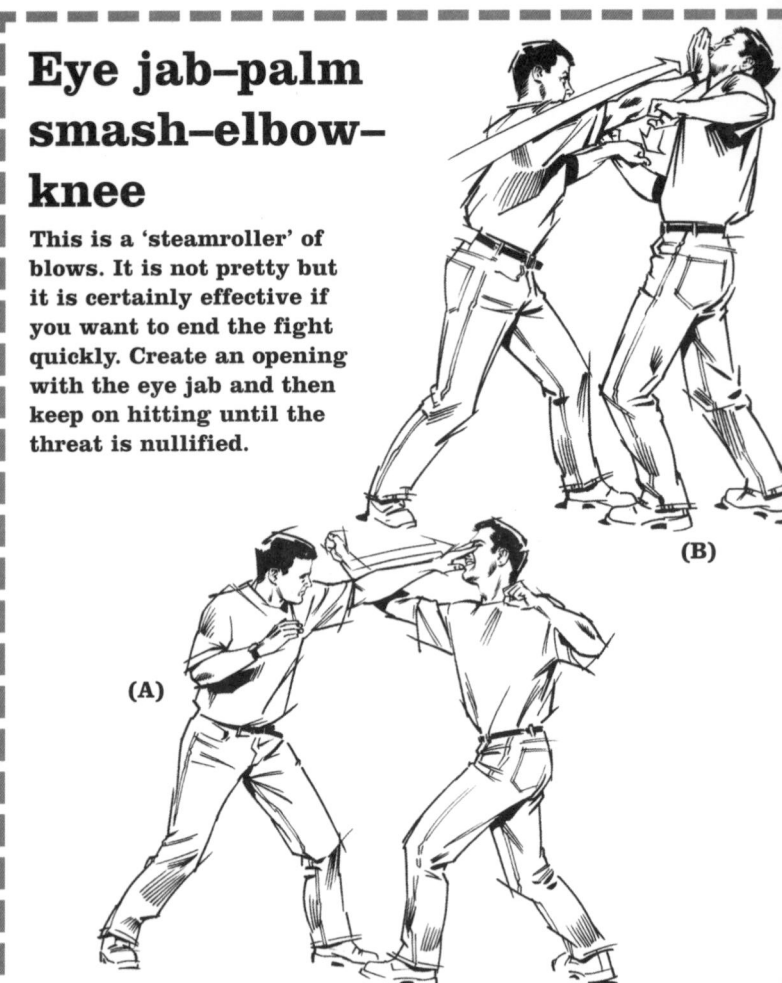

(A)

(B)

Set-Piece 3: Eye Jab–Palm Smash–Elbow–Knee

Interrupt whatever the attacker is doing (probably throwing a wild haymaker) with a fast lead-hand eye jab to gain the initiative. Follow up with a strong-hand palm strike to the jaw. If this does not end the matter,

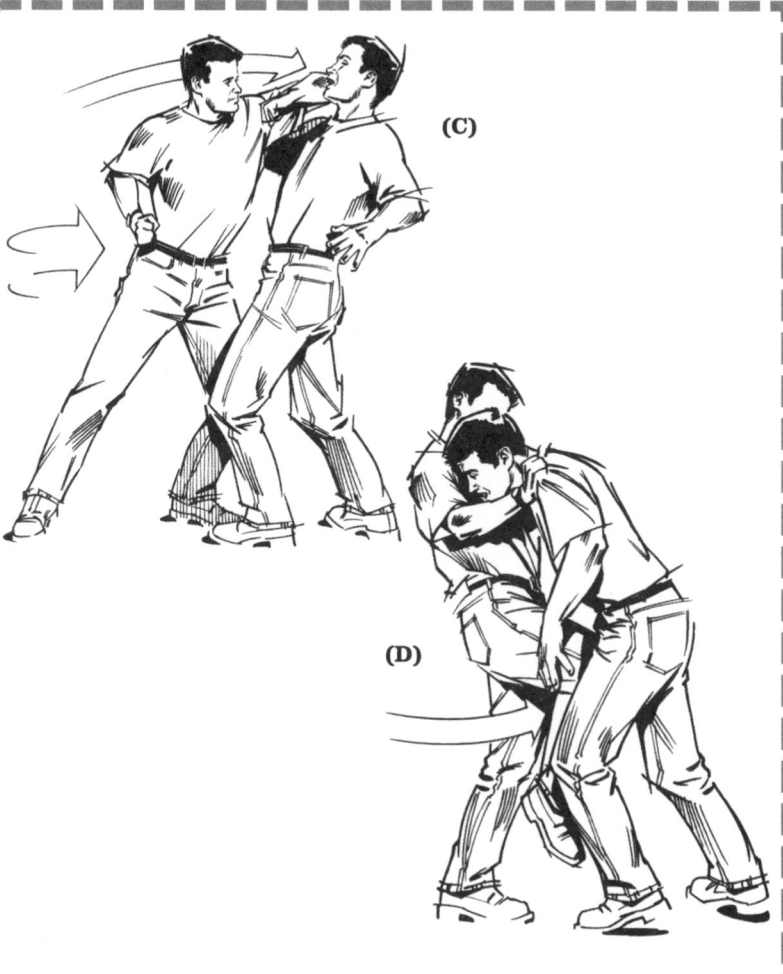

(C)

(D)

attack again with a hooking elbow using your lead arm. Target the jaw if you can but anywhere on the head is good. This is followed up if necessary by grabbing the assailant and delivering a knee strike.

Set-Piece 4: Body Shot–Takedown–Knee Drop

Bring the opponent's head down with a body shot, and grab him around the back of the head, pulling down and forward as you pivot to the side. Do not just pull with your arms, use your bodyweight. The finish is a knee drop into the ribs, followed by strikes to the head if necessary.

Set-Piece 5: Hook Punch Defence with Guillotine Choke

As the assailant launches his attack, interrupt it by lunging forward to smother the blow. Using your left arm to trap his punching arm, shoot your right over his shoulder and use it to drag his head down onto your hip, looping your arm through under his throat for a guillotine choke. From this position, launch knee strikes into his body. Knee from the back foot and drive right through. Even if your choke is not fully on, you will push the air out of the assailant's lungs and the choke will make it hard to get more in.

After a couple of strikes, the opponent will start to defend himself with his arms or elbows, so it will be time for you to change tactics.

Body shot and takedown

The body shot brings the attacker's head down. Exploit this movement by pulling his head down and forward, in the direction he is already going.

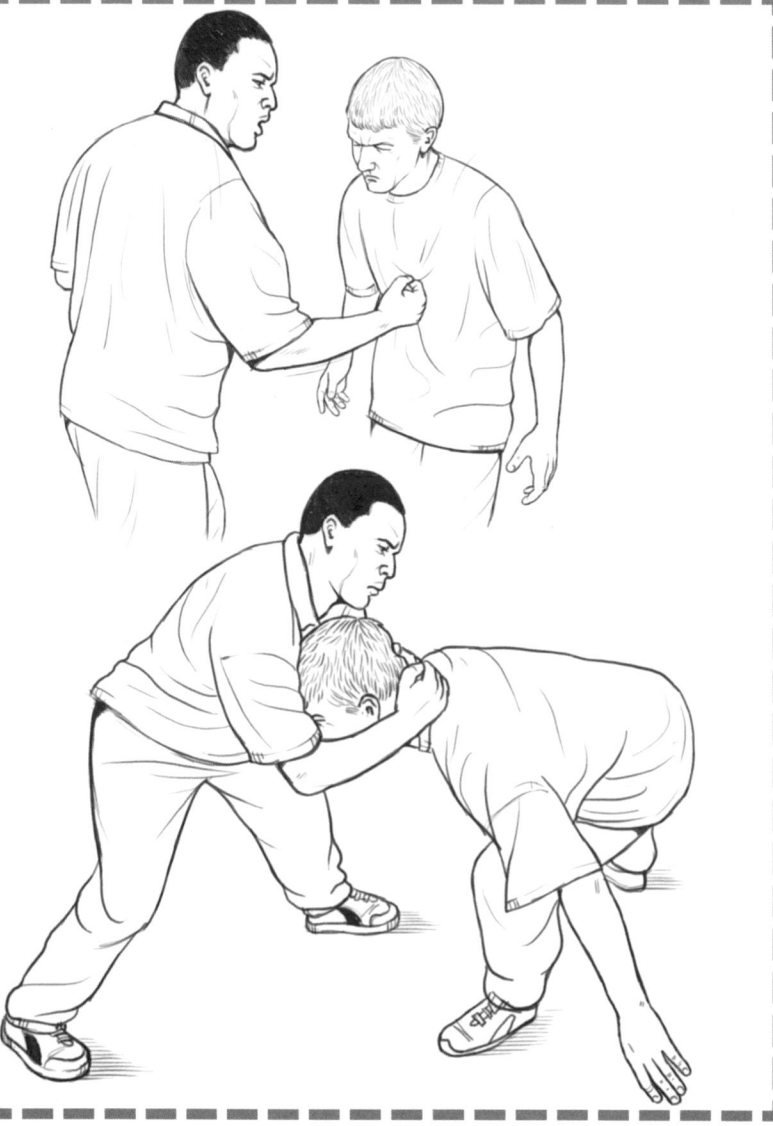

Hook punch defence with guillotine choke

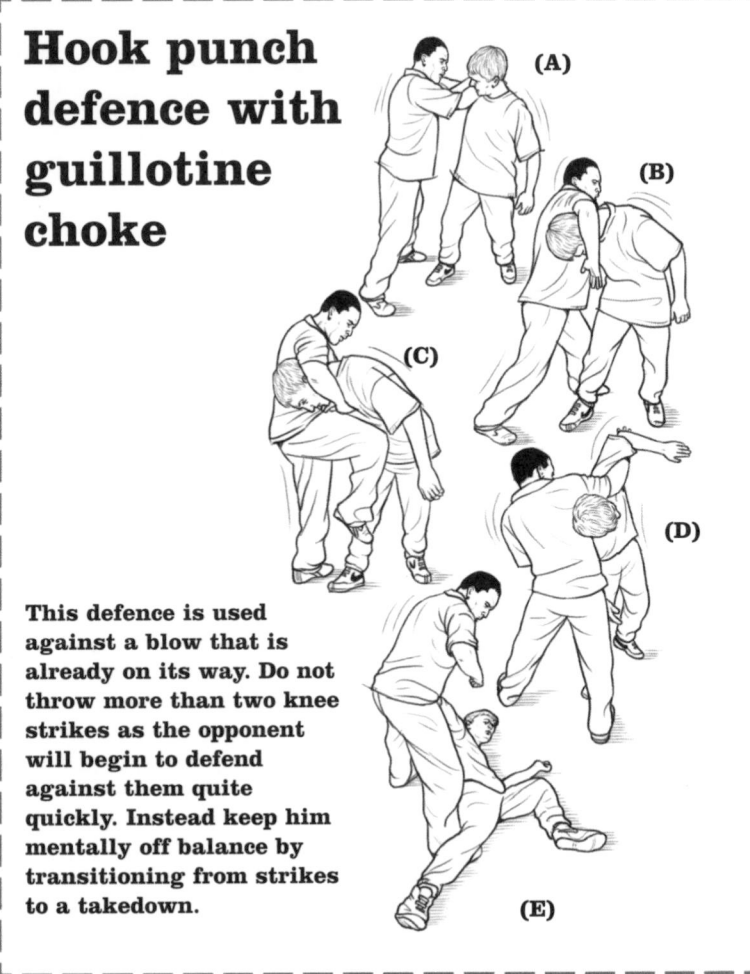

(A)
(B)
(C)
(D)
(E)

This defence is used against a blow that is already on its way. Do not throw more than two knee strikes as the opponent will begin to defend against them quite quickly. Instead keep him mentally off balance by transitioning from strikes to a takedown.

Take him down by lifting one shoulder up and pushing the other down while pivoting away, and finish with a knee drop.

Set-Piece 6: Hook Punch Defence with Outer Reap Takedown
As the assailant throws a hook punch, lunge forward and jam it,

Hook punch defence with outer reap takedown

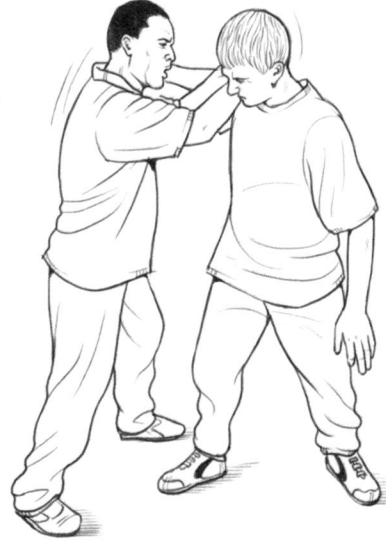

Make sure you crash into the opponent hard enough to make him recoil and lose his balance. This will enable you to take him down hard.

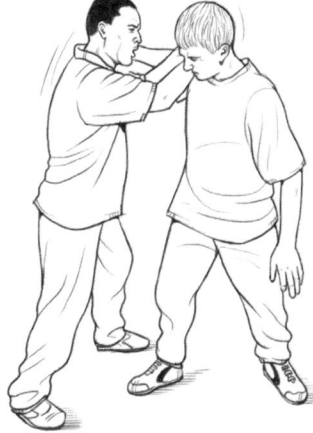

slamming your elbows or forearms hard into his biceps and chest to drive him back, knocking him off balance. Now push forward, shoving his head back, and sweep his foot away from under him. As the assailant crashes to the floor, you can depart swiftly.

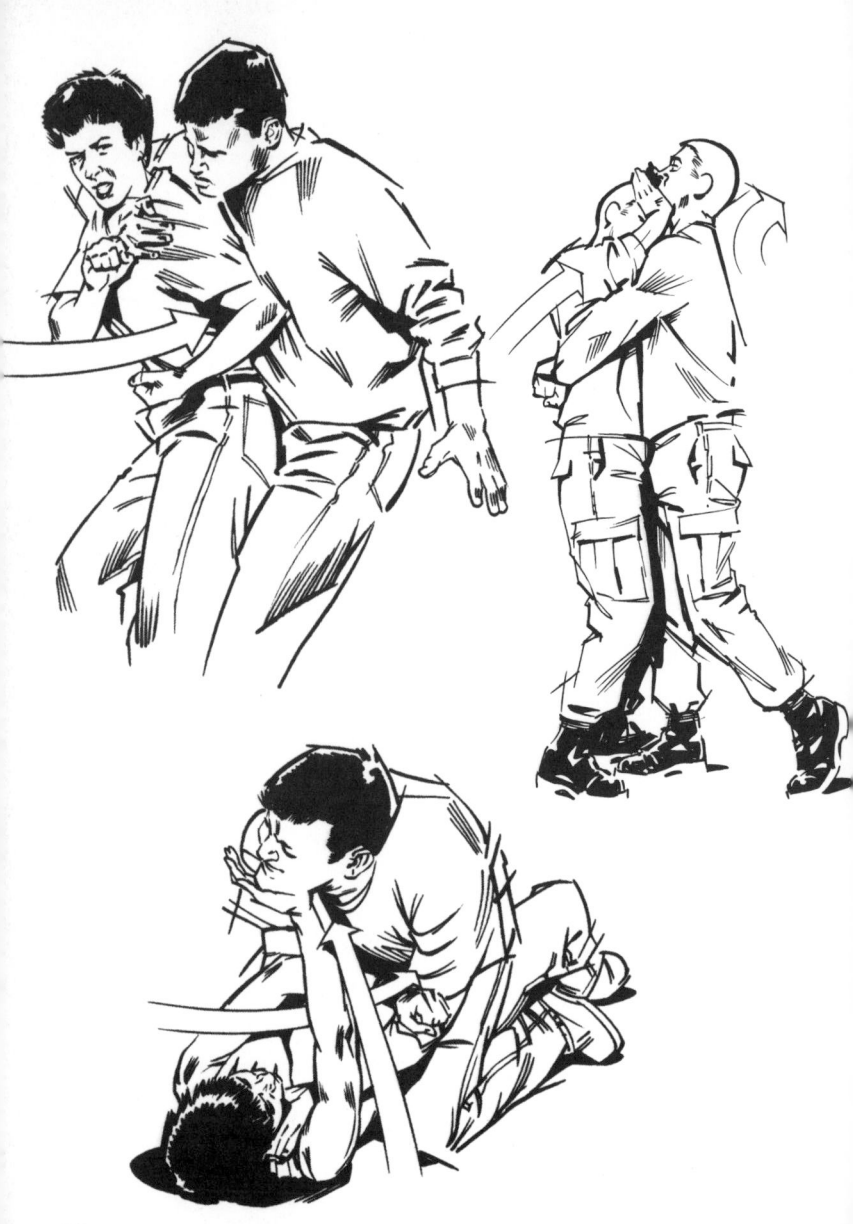

By far the most likely threat faced by civilians is that of an unarmed assailant. Ideally, you can pre-empt the opponent before he launches his attack, for example while he is posturing and threatening you. This has the advantage that it can catch him mentally off guard. He has not yet made the decision to 'go' and is expecting a defensive response from you. He might half-expect you to start posturing and shouting much as he is, but a sudden and decisive action will almost certainly catch him by surprise.

OPEN-HAND THREAT

The opponent is behaving aggressively, perhaps working up to attacking you, but has not yet committed himself. He may have his fists up in something like a boxer's guard, or may point his finger at you. If he is foolish enough to stand within punching range with his hands splayed to make himself look big and threatening, you have a clear shot at his head and should take it for all it is worth.

Elbow Scoop

Grab whichever of the opponent's arms is closest to you, 'scooping' it

....

Left: Most attacks will come from unarmed assailants, which can be defended against with learned techniques.

10

An attack with fists or feet can be just as life-threatening as an assault with a lethal weapon.

In Action
Defeating Unarmed Attacks

Elbow scoop

Grab the elbow and pull towards your opposite shoulder, stepping forward and out to the side as you do. The combination of your movement and spinning the opponent will place you behind him, making a choke or restraint easy.

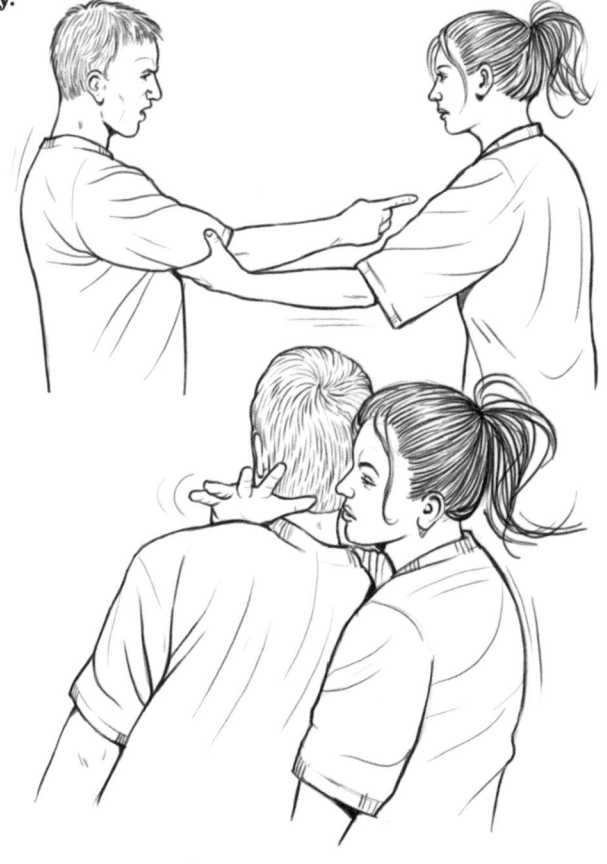

Straight left

While the opponent is waving his arms about and 'posturing', he is no real threat. If he looks like he is about to launch an attack, you can beat him to the punch with a fast lead-hand shot to the jaw.

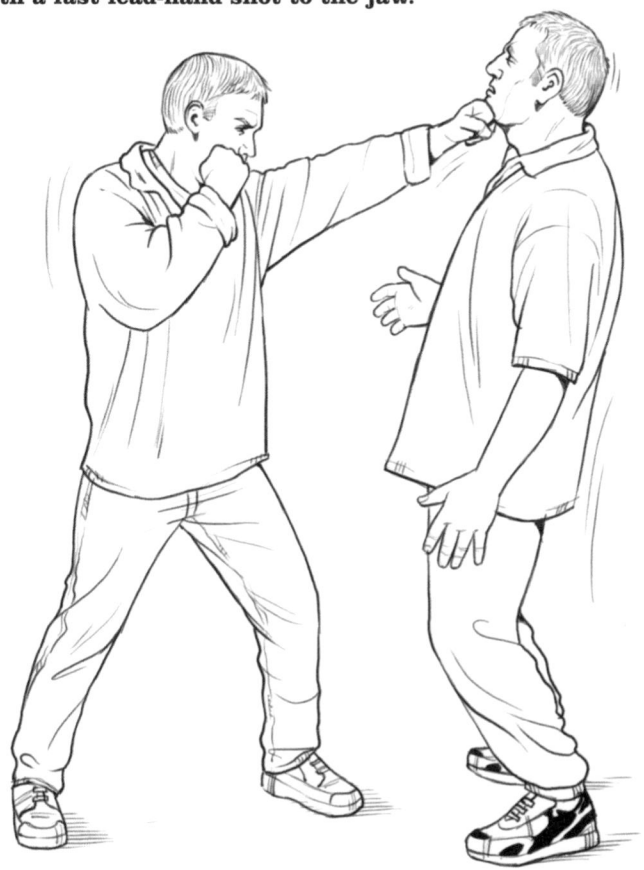

Elbow strikes

If the opponent reaches for you, you can bat his arm aside with your lead hand and throw an elbow strike into his jaw. Alternatively, use his forward movement to your advantage by intercepting him with an elbow strike to the face.

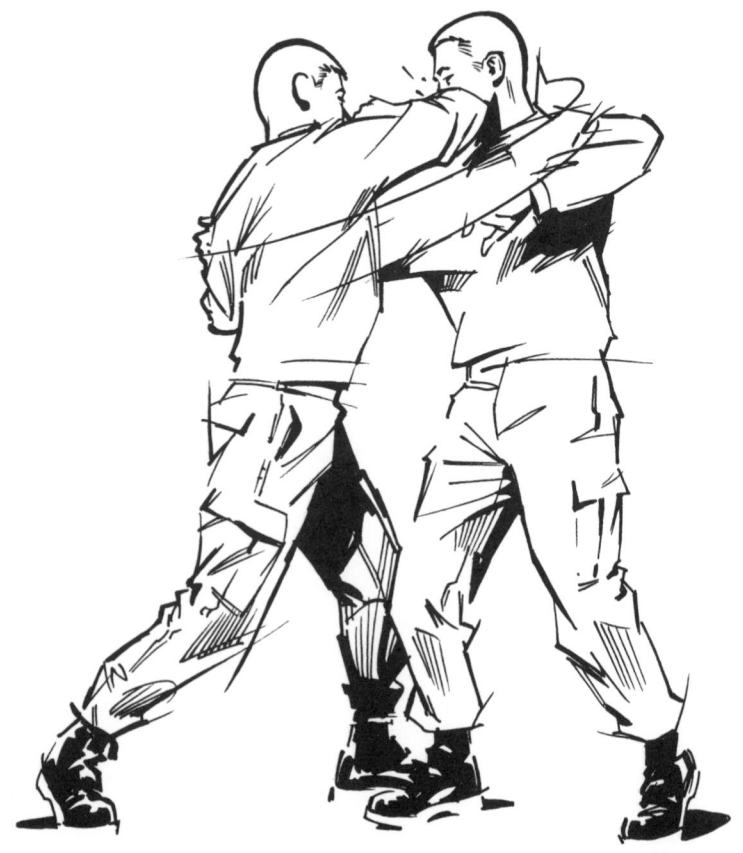

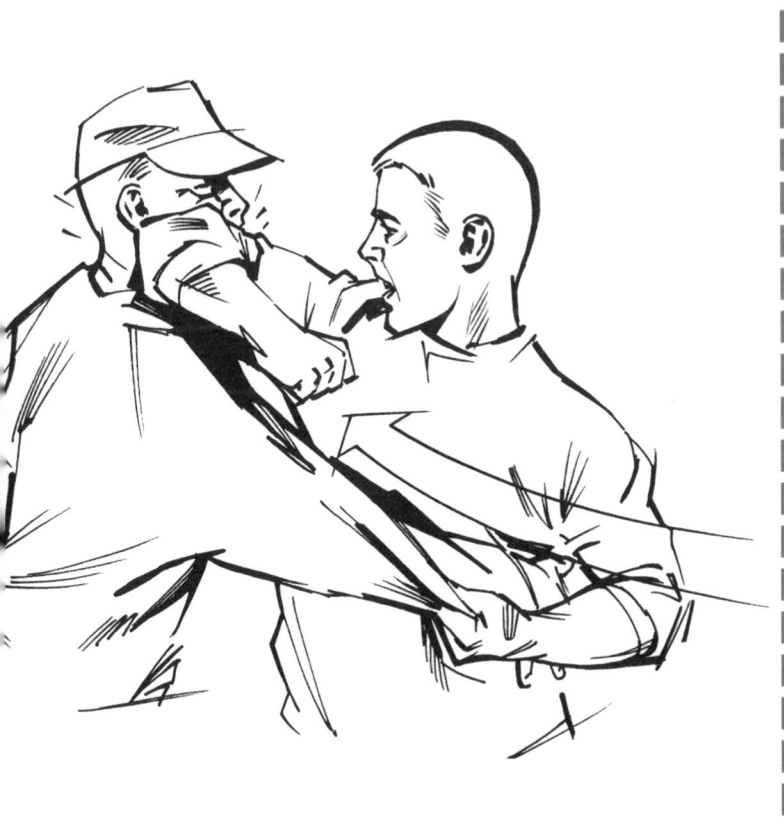

towards you and across your front with your outside hand. At the same time, step out to the side and forward. Your aim is to spin the opponent round and move behind him, allowing you to apply a rear choke. This can be used to restrain him, to render him unconscious or to move him where you want, perhaps as a human shield against his friends.

Pull Down Guard
Against an opponent who has a guard up, pull his hands down and forward, and fire a right cross over the top into his jaw. His instinctive resistance to the pull should cause his head to come forward, dragging him into your strike.

STRAIGHT PUNCHES
Straight punches are fairly rare on the street, but they do happen. Straight shots come in fast and can be hard to stop, but they offer the defender many opportunities for a counterattack. The following defences all work equally well against a lead-hand or rear-hand punch. The key in each case is to move as well as deflect the punch.

Deflect and Elbow
Step to the outside and deflect the blow away from you. Against a lead-hand (left hand in most cases) punch you will change leads by stepping through and turning to face the assailant, placing you outside the area where he can hit you without turning to face you. Prevent him from doing so by using your rear hand to push against his arm while you deliver a hooked elbow shot just behind his ear. This is one of the best spots to achieve a knockout.

Arm Break
Step out to the side and forward, trapping the assailant's arm with one of yours. Strike just above his elbow with your other forearm, as close to your own elbow as you can. Your aim is to dislocate his elbow. If this fails, you can still strike from this position or grab and knee him.

Deflect and Stomp Kick
Bat the strike aside as you step forward without turning to face the assailant. Deliver a sideways stomp kick to the side of his knee. Try to push right through so that your foot reaches the ground. This will cause massive – probably permanent – damage to the assailant's knee so should be reserved for a very serious threat.

HOOKED PUNCHES
Most aggressors will simply wade forward, launching big, wide swings with each arm alternately. Any one of these shots can knock you out, but fortunately they are easy to see coming and to deal with. These defences can be used against the first or any subsequent hook punch.

Cross-guard and elbow strike

The cross-guard is highly effective against hooked punches as the opponent tends to strike your elbows with his fists. Use the cross-guard to protect yourself as you close in for an elbow strike.

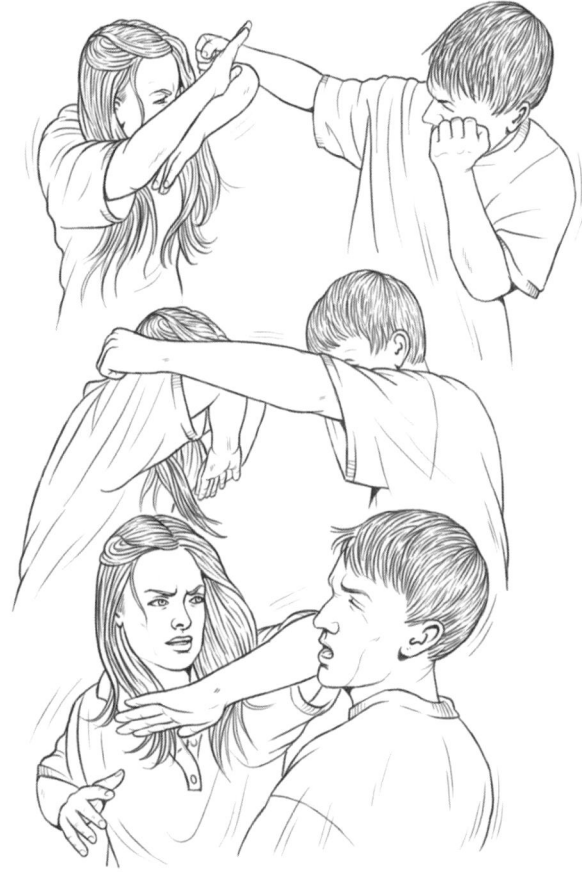

Cross-Guard and Elbow Strikes

Raise your elbow and let the assailant smash his hand or arm into it. If the next punch is coming fast, use the other elbow to protect you. Look through the gaps in your guard and drive forwards, ramming your elbow into the opponent's chest or face. Once in close you can finish by ramming his head back and sweeping his foot away for an outer reap takedown.

Trap Arm and Grab Throat

Cover your head and move forward, wrapping the opponent's arm as soon as it hits your cover. Grab his throat in a 'C-grip' around the larynx and squeeze. Alternatively, you can elbow or strike the opponent in the head while you have his arm trapped, then transition into a takedown. The inner and outer reap takedowns are very accessible from this position.

Duck and Elbow

Duck under the swinging strike, stepping forward and out to the side. As you do so, fire a hooking elbow strike into the opponent's ribs. Once past his strike, turn and finish him off. If he is still upright, apply a rear choke. Alternatively you can perform a rear takedown by grabbing his head or shoulders and pulling back while you kick one of his feet out from under him.

KICKS

Very few 'street' attackers can kick effectively. Most will throw a swinging 'football' style kick at your legs or groin. This is defended in much the same way as a martial arts style front kick. Most kicks can be countered by simply not letting the attacker have room to throw them – if you are driving forward into him throwing strikes of your own, he will not have the time and space needed to launch a kick.

Evade and Kick

Most kicks are 'telegraphed', i.e. the attacker gives away his intentions by the movements he makes when setting up the kick. This should give you ample time to evade the kick. Sidestep and launch a stomping side kick of your own into whichever of the attacker's legs he is standing on. With all of his weight on it, this leg will be firmly anchored and will be severely damaged by your kick.

Catch and Takedown

Evade a little less widely, but enough to make the kick miss you, and catch the opponent's leg. Lift it up and towards his face as you move in and sweep his other leg. You will dump him on his back from a great height, probably ending the matter.

DEFEATING GRABS AND TACKLES

Most fights involve grabs and grappling at some point, even if they start out as punching matches. It is very rare for someone to grab and simply hold; most grabs are followed

Defensive side kick

As the opponent begins to move in, 'chamber' your lead leg and launch a side kick into his midsection. You will need to lean back a little to maintain your balance, but not too far or the impact will push you over.

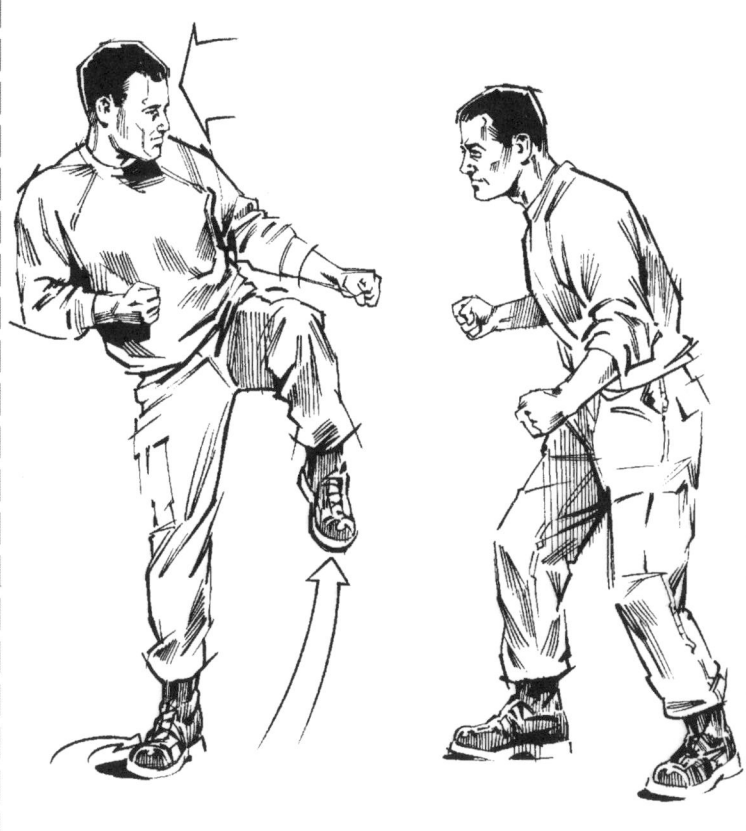

Catch and takedown

As the opponent kicks, move to the side and catch his leg. The simplest counter is to push him over, but for a fight-ending takedown, hook his other foot away from under him as you push his shoulder back.

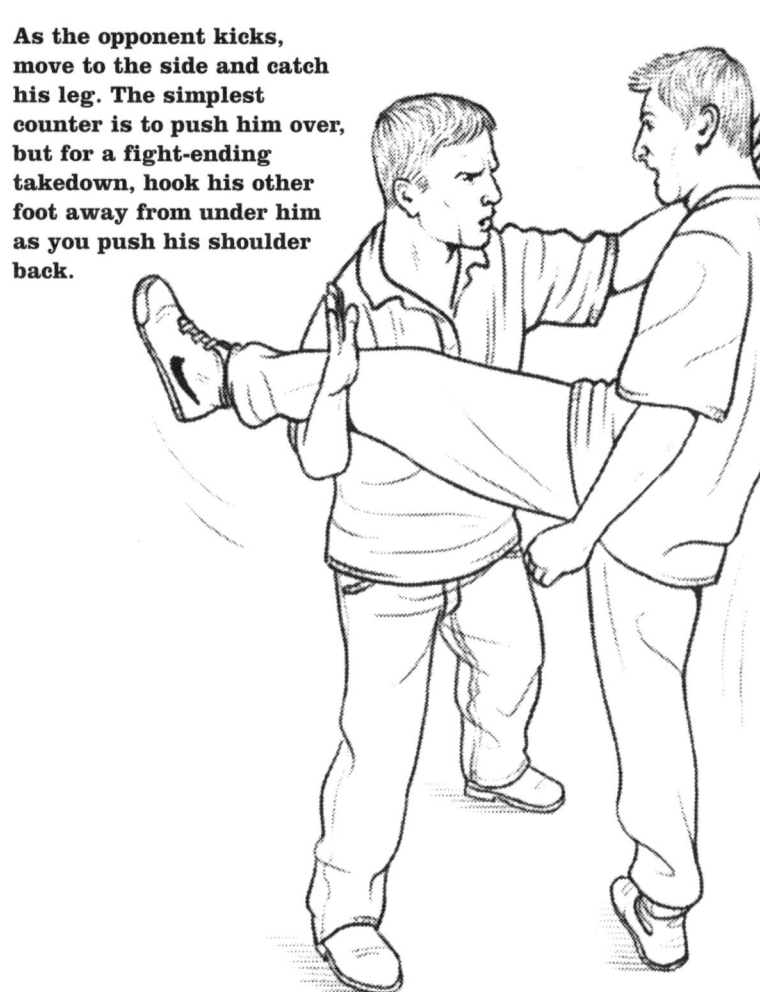

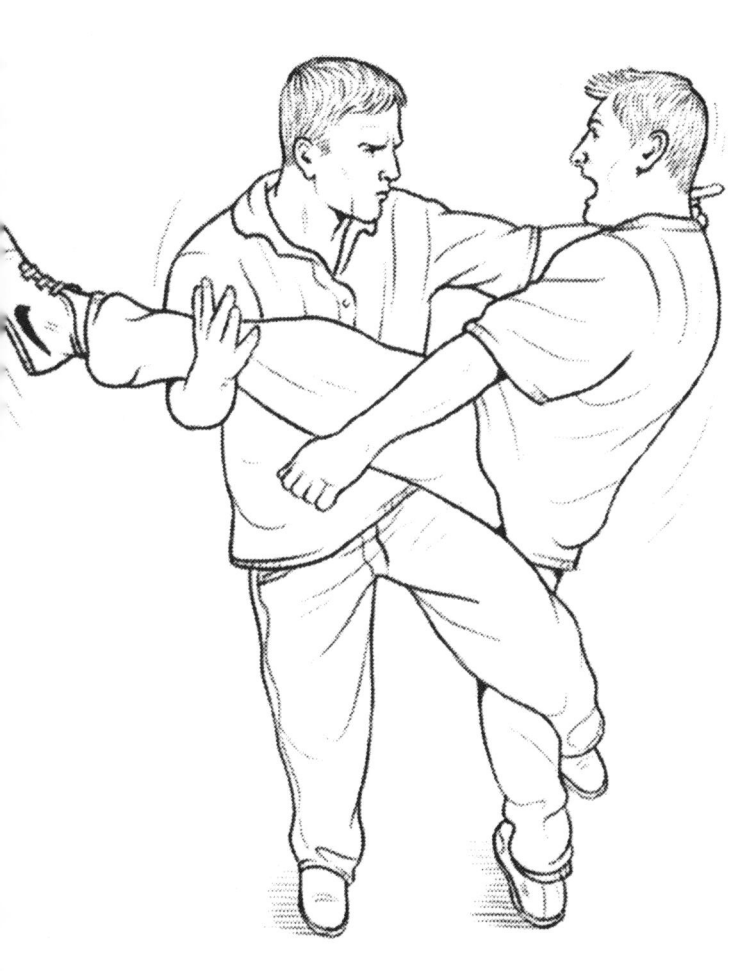

Mutual grab

There is a tendency to 'mirror' whatever the opponent does, which means that you can end up in a position like this where nobody has an advantage. Just because someone is trying to grab you does not mean you must wrestle with him. Striking may be a better option, so play to your strengths and not his!

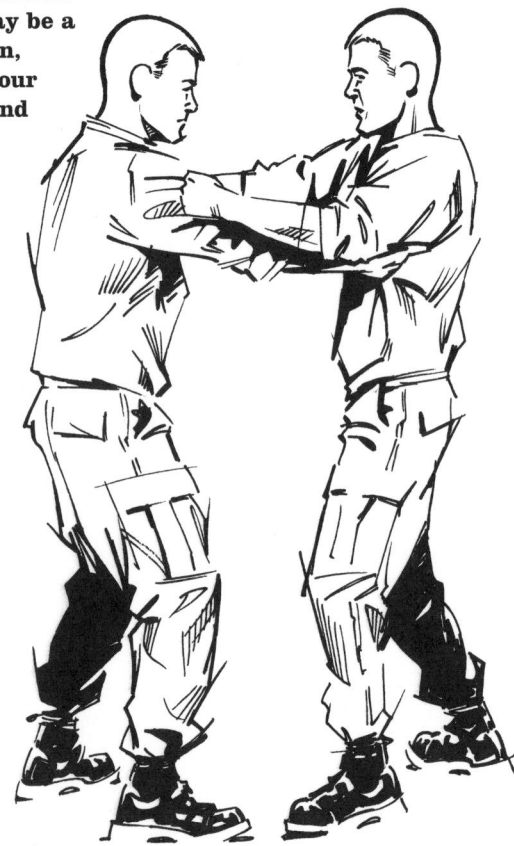

by a blow, or an attempt to exert dominance by ragging the victim about, bashing them into things or at the very least a verbal assault.

This means that many of the traditional martial arts techniques for dealing with grabs, while theoretically valid, are virtually impossible to use against a determined opponent. Simpler measures are generally more effective.

THREE STAGES OF A GRAB

There are three stages to a grab attack: when it is 'in progress', i.e. the bad guy is reaching in to get hold but has not secured a grip yet; when it is 'on', i.e. the bad guy has a grip on you; and when it is 'really on'. The latter stage occurs when someone properly anchors his grip, e.g. by twisting his hand into your clothing.

Grabs are ideally defeated before they are properly established. Once a grab is fully anchored, you will not be able to prise it off. Struggling with the attacker's grabbing hand simply makes you vulnerable to whatever else he wants to do, such as hitting you with his other hand. You may, however, be able to induce the opponent to let go of you, say by hitting him or causing him pain.

ONE-HANDED GRABS

One-handed grabs are normally aimed at clothing, usually the lapels. The assailant keeps one hand free for

TIP: USES OF GRABS

It is instinctive to grab an opponent, and many aggressors will do it without really having a plan in mind. Generally speaking, someone who grabs you with their strong hand means to exert dominance by means of the grab. A weak-hand grab is normally used to immobilize the victim for a blow with the strong hand. Deeper grabs and tackles are normally used in an attempt to take the fight to the ground.

whatever else he has in mind, which might be no more than wagging a finger at you but is probably more serious. However, nobody ever died of a clothing grab, so getting the attacker's hand off you may be less important than stopping him from doing whatever he plans to do next.

Grab in Progress

As the assailant reaches for you, you have an opportunity to prevent him from getting hold. The straight punch

Preventing a grab

The simplest way to defeat a grab is to knock the attacker's arms away. It is generally more advantageous to push his arms across your body, so that you end up 'outside' instead of directly in front of him, between his arms. In either case, take the initiative with strikes rather than waiting to see what happens next.

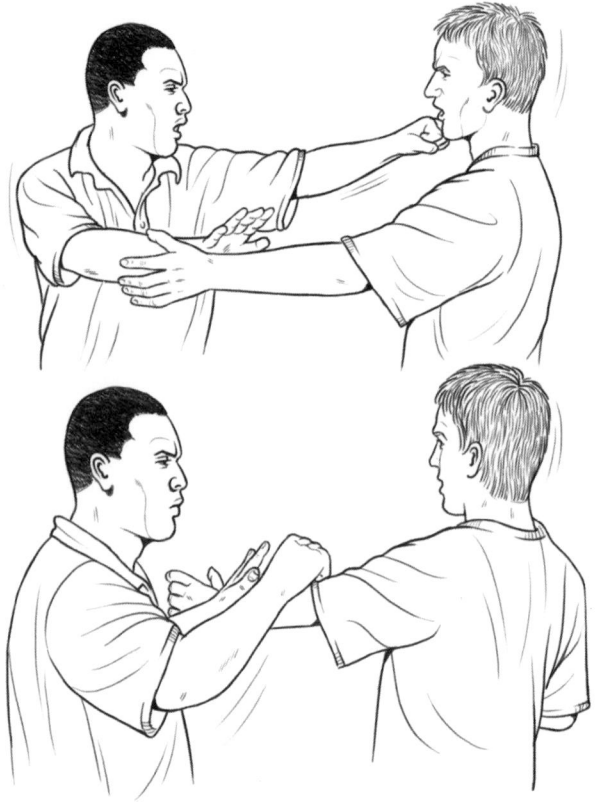

defences covered earlier work fine, or you could bat the grabbing hand away and punch him in the face. There is no need for a big Karate-style block; just knock the grabbing arm to the side and launch a counter-attack. You can deflect the grab to either side; the most important thing is to prevent it from reaching you.

Grab in Place

If the grab is in place but not firmly on, for example because the attacker has failed to get a good hold on you, it may be possible to peel it off and apply a wrist lock. However this is hard to do under combat conditions, i.e. while someone is punching you in the head. Instead, you must induce the attacker to let go by hurting him, or use the grab to your advantage. After all, someone who has hold of you has just immobilized one of his hands while both of yours remain free.

Pull In and Counter

Drop your forearm into the crook of the grabbing arm and push down, leaning your weight forward over the top to increase the force. It is unlikely that the assailant will let go, but that would be a success in its own right. More likely, you will pull him forward and trap his arm while you strike him with your free hand.

Counterstrikes

An attacker will normally pull you in close, bending his arm. If for some reason he has his arm out straight, perhaps to keep you out of reach because you keep clawing at his face or poking at his eyes, you can strike his elbow with your palm, knocking it upwards. In theory this can dislocate the elbow but you are more likely just to cause some pain – which may induce the attacker to let go or to pull you in close where you can recommence sticking your thumb in his eye socket.

Alternatively, strike hard and deep into his shoulder with your opposite hand. Use a vertical fist and aim to drive into the crease of the shoulder joint. This often causes the assailant to let go involuntarily as a result of sudden pain, and also drives him back, jerking the grab off you.

TWO-HANDED GRABS AND STRANGLES

There are not many reasons why an attacker would grab you with both hands. He might want to shake you around as part of an attempt to dominate you, or to pull you forward for a headbutt. There is an outside possibility that he might want to strangle you, but this is relatively rare. When it does happen, it tends to be in a 'domestic' situation, with a more powerful individual attacking a weaker one.

It is possible to deal with most two-handed grabs before they land by sidestepping and batting the arms aside, much as with one-handed

Pull in and counter

There is no point trying to get a firmly fixed grab off you. Instead, drop your forearm into the crook of the opponent's grabbing arm and push down to pull him in. Follow up with blows to the head.

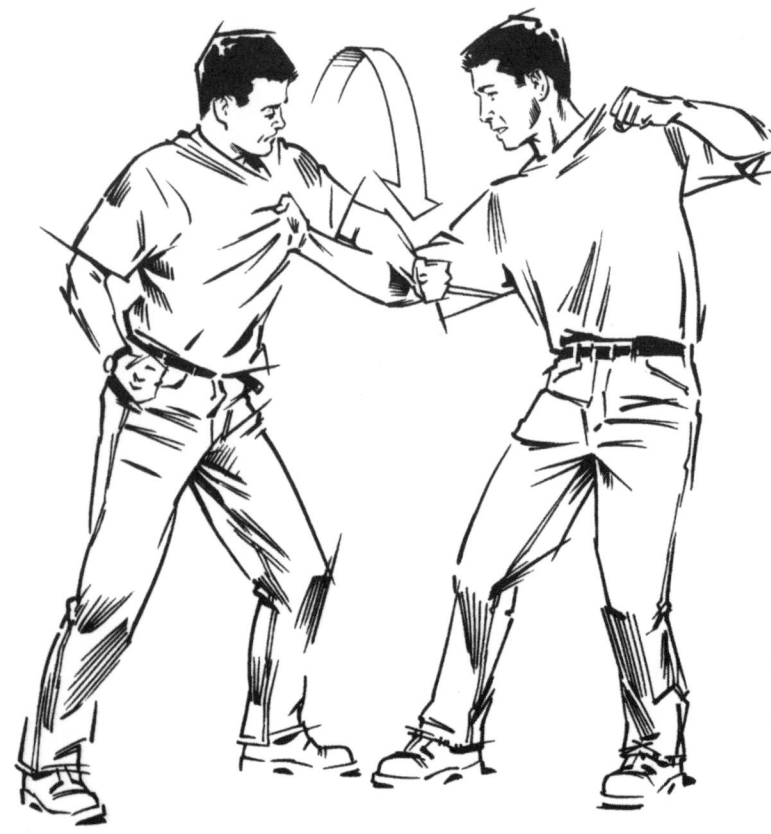

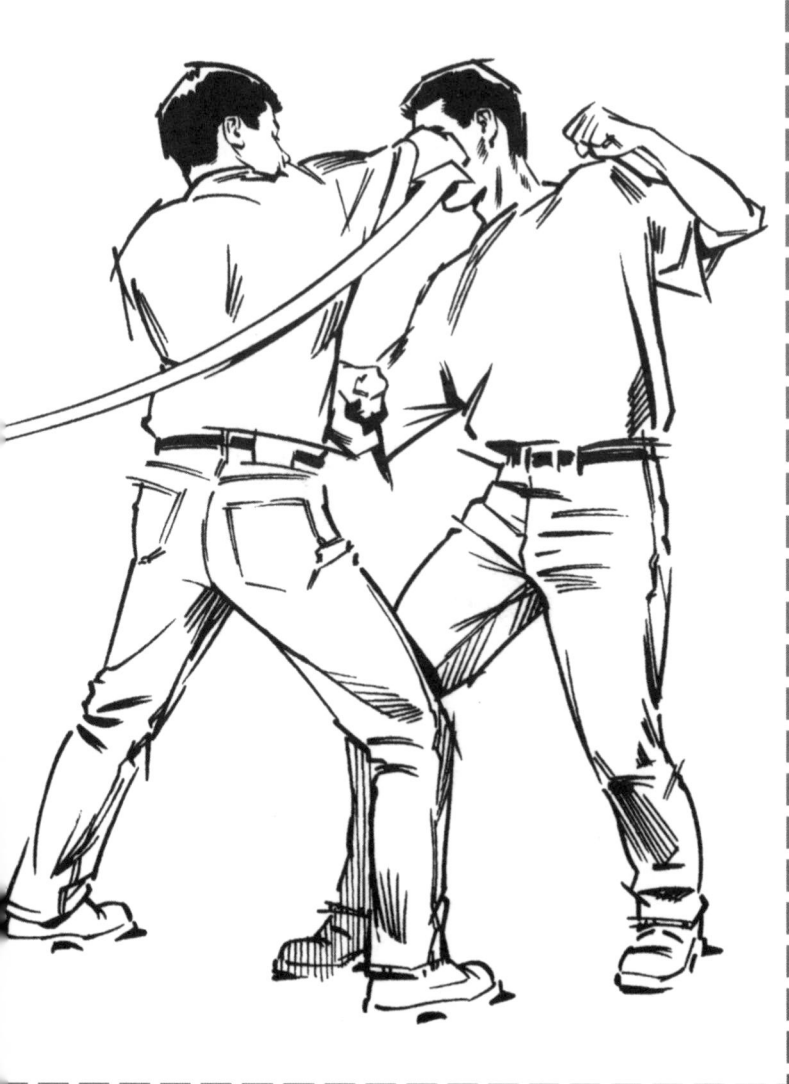

Defeating a lapel grab

Drag the opponent forward and off balance by throwing your arm over his and twisting downwards, then uncoil in the opposite direction to slam an elbow into his head.

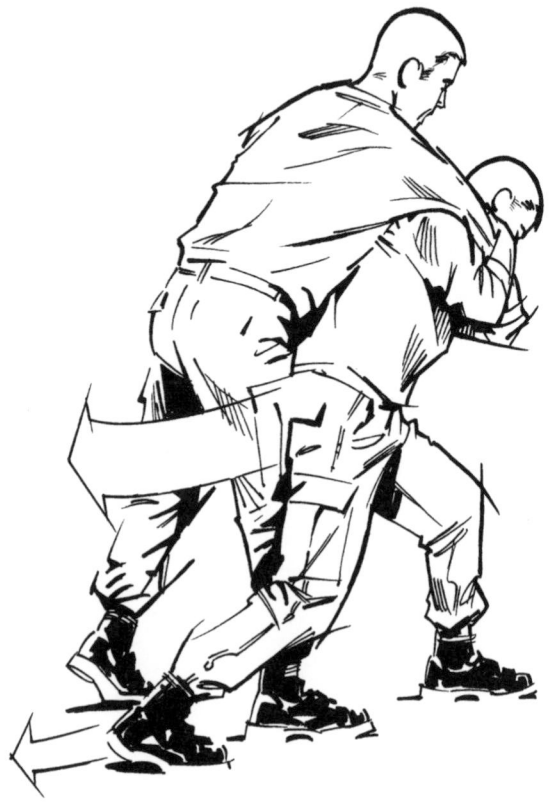

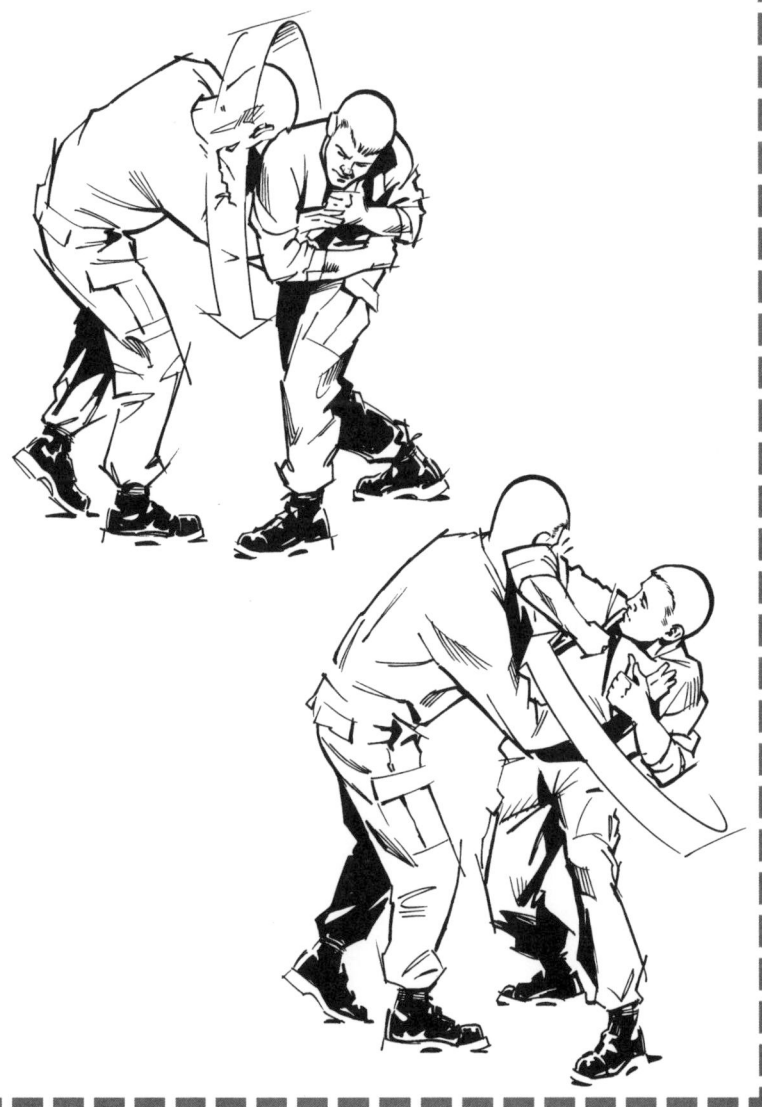

grabs. Obviously, if someone is reaching for your throat then you are looking at a likely attempt to murder you. Half-measures at this point could literally get you killed, so if the hands are coming at your throat rather than your clothing, treat the situation as utterly desperate and act accordingly.

Two-handed grabs to the lapels and two-handed strangles use much the same hand position, though higher and lower according to the intent. The hands come in along much the same path in both cases, and the same countermeasures are useful.

Headbutt defence (alternative)

A headbutt to the chest might seem like a strange idea, but it does inflict considerable pain. This can be doubled up by whipping your head back up under the attacker's jaw.

'Wedge' and Knee Strike

Bring your hands up between those of the aggressor, pushing them rapidly up and outwards to shove his hands apart before the grab can reach you. A headbutt to his nose is an option at this point. Whether this is done or not, grab him round the back of the neck and deliver a knee strike to his groin.

Headbutt Defence

A two-handed grab of this sort is often used to pull the victim in for a headbutt. Defeat the butt by either putting one hand on the attacker's

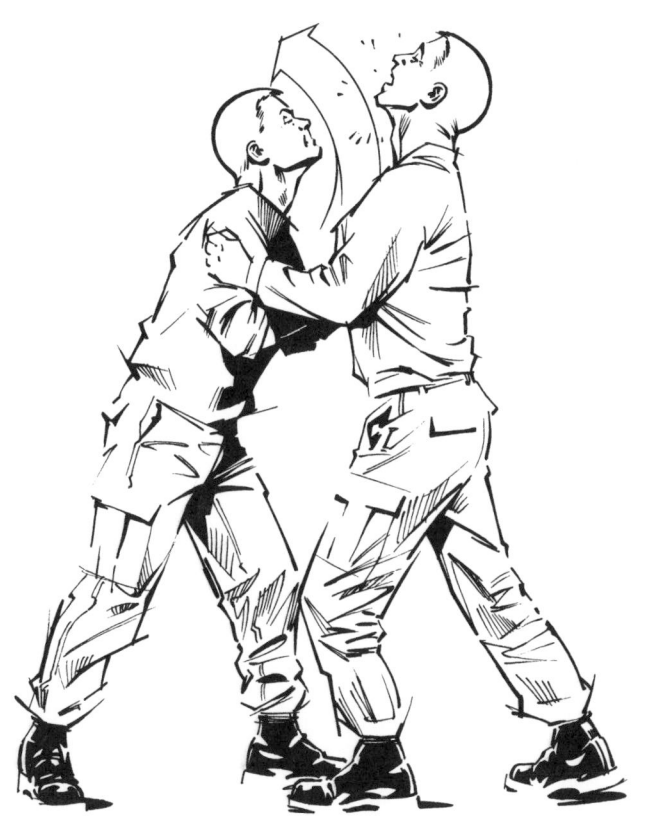

TIP:
WRIST GRABS

Many martial arts seem obsessed with wrist grabs. This reflects their origins, in a time when grabbing the sword arm was a common way to prevent a warrior from deploying his weapon. The reality of modern self-defence is that wrist grabs occur for two reasons:

- Dominance in a domestic confrontation, i.e. a stronger individual trying to control a weaker one.
- Where someone is carrying a sidearm and the attacker seeks to stop it from being drawn.

Thus learning to deal with them is useful, but they are extremely uncommon in an all-out fight situation. And nobody ever charged up to their victim, grabbed their wrist and stood there waiting to be dealt with. Training must be realistic if it is to be any use in a real situation.

forehead or your forearm across in front of your face. Since the attacker has obligingly brought his head close to you, launch a series of face attacks as detailed under 'shutdown techniques' in Chapter 8. This should induce him to let you go or may create an opportunity for other attacks.

WRIST GRABS

Wrist grabs are more common in a domestic context than in a fight. Someone who really means you harm will hit you or wrestle you to the ground rather than grabbing your wrist, and if you are actively resisting, e.g. hitting him, he will find it very difficult to catch hold of your wrist.

An attacker might grab one or both of your wrists, and might reach across (e.g. right hand to right wrist) or grab on the same side (e.g. left hand to right wrist). Similar measures work against all wrist grabs and in the case where both wrists have been grabbed, if you free one and start hitting the assailant, he will usually let go of the other.

It is necessary to remember, however, that getting a wrist grab off you will not end the situation. You make have to strike the attacker, flee, or put up a fence and deter him verbally. Whatever you do, do not just break a wrist grab and stand there feeling good about your victory, because you have not won yet and might get punched in the face.

Breaking fingers and thumbs

Most grabs can be effectively dislodged by grabbing the attacker's fingers or thumb and snapping them. It is hard to do this while he is hitting you, however, so do not fixate on the grab.

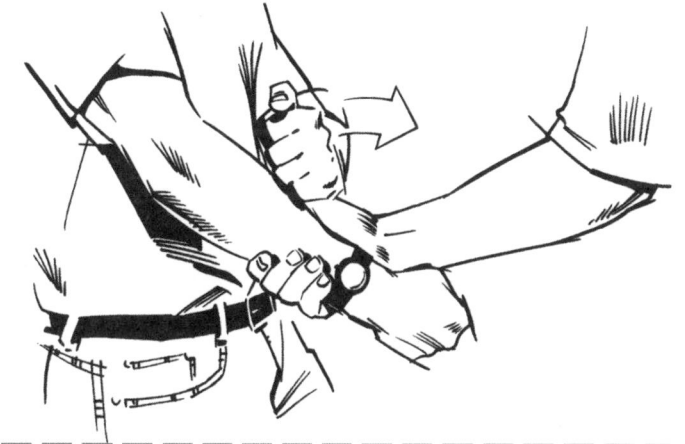

Thumb Break

If you can grab the attacker's fingers or thumb and yank hard, you may break them. To avoid this, he will usually let go of your wrist, which is what you wanted all along.

Twist and Pull

Twist your wrist hard and pull it back, or back and up. This should break most grips, though you will need to follow up with some kind of counter-attack to avoid the opponent just grabbing you once again, or escalating to hitting you.

BEAR HUGS

Bear hugs can be performed from in front or behind. There is nothing scientific about this; the attacker grabs you around the body, over or under the arms, and squeezes. If he is very strong he can stop you from breathing, but most of the time all he

Defending a rear bear hug

A well-anchored bear hug is hard to dislodge. You can make yourself very unpleasant to hold on to by stamping on the opponent's feet and kicking backwards as you try to loosen his grip.

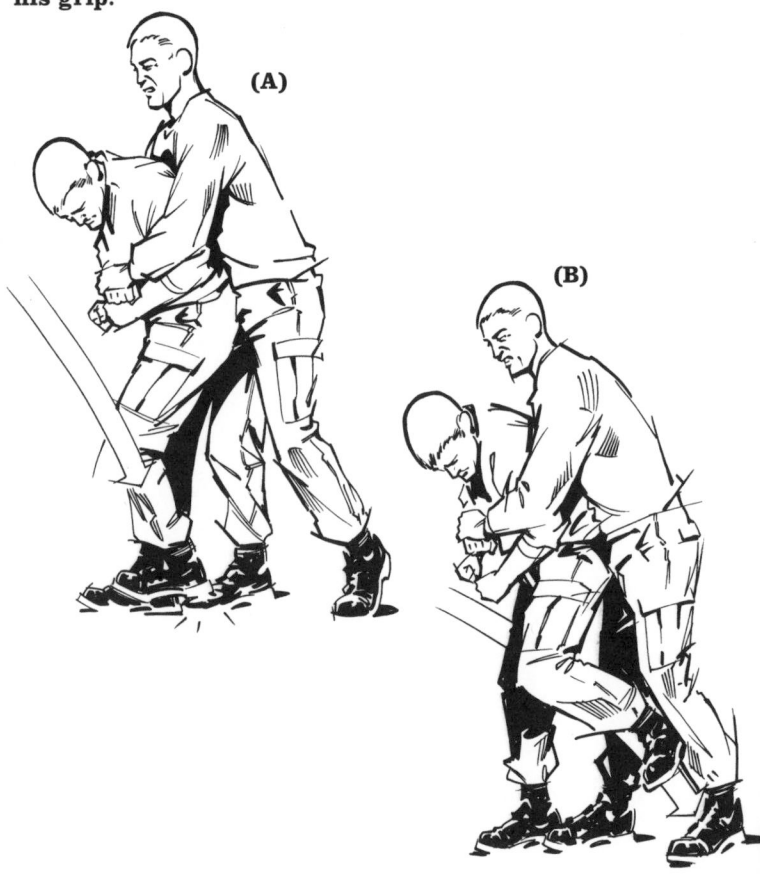

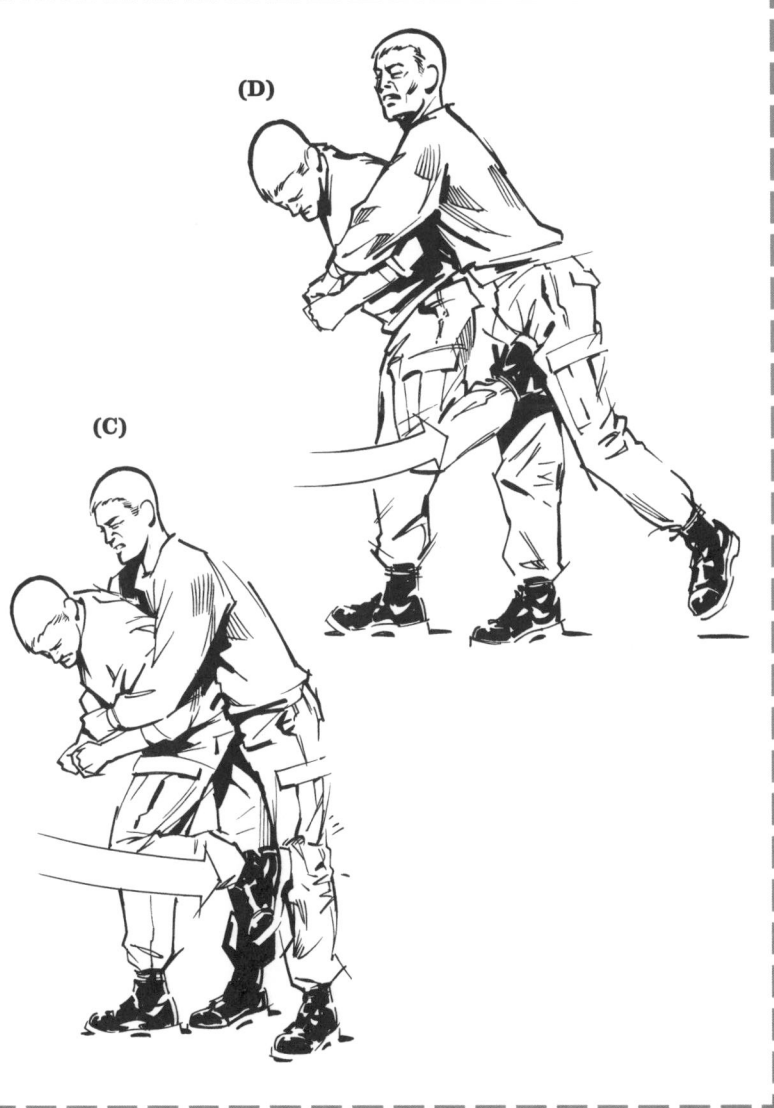

(D)

(C)

can do is hold you or pick you up and move you. He will have to let go to do anything else.

An attacker might pick up the victim with a bear hug and then throw them to the ground. He will expect the victim to be stunned and hurt by this; if you keep your wits then you have an opportunity to counterattack.

General Bear Hug Defences

The aim is to make yourself difficult to keep hold of while inflicting pain on the attacker. If he is in front of you, you can headbutt, bite, and kick at his shins. If grabbed from behind, you can kick or butt backwards. It may be counterintuitive, but one of the best ways to make yourself hard to hold is to jump up and jerk and kick violently. This means the attacker must hold your entire weight, which is bouncing around unpredictably. If you can grab the attacker's hands, breaking fingers by pulling them back or sideways will effect a release, either from pain or when he runs out of fingers to grip with.

Front Bear Hug

If you are grabbed under the arms, you can free yourself by twisting the attacker's head. Grab his chin and the back of his head and twist hard. This often causes an attacker to fall. If he stays upright, hit him as hard as you can as soon as you are free of

his grip, and keep attacking until you are sure there is no chance he can grab you again. If you can only get one hand out, it is still possible to release yourself by using 'shutdown

Defending a front bear hug

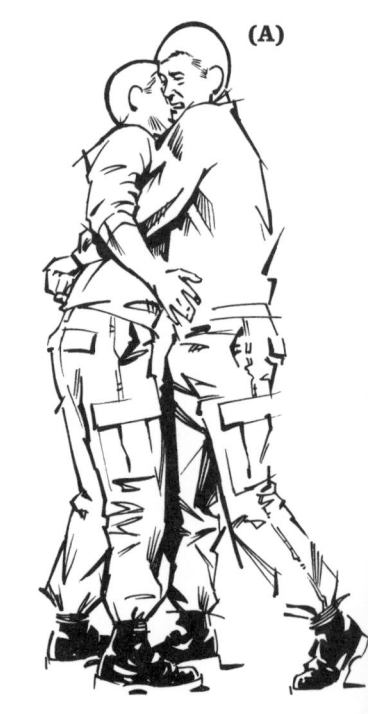

(A)

techniques' to make the attacker want to put some distance between you, or by striking him hard under the chin and then shoving his head up and back to lever him off you.

Rear Bear Hug

As soon as the attacker's arms start to go around you, drop your weight and make yourself as big as possible by pushing out your arms.

If only one of your arms is free, one option is to strike the opponent under the jaw and push his head back, levering him off you. However strong his arms may be, he will have to let go once his head is pushed far enough backwards.

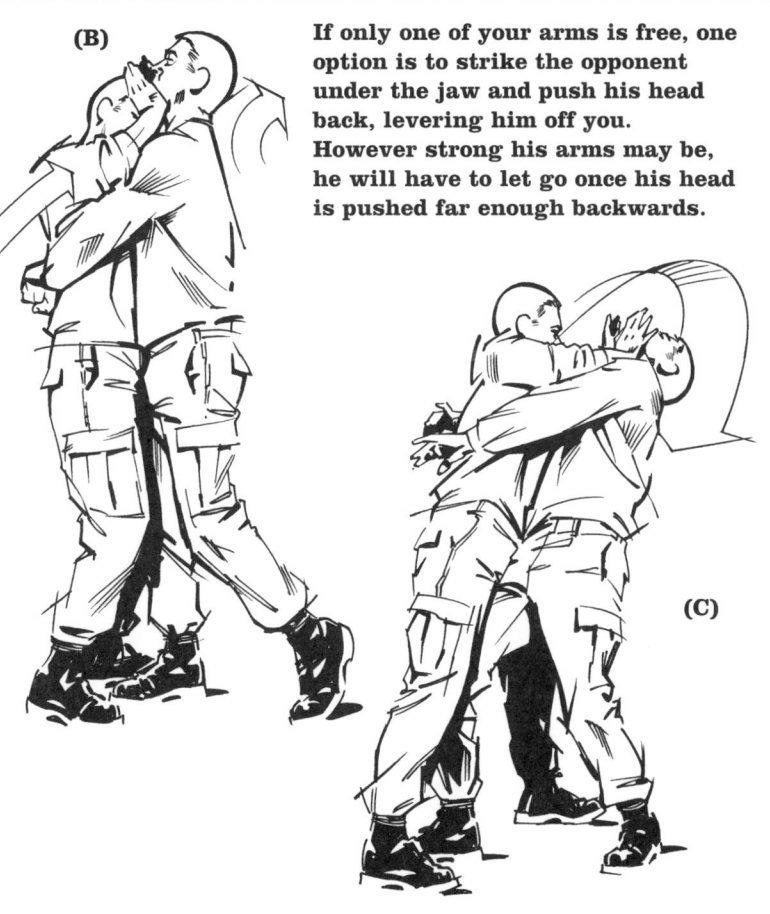

(B)

(C)

If you can prevent the attacker's hands from meeting, you will be able to peel one of them off you and escape through the gap. Alternatively you can sharply push the opponent's arms up and duck out between them. As another option, you may be able to throw the attacker by grabbing one of his arms, twisting to the side and bending sharply forwards, essentially performing a hip throw.

TACKLES

It is not uncommon for an attacker to launch a waist-height tackle. This can be used as a takedown or to run the victim backwards into something. It also happens from time to time when an attacker gets hit and instinctively closes in while he collects his wits. Fortunately tackles of this sort are fairly easy to deal with.

Far more dangerous is a low 'shoot' of the sort used in Mixed Martial Arts. Here, the attacker comes in very low and grabs the victim around the legs, resulting in an extremely hard takedown. It is possible to counter a waist tackle in various ways, such as kneeing the attacker in the face as he comes in, but if you see an opponent go very low to shoot in, you must use a sprawl to defend. The sprawl is the only reliable defence against a deep shoot, and you cannot afford to risk failure.

Jamming a Tackle

As the opponent rushes in, drive forward and meet him, keeping your rear foot well back to act as a brace. This also prevents the opponent from getting hold of your legs. A tackle around the waist is above your centre of gravity and can be jammed, but if the assailant can grab your legs and pull them forward as he pushes at waist height, you will go down. Follow up quickly with a guillotine choke or an elbow into the back of the neck or the back.

Dumping a Tackle

If the opponent rushes in with his head down, he is off balance. Step quickly back, bringing your hands down on the back of his neck. Imagine you are dropping an anvil on him; your hands must be as 'heavy' as you can make them. If you hit him hard enough, he will crash to the ground where you were just standing.

Sprawling

If in any doubt, use a sprawl. True, it will take you to the ground but at least you will be on top – and better off than if you had attempted a different defence and failed. As the opponent shoots in, skip both your feet well back so that you more or less fall onto his back. Grab him around the floating ribs area and squeeze as hard as you can. Your weight combined with his should drive him down, but you can help the

Sprawl defence

Against a deep tackle, the most reliable defence is the 'sprawl'. Skip your feet back and allow your self to fall onto the attacker's back, driving him to the floor.

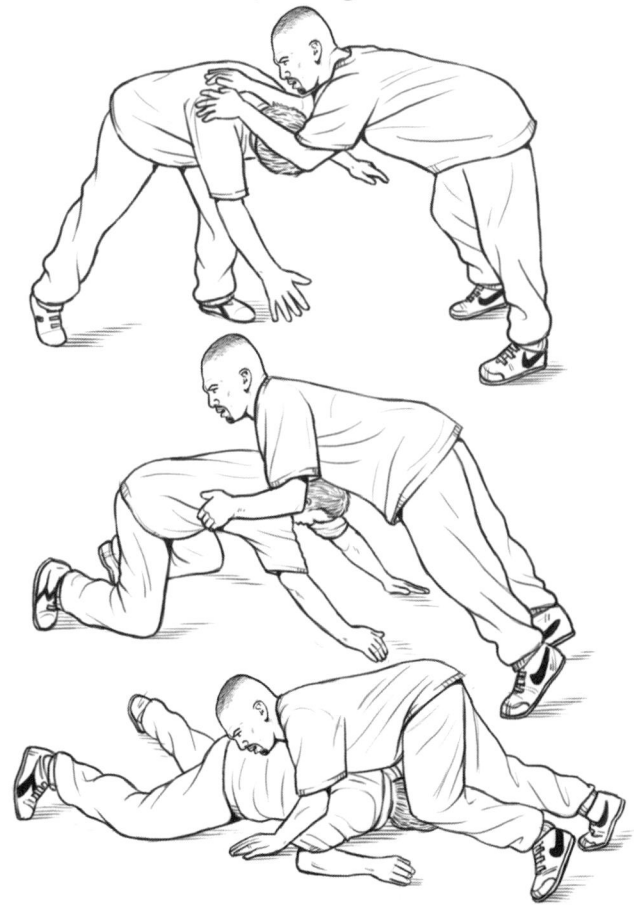

Defeating a waist tackle

Against a waist-height tackle, an effective defence is to lengthen your stance, drive forward and push the attacker's head down, dropping an elbow into his back, neck or head.

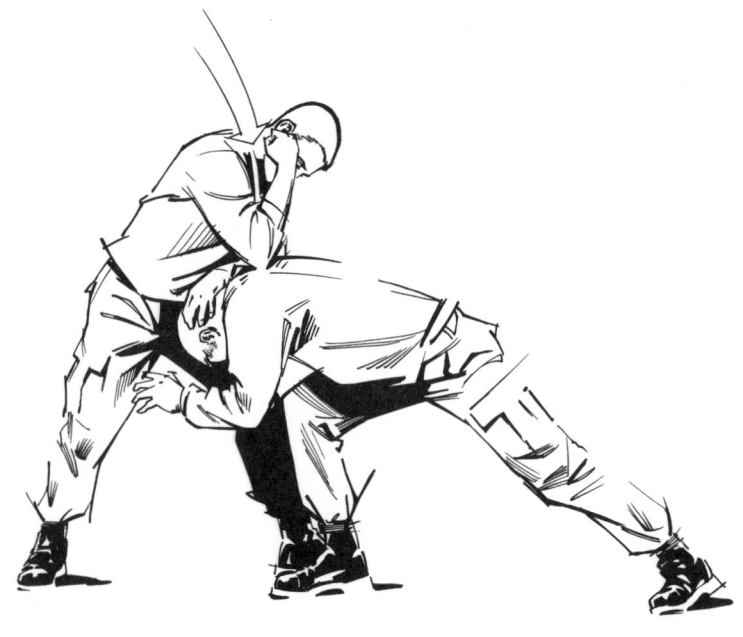

process by shaking him violently from side to side.

Land on top of him and keep your weight on his back as you begin your next move. You might be able to knee him in the top of the head, or you may have to begin ground-

fighting. Groundfighting is covered in Chapter 13.

REAR GRABS AND CHOKES

An attacker who grabs you from the rear has three options: drag you off

Rear choke

Special forces soldiers are known to use this move, especially when wanting to neutralize an opponent silently. One arm is wrapped fully around the opponent's neck, bringing the hand inside the crook of the other elbow to form a choke.

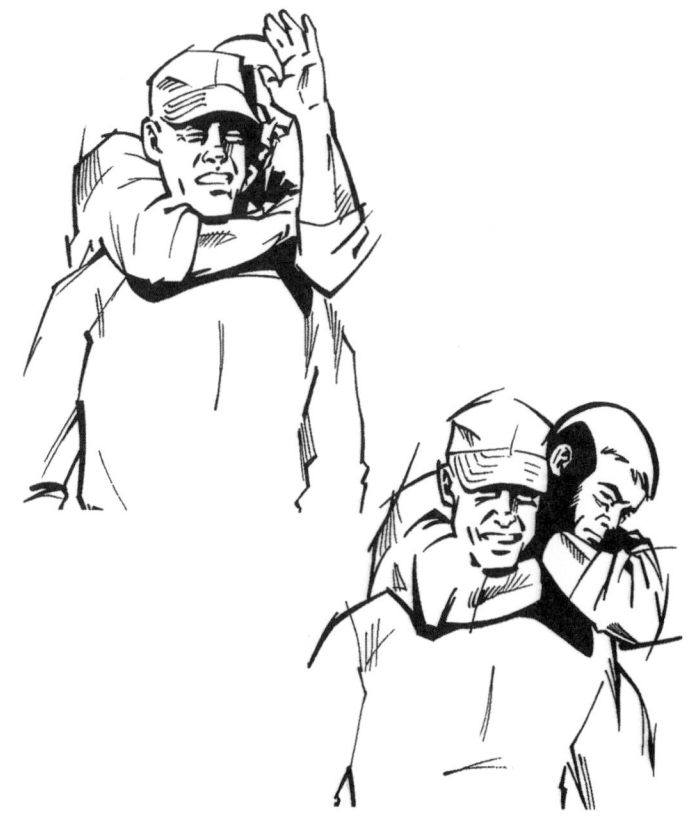

somewhere, choke you, or spin you round so he can hit you. Most grabs for the purpose of dragging you are likely to be variations on the bear hug and have thus already been covered.

Shoulder Grab and Turn

The assailant grabs you by the shoulder and pulls, wishing to spin you around into the punch he is about to throw. The grab puts him

Defending a rear choke

Grab the attacker's fingers and break them while firing elbow strikes back into his solar plexus. You can also weaken the hold by stamping on the attacker's foot.

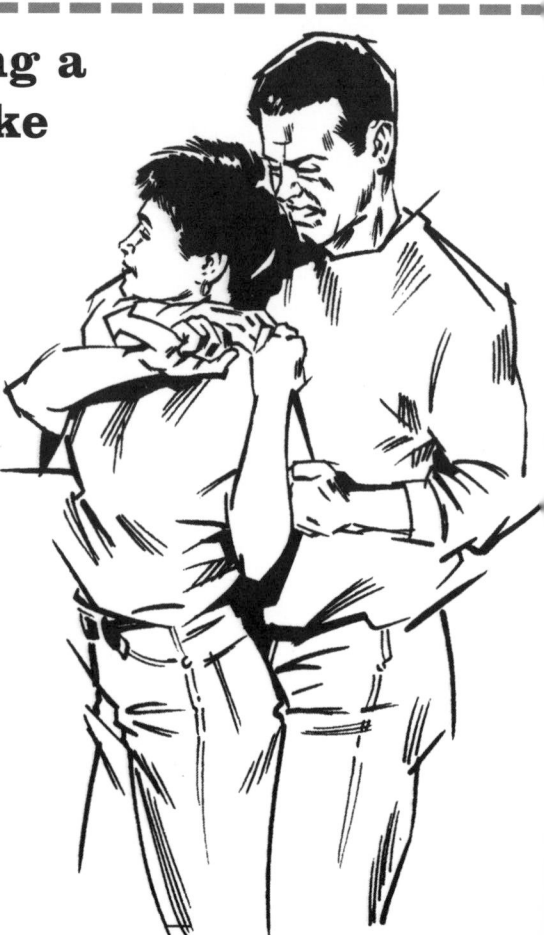

at an ideal distance to hit you. To avoid this, step away as you turn and grab his arm, pulling him off balance. You have many good options from this position.

Rear Choke

A rear choke can be used to actually choke you, to control you for another assailant to hit, or to drag you somewhere. In any case it

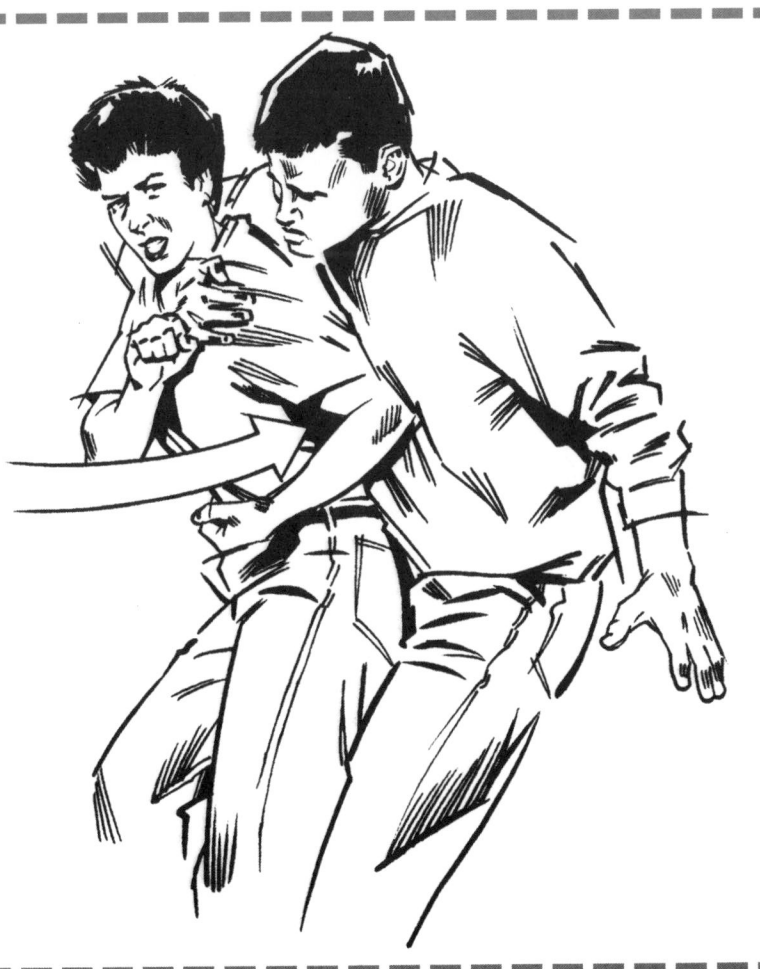

is important to act quickly. It is sometimes possible to grab fingers and break them to effect a release, but if the choke is well anchored this is unlikely. Relieve the pressure on your windpipe by turning your chin into the crook of the attacker's elbow and pull the choke off. If you cannot get it off completely you can relieve the pressure somewhat. Drive your elbow hard backwards into the assailant as you pull at the choke. Rather than a steady pull, a series of sudden jerks can work better.

If you can, get your chin down to prevent the choke pressing on your throat. Bite the attacker's arm if you can. You can also stamp on his feet. The aim, as with bear hugs, is to make yourself both difficult and painful to hold on to.

Alternatively, you may be able to dislodge the attacker by grabbing his arm and dropping forward, rolling your shoulder down on the same side as the arm you have grabbed. This will throw him over your shoulder to land in front of you.

HEADLOCKS

Headlocks are among the commonest grappling positions. They occur by accident as often as deliberately, as combatants instinctively grab at one another's head. A headlock might or might not choke you. Again, this happens by accident as often as by design.

The most accessible target from this position is the opponent's groin. Strike or grab his testicles and try to pull the headlock off you. You may be able to loosen his grip and pop

Extreme close quarters

You have many options at very close quarters, other than grappling. Short, hard strikes to the head or groin are effective, and even if you have no other options you can still bite. None of these are fight-ending techniques but they will open up some space to deliver something more decisive.

backwards out of the lock. If not, bring your hand up and drive the edge of it under his nose, causing considerable pain. Tip the opponent's head back to overbalance him, driving forward with your leg to give him something to fall over. Further blows to the groin will distract him or encourage him to let you go of his own accord.

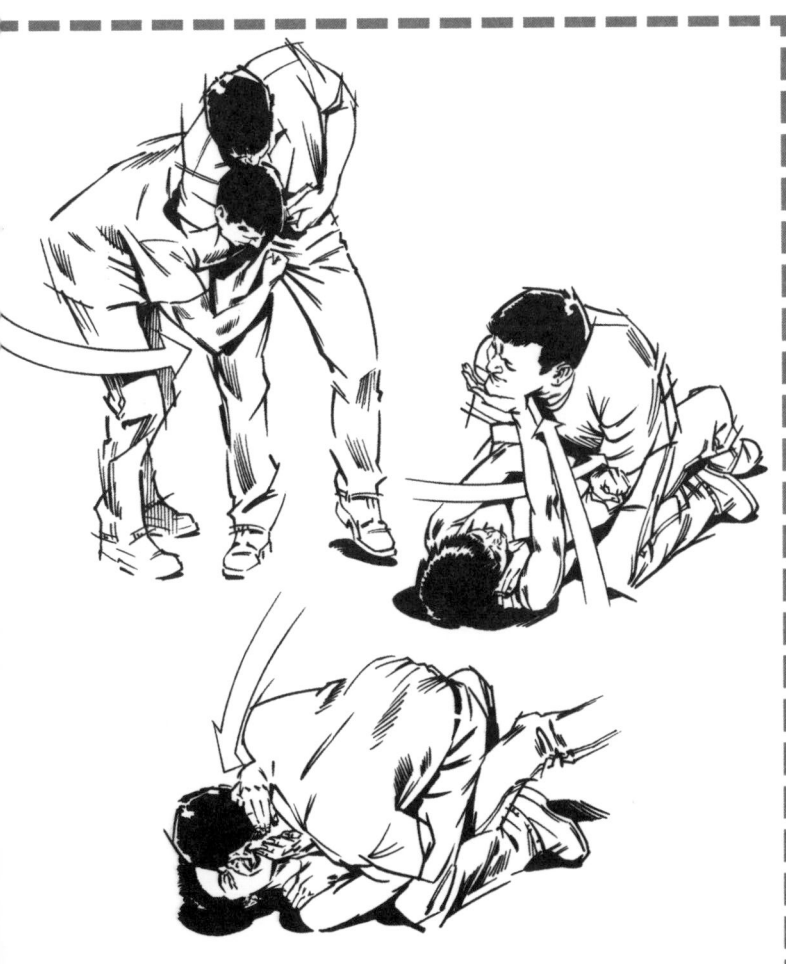

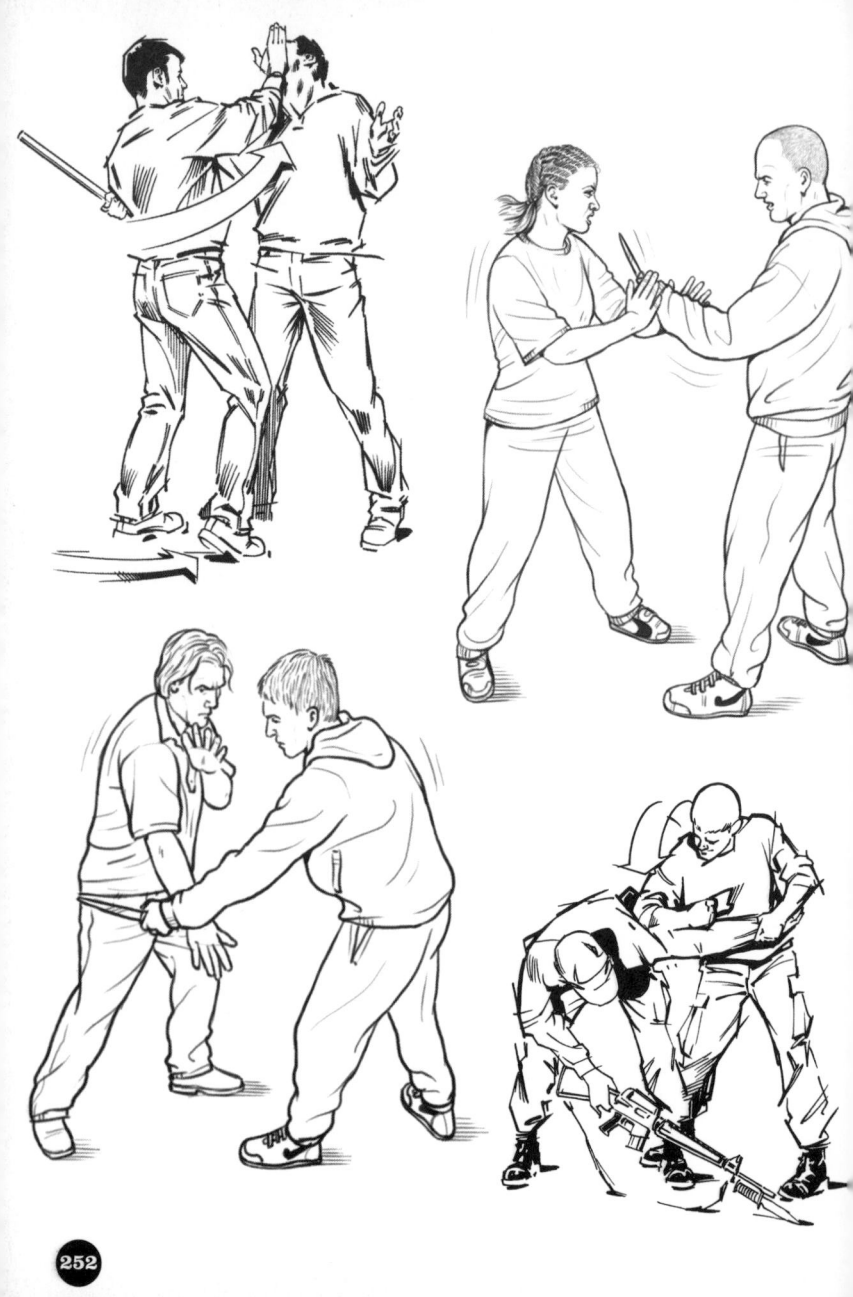

A ny weapon is a very serious threat to your life. Or more accurately, the person wielding the weapon is a serious threat. A knife or baseball bat cannot kill you whilst lying on the floor, but an assailant who has lost his weapon can still beat you senseless then pick up his weapon again to finish you off. Thus, although specialist disarming techniques are taught to the military, merely getting his weapon away from the assailant is not the goal. There is nothing to stop a disarmed enemy from continuing to fight and possibly regaining his weapon. Thus the aim is to nullify the threat posed by an armed assailant, not to create a disarmed but still dangerous opponent.

Tackling a knife or other weapon is very much a last resort. There is a strong possibility that you will be cut or stabbed even if you win the fight. Thus it is best to deal with the situation using other means if possible – surrendering property perhaps. However, some assailants will cut you even if you comply with their demands, and others simply want to harm you.

If you do have to tackle a knife or other weapon, you are facing a lethal threat and must not take half-

....

Left: When a weapon is used in an attack the stakes are higher.

11

The measures used to deal with armed attacks are not very different from those used to counter punches and grabs.

In Action

Defeating Hand-Held Weapon Attacks

TIP: THREATS AND ATTACKS

Sharp weapons are often used as a way of threatening someone, usually to obtain money or property. To pose a credible threat, the attacker has to brandish the weapon. On the other hand, a serious attacker who knows what he is doing will tend to conceal the weapon until he intends to use it.

Many knife attacks are not really 'fights' at all. They more closely resemble assassinations, with the victim unaware of the weapon until after they have been stabbed. It is thus vital to be aware of your surroundings and to prevent suspect people from getting close to you.

measures. In the midst of a fight, even an opponent who did not really intend to use his weapon will do so unless you can stop him. So you must make sure that the attacker is disabled or you are safe before you stop.

KNIFE THREAT FRONT

It is rare for someone to wander around with a knife in their hand. More likely they will deploy it from wherever it is being carried as they approach. Or, they might decide they need a weapon in the middle of a confrontation and reach for it.

Your best chance to deal with the threat is as the weapon is drawn. Once it is out, you will need to decide whether it is likely to be used or not. If you believe that the attacker is going to use his weapon, or he is demanding something unacceptable, such as wanting you to go somewhere with him, then tackling him while he is waving his knife about making threats is a better option than dealing with a committed attack.

Foul Draw Front

The assailant reaches into the front pocket of his clothing, e.g. a hoodie, and you believe he is going for a knife. Lunge forward and jam his arm against his body with your lead hand while unleashing a barrage of strikes with the other.

Foul Draw Rear

The assailant reaches into a rear pocket or his waistband. Push one arm through under his weapon hand and pull up. Reach over his opposite shoulder and reach down,

Hidden knife

A knife is easy to conceal. It is wise not to let suspect people get close to you, and to assume that any hand you cannot see to be currently empty may contain a weapon.

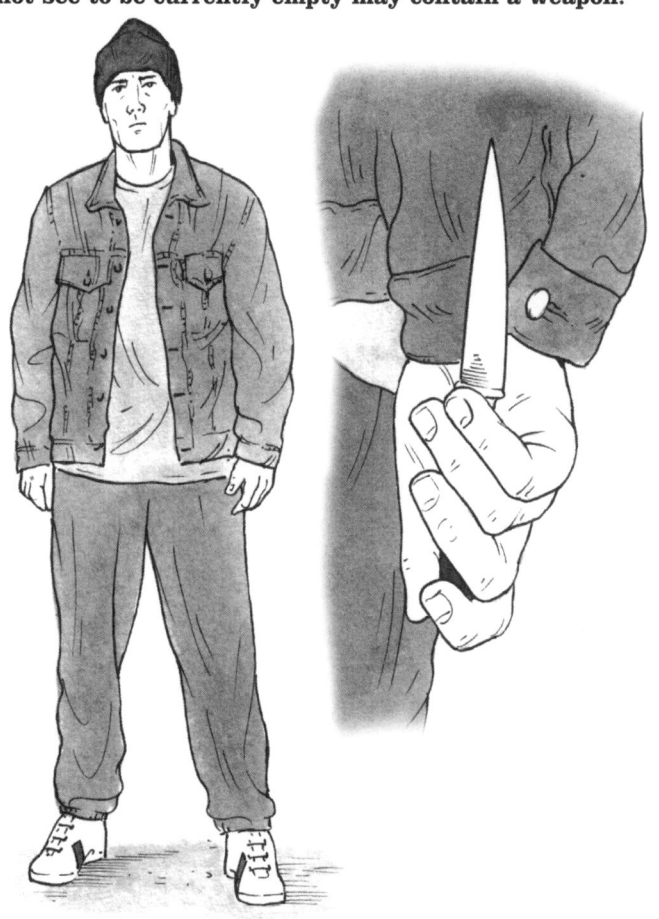

TIP:
WATCH THE HANDS

It is instinctive when in a confrontation, to keep your hands in front of you as weapons or to splay them out to make yourself seem bigger. If a hand disappears under clothing in such a situation, there is usually a reason.

You should always be aware that a hand you cannot see to be empty may contain a weapon, and if that hand goes 'out of play' during a situation where it would be instinctive to keep it in view, be prepared to deal with an armed attack.

Military disarm

If you manage to grab the knife hand, pivot so that you are facing the same way as the attacker. Wrench his arm up and across your body to break it.

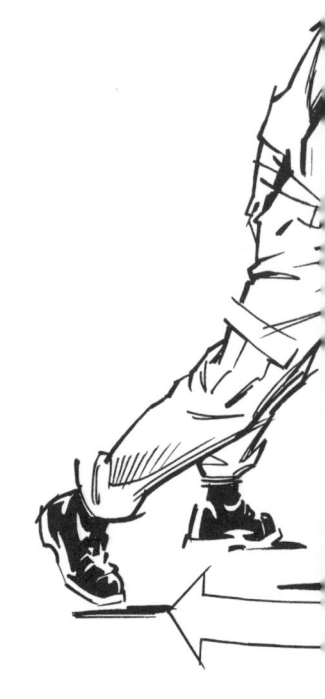

locking your hands together. Drive forward and trip the assailant with an inner reap as per Chapter 7, forcing him down with his weapon hand under him.

Strike to Disarm
The assailant is holding the weapon out towards you. Strike with both hands just in front of and behind the wrist, flipping it sharply around. This

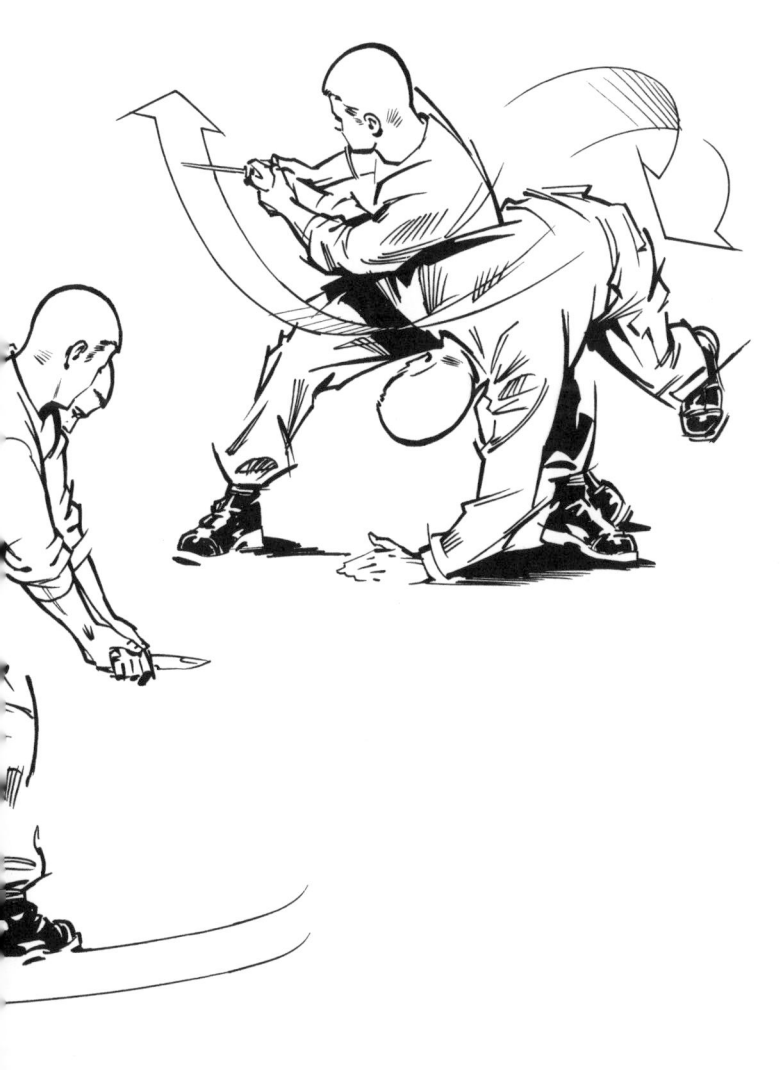

Strike to disarm

Strike the back of the attacker's hand and the inside of his wrist simultaneously, causing the hand to whip around. Often the weapon will fly out of the attacker's hand. However, this strike must be made suddenly and with total commitment.

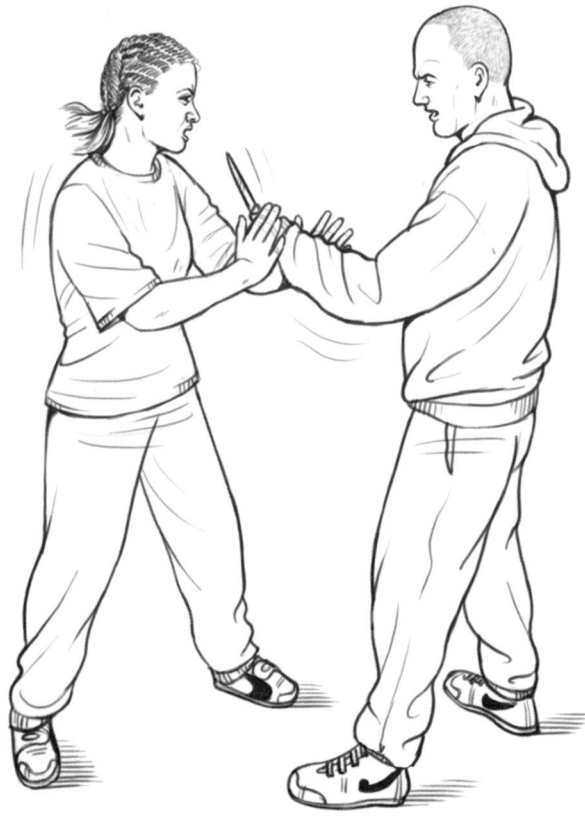

can cause the knife to fly out of the assailant's hand or just twist around so it is not pointing at you. Either way, strike him immediately to end the situation; he is still dangerous even without his weapon.

Deflect and Strike

The assailant is holding the weapon out towards you. Knock it to one side with your lead hand and strike him with your strong hand. Bring your lead hand around to the same side of his arm as your strong hand, enabling you to push him into a position from which it is difficult to attack you.

Deflect and Control

The assailant has a knife with its edge pressed to your throat. Make sure you know where the sharp edge is (his hand position will tell you), and push the blade away from you. Going the wrong way will cut your own throat. As you push the weapon away, step forward and round so that you are facing the same way as the attacker. Grab his arm and yank it across your body, driving forward to shove him to the ground.

KNIFE THREAT REAR

The assailant has a knife to your throat from behind. Pull his arm away from your throat and bend forward, turning your shoulder to perform a shoulder throw. Do not lose control of the knife arm; pin it and deliver strikes to subdue the attacker.

TIP: CUTS AND STABS

Most people who stab will thrust the weapon towards the body, usually in a somewhat upwards direction. Slashes tend to be directed at the head and neck. Stabs tend to be more lethal but are in many ways easier to defend against than cuts or slashes.

You can usually see what someone is planning to do by the position of their weapon. If it is raised, a slash is likely. If it is held lower, with the point towards you then the intent is probably to stab.

Many assailants will grab and pull the victim onto the weapon, making repeated pumping actions with the weapon to deliver several stab wounds.

KNIFE THRUST TO BODY

As the assailant begins his thrust, move to the side and angle your body so that the blade of the weapon

Rear knife defence

The first priority is to get the knife away from your throat. Grab the knife arm and pull down and forward, bending forward to throw the opponent over your shoulder. Pin his knife arm and finish him with either a knee drop or strikes to the head.

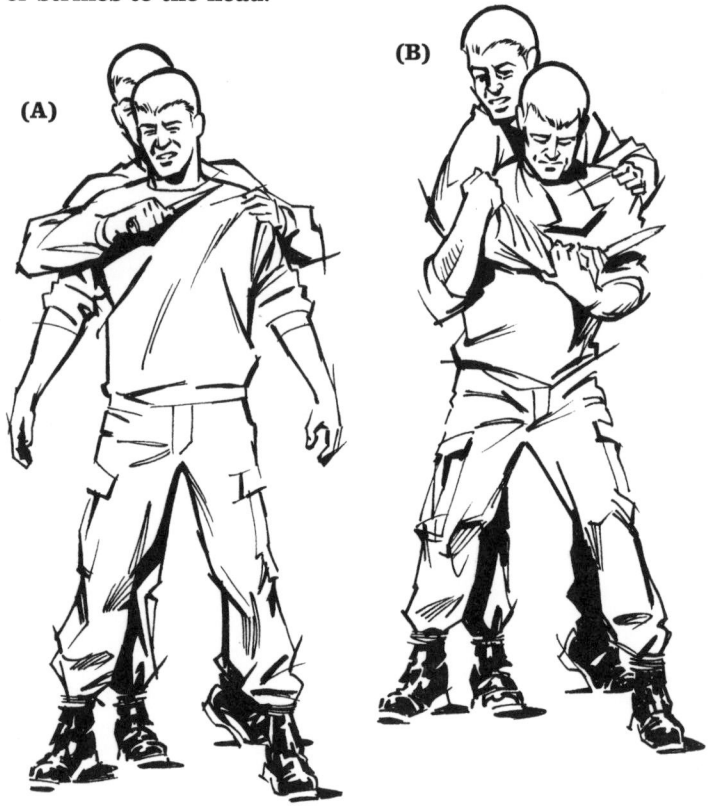

(A)

(B)

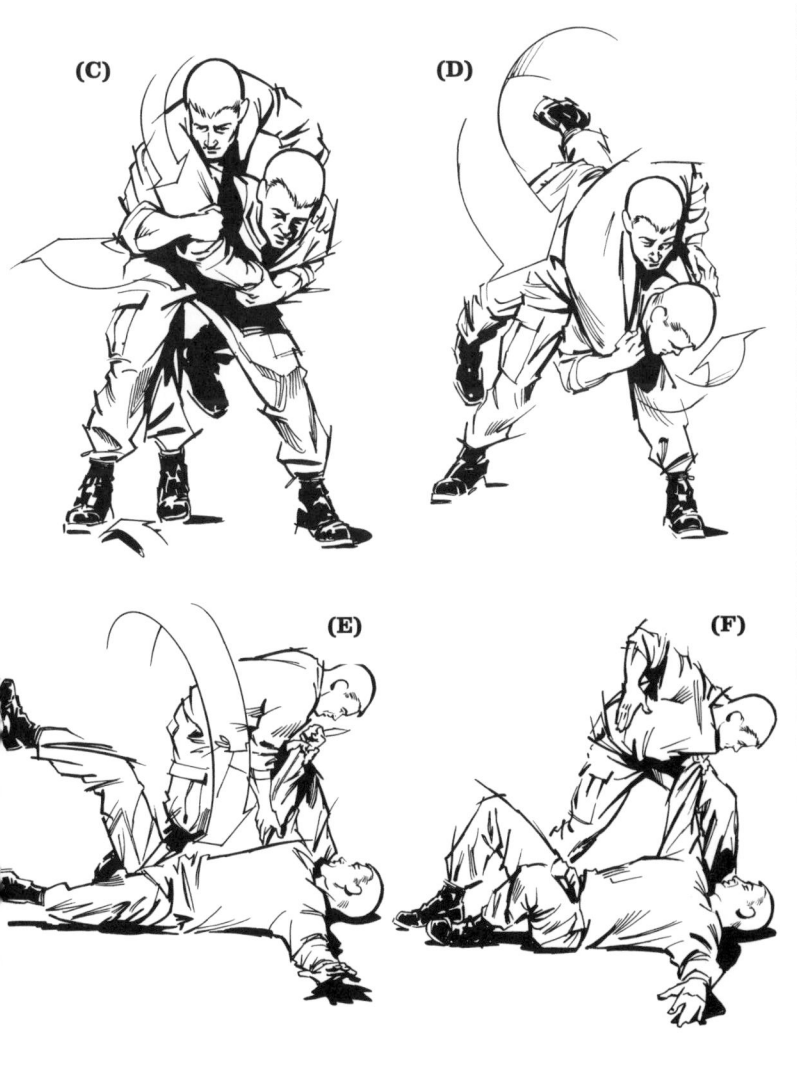

TIP: KICKS AND X-BLOCKS

Many martial arts teach their students to kick knives away or to defeat stabs with a crossed-wrist 'X-block'. It is possible that someone, somewhere has made this work, but both measures are ineffective and likely to result in you being stabbed.

goes past you. At the same time deflect the thrusting arm to the side. Step in and deliver strikes. If you can get the knife arm under control or break it, do so. If you cannot, keep hitting the opponent to prevent him regaining the initiative and stabbing you.

BAYONET THRUST TO BODY

A bayonet attack can be countered in much the same way as a knife thrust. Move to the side and deflect the weapon away from you. Grab the attacker's weapon or wrist and deliver an arm-breaking elbow strike. Follow up with a second elbow strike

and push into the shoulder to bring him down, and finish with a kick to the face.

KNIFE SLASH TO HEAD OR NECK

A slash with a blade follows a similar path to a hooked punch. Moving back out of reach is a temporary measure at best. Instead move inside the slash and stop the arm, wrapping it with your own arm to immobilize the weapon. This places the knife close to you, but it cannot harm you if it cannot move. Deliver a web-hand strike to the throat, and/or pull the attacker in close and knee him into submission.

PRE-EMPTIVE KICK

At any time when you have a chance to act – perhaps as the attacker is threatening you, or just before he stabs – you can gain the initiative by kicking him in the knee. This keeps your body out of reach of the knife. Follow up immediately by shoving the knife hand to the side – it does not matter where it goes, so long as it is not pointed at you – and close in to deliver strikes. From here, you must 'steamroller' the assailant with constant attacks and make sure he does not get the chance to stab you.

DEFEATING BLUNT WEAPON ATTACKS

Blunt weapons come in all shapes and sizes. Virtually any object can be

Pre-emptive kick

A kick to the knee may gain you time to get close and continue attacking the knife-wielder. It will not end the matter on its own, so shove the knife arm aside and deliver more strikes until you are sure you are safe.

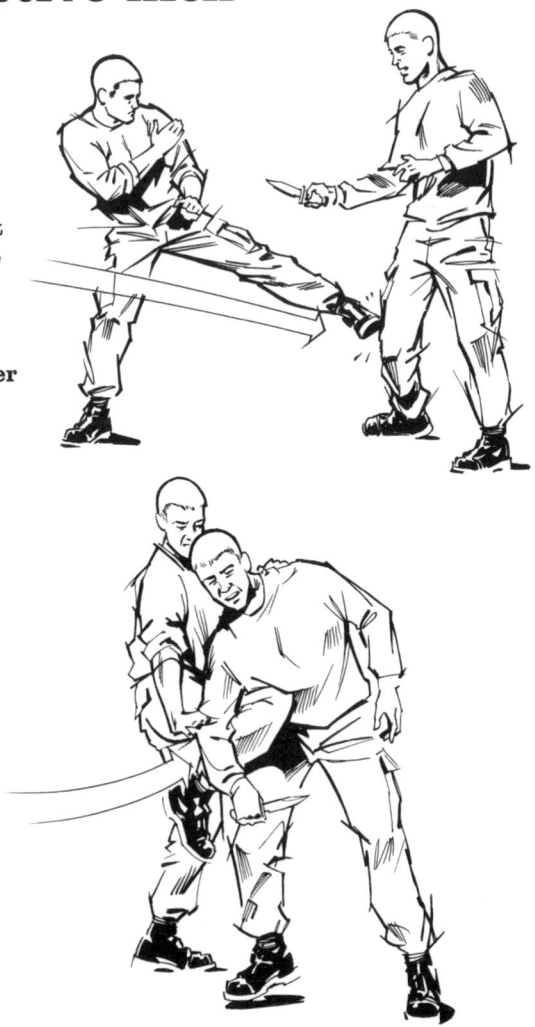

TIP: SECURE THE WEAPON!

In all cases where you face an armed attack, deal with the assailant rather than the weapon. However, as soon as the situation is over, get control of the weapon. Do not leave guns, knives, sticks and so forth lying around for the attacker you thought was finished to pick up and use against you.

Deflect and counterattack

The 'downward X-block' taught in many martial arts is ineffective. Attempting to stop a knife this way will probably get you killed. Instead, deflect the thrust with one arm and follow up any way you can. It may be possible to trap the knife arm and break it, or you may simply have to pin the arm as best you can and unload a barrage of strikes until the attacker is disabled.

picked up to use as a clubbing tool, though some are more useful than others. Generally speaking, an aggressor will swing a blunt instrument forehand, i.e. inwards and downwards from the side it is being held on. Backhand blows, chambered across the body, are less common as an initial strike but often follow up a forehand strike.

Overhead blows, straight down, are normally used with two-handed weapons such as a baseball bat, or large unwieldy objects such as chairs. Note that to be any real threat, a blunt object must be moving. The further it

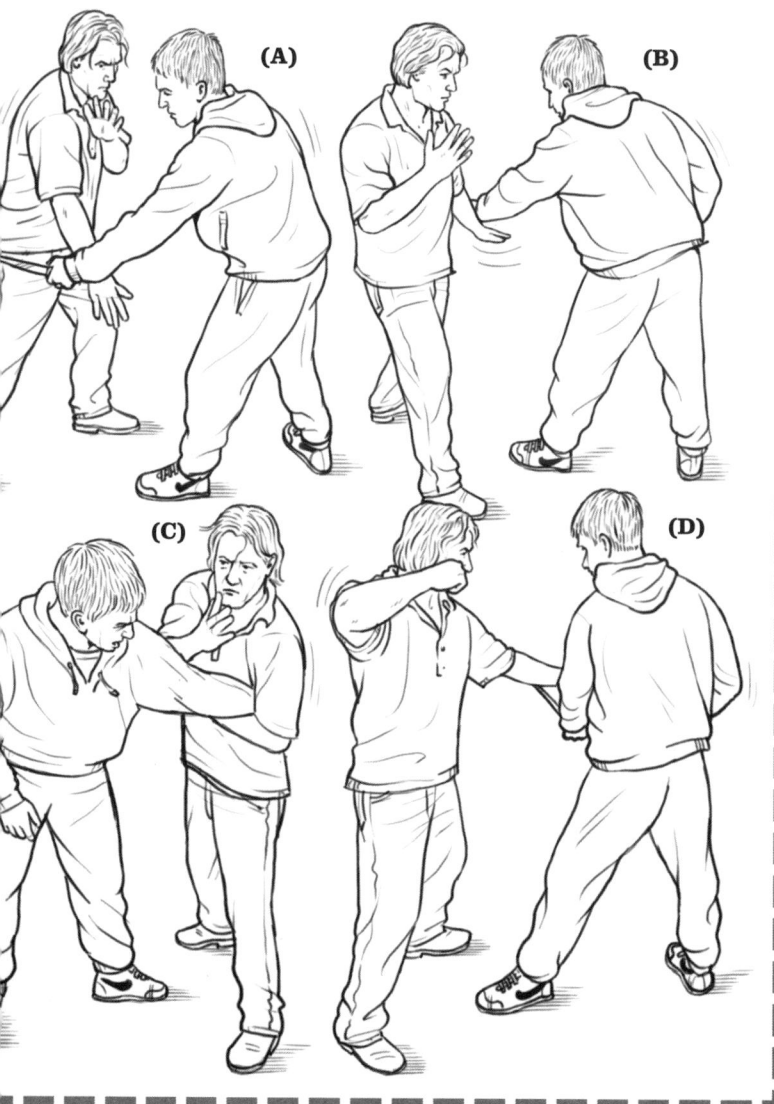

Defeating a bayonet attack

As the attacker commits himself to the attack, bat the weapon aside and close in, disabling his arm with strikes to take the weapon out of the equation before finishing him off with a kick to the head.

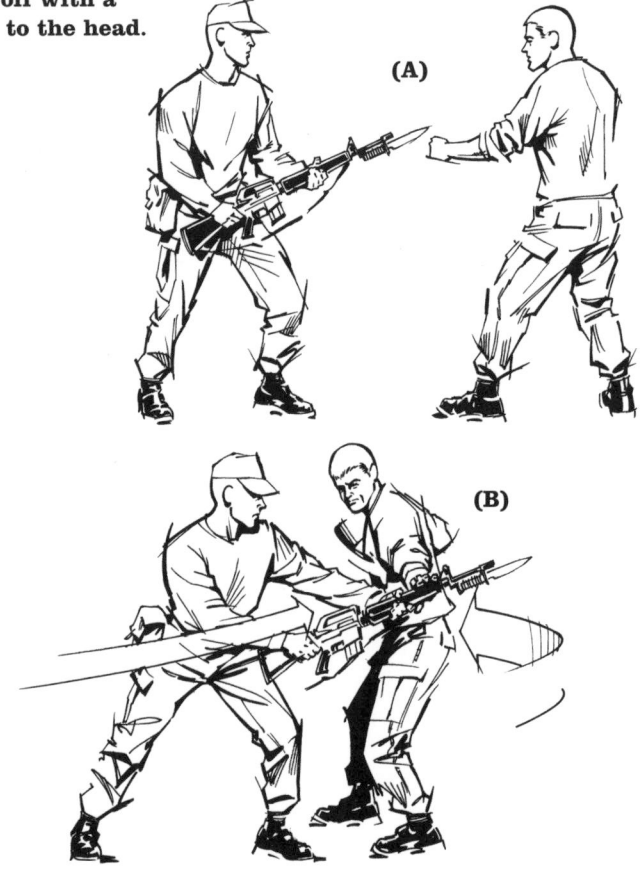

(A)

(B)

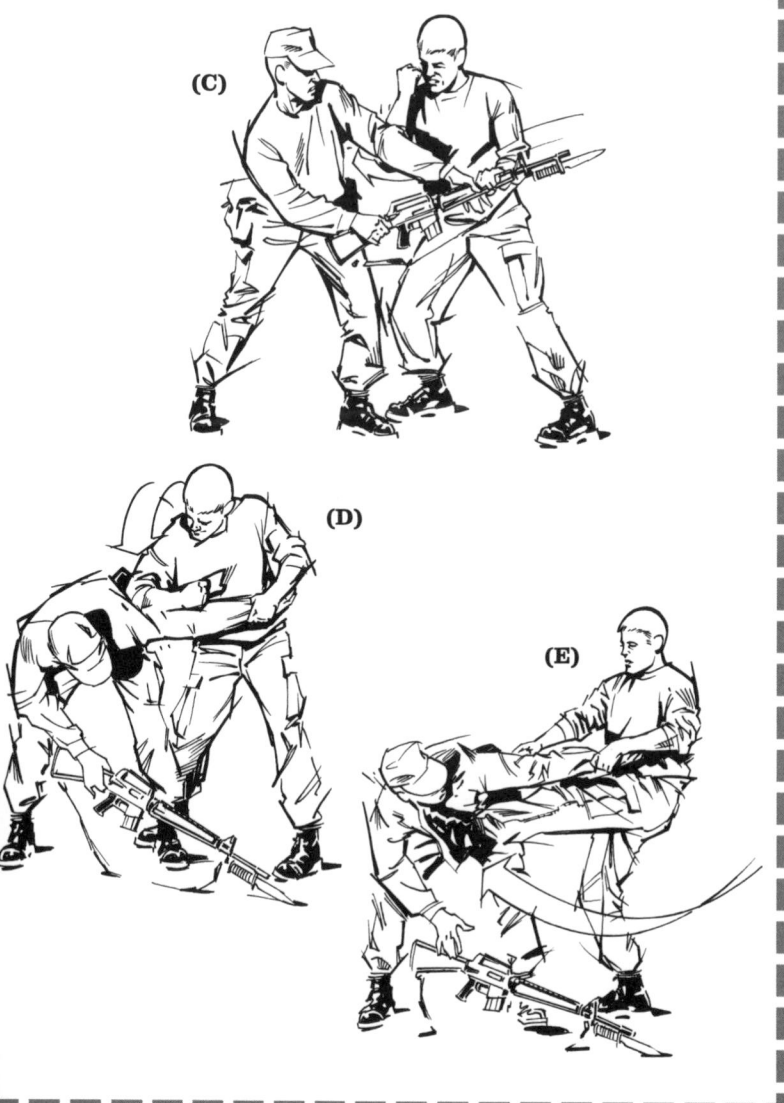

travels before striking the target, the greater the force it will deliver. The closer you are to most blunt weapons, the safer you will be.

Forehand Defence with Takedown

The assailant has a roughly baton-sized object and swings it forehand at you. Move in and jam the attack just as you would with a hook punch, driving one forearm into the crook of the attacker's elbow and one into the shoulder. Wrap the striking arm to prevent another blow and push through for an outer reap takedown.

Keep the assailant's weapon arm under control as you dump him on his back, and finish him off with strikes. It is sometimes possible to 'strip' the weapon out of his hand by sliding your wrapping arm up towards and past his hand, but it is more important to subdue the attacker than take away his weapon.

Throat strike

Deflect the knife out and strike the assailant in the throat with the web of your hand. This can kill, but when you are being attacked with a knife virtually any degree of force is justified.

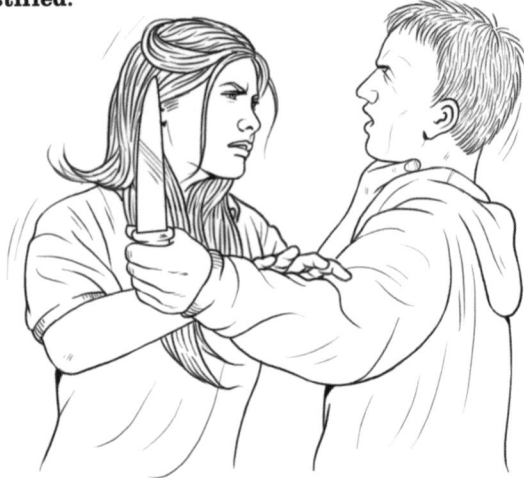

Forehand Defence with Strikes
Jam the strike as described above and wrap the attacker's arm. Deliver a palm strike to his head. You may be able to push his head back for a takedown at this point. If not, keep hitting him. Instead of the palm blow, you could also pull the assailant's head down and begin kneeing him.

Forehand Defence with Kick
As the assailant begins his swing, duck under it and step forward so that you are to his side. Deliver a side stomp kick into his knee. This option is risky for two reasons – if you mistime the duck you will be hit in the head, and if the kick misses you are no better off. However, it does allow you to take out an armed

Forehand defence with takedown

A swinging strike can be jammed just like a hook punch. Wrap the arm to immobilize the weapon and take the opponent down with an outer reap.

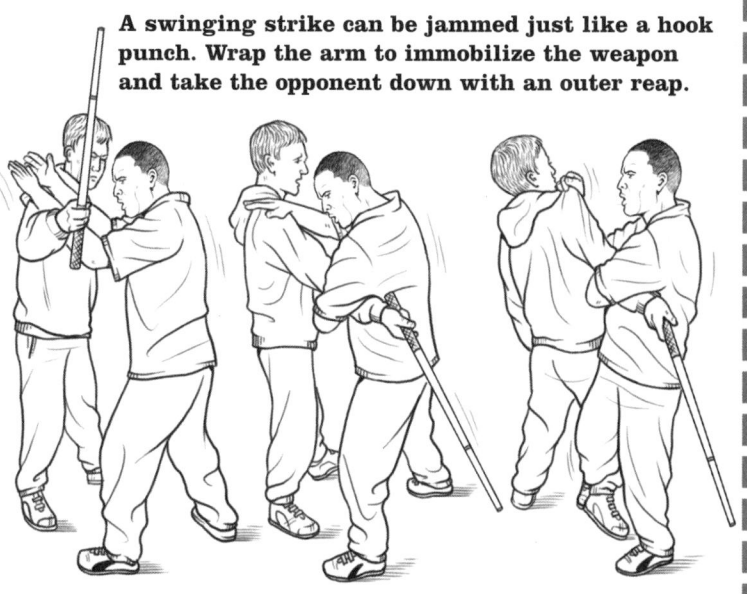

opponent 'in passing' and make off before his friends get involved.

Backhand Defence with Strikes

As the assailant 'chambers' his strike, push his weapon arm into his body to prevent it being swung at you. Drive forward, keeping the weapon trapped, and deliver strikes with your knees and other hand. The attacker will try to move away from you, in order to open up distance for a swing. Stay with him and keep attacking until he is subdued or falls over something.

Backhand Defence with Weapon Headlock

As the assailant chambers his swing, push his weapon arm into his body and reach over his shoulder, grabbing

Forehand defence with kick

Duck under the strike and step forward, delivering a side thrust kick to the side of the attacker's knee. Be prepared to turn towards him and follow up with more strikes, but if your kick connects properly you will not need to.

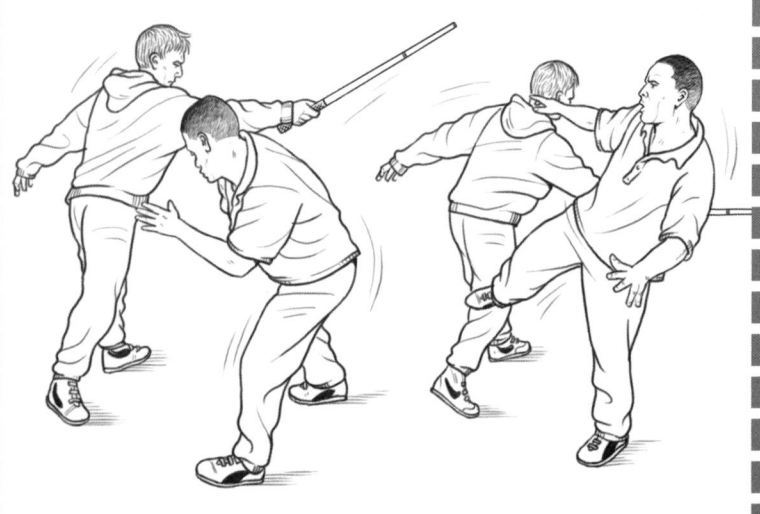

the other end of his weapon. Jam his weapon arm with your chest and transfer your grip so that you are holding both ends of his weapon, Pull it hard towards you and push your chest forward, digging the weapon in to the back of his neck. When you are ready, pull one end of the weapon and push the other, pivoting your body as you do for a takedown.

The assailant might let go of his weapon to relieve the pressure on his neck. If he does, you have hold of it and can now use it against him.

Overhead Defence by Evasion

If the assailant starts to swing overhead, probably with a two-handed grip on his weapon, move to the side and bat the weapon down as it goes past. Coupled with the force of the swing this will cause the attacker to stumble forward. Until he regains his balance he is very vulnerable. Close in, grab his shoulder and pull him onto a knee strike to the thigh muscle. Follow up with additional strikes.

Backhand strike defence

Jam the strike by pushing the attacker's arm into his body. Reach through and grab the weapon, using it as a lever to spin him to the ground.

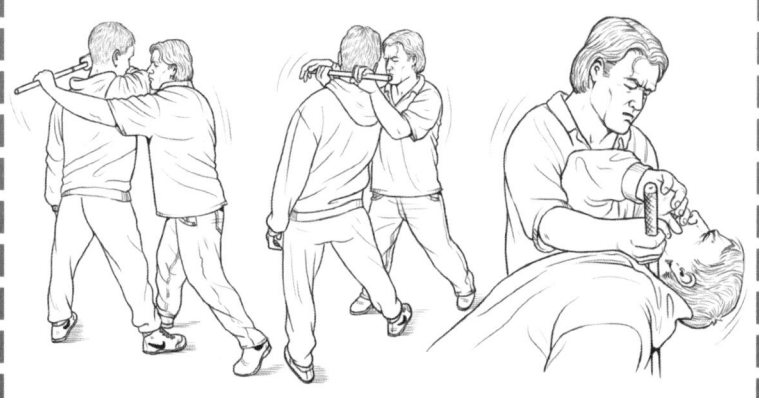

Immobilize the weapon

A blunt weapon cannot harm you if it cannot move. The arm-wrap technique is an effective way to ensure this. Knees, elbows, palm strikes and headbutts can be delivered from this position. Often the attacker will fixate on his weapon, struggling to free it, and give you time to strike him repeatedly.

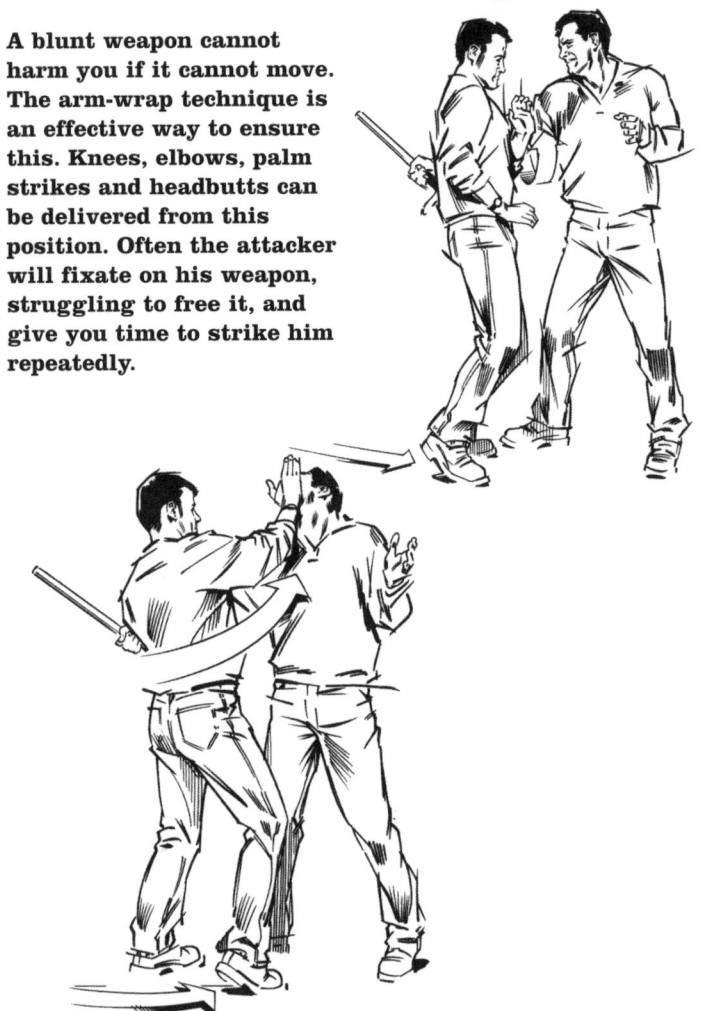

TIP:
SHOULD YOU FIGHT BACK?

It can be difficult to decide in a split second, especially if you are confronted with a weapon, whether you should fight back or not. Instinct and training are your guide here. If you think that your best option is to take a beating rather than being killed, or to hand over property rather than fight, then do so.

However, compliance does not guarantee safety – muggers have been known to kill their victims after getting what they want, for example. People who fought back, even if they lost, tend to make a better mental and emotional recovery than those that did not.

In a study a few years ago, the British Home Office determined that in the case of attempted rape, women who fought back or made a lot of noise were 50 per cent likely to escape completely unharmed. Those that both made a lot of noise and fought back escaped unharmed 90 per cent of the time.

This is a decision that only you can make, but on balance it seems to be better to fight for your safety than to hope the attacker only wants to hurt you a bit.

Horizontal Butt Stroke

Most people would not think of thrusting with a blunt weapon, but this is a very effective form of attack. For example, soldiers are trained to use their rifle butts in this manner.

Step to the side and deflect the blow away from you, turning to deliver an elbow strike to the side of the head. Yank the attacker's arm down and backwards as you step around behind him. Wrap your other arm around his throat and choke him, or pull back and kick one of his feet away for a rear takedown.

Vertical Butt Stroke

Against an attacker striking down and forwards with a rifle butt or similar implement, move to the side and deflect the stroke down and away from you. However, if the attack is very committed the assailant might move forward out of your reach. Turn and step after him, throwing a low roundhouse kick into the back of his leg just below the knee. This will cause him to fall on his back in front of you where he is vulnerable.

Heavy Blunt Objects

Against an opponent who raises a heavy object – for example a fire extinguisher – over his head, you must get out of the way. Imagine you are standing on the bottom leg of a letter 'Y' and the attacker is at the fork. Move up either arm of the Y, out of the way of the weapon, and turn to engage the attacker with strikes before he regains control. You may be able to simply push him so that he falls over his weapon. Note: If you hit him while he is holding the weapon over his head, it may fall on his head – or yours. Do not take the risk.

Defending against heavy blunt objects

Never try to stop a heavy object from falling on you. Instead, get out of the way by moving forward and to the side. Gain the initiative with strikes before the attacker can recover.

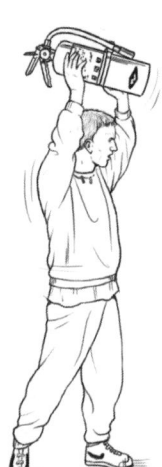
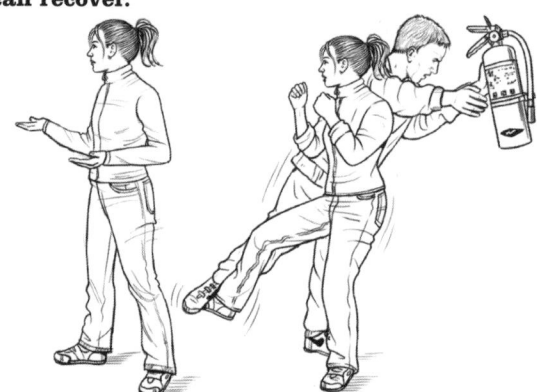

Ineffective blocks

It is pointless to try to stop a weapon by blocking with an arm like this. Chances are the strike will crash right through and hit you anyway. If the attacker's arm bends at the elbow the weapon will whip down and smack you in the head. Jam the strike as shown previously, or duck under it, but do not bet your survival on ineffective blocks like this one.

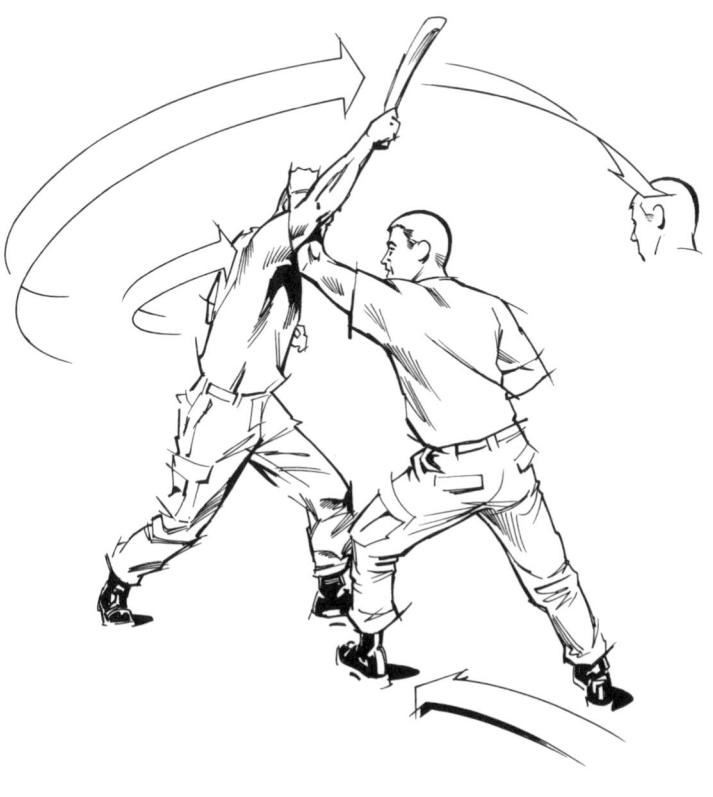

Defending an overhead strike

Against a downward jab or two-handed overhead swing, e.g. with a baseball bat, step to the side and slap the attacker's arm down and away from you. This will pull him off balance. A roundhouse kick to the rear of the attacker's leg will then bring him down and may disable his leg.

(A)

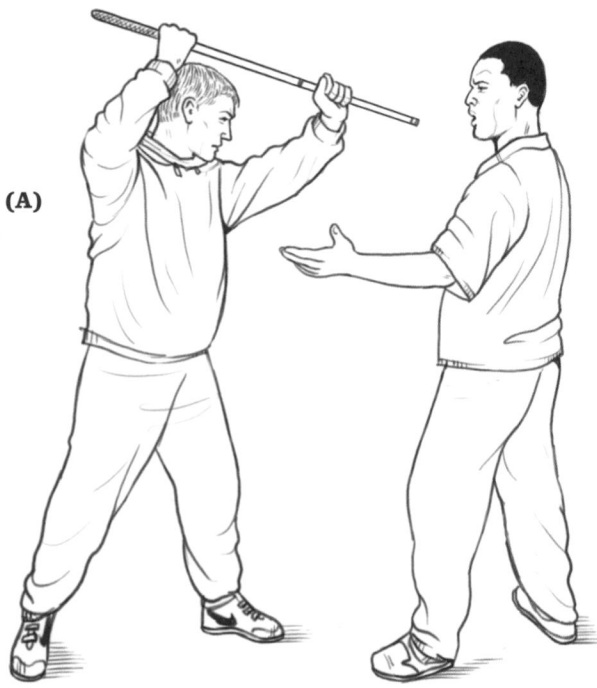

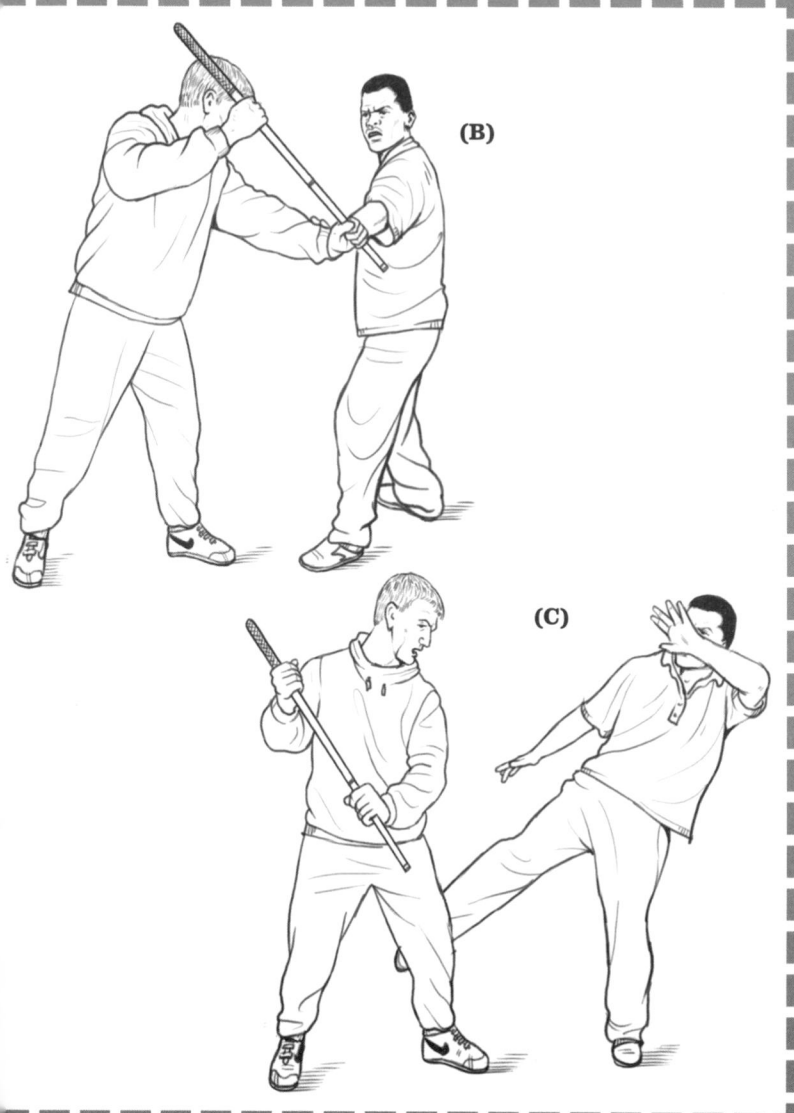

(B)

(C)

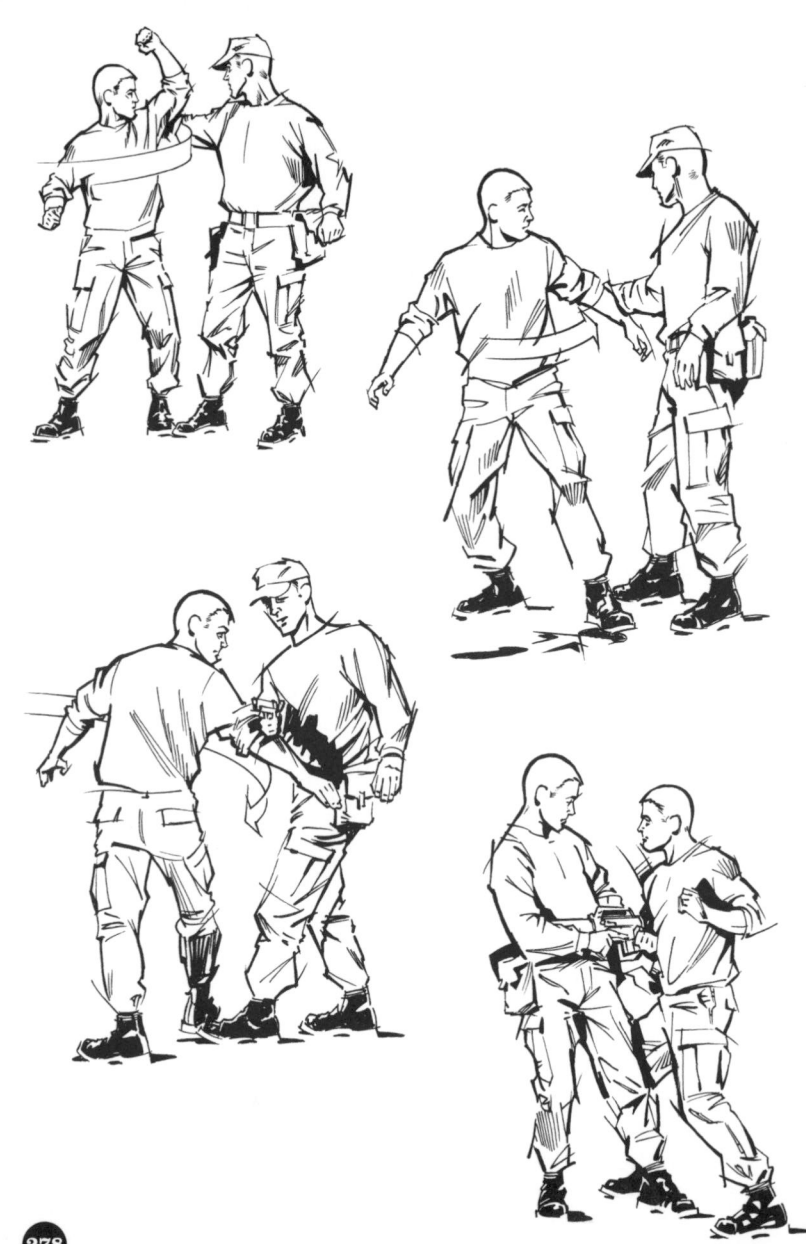

F irearms are all extremely dangerous, though some are more lethal than others. As a general rule, it is wise to comply with anyone who has a gun. However, if you think you are going to be killed, or the situation becomes unacceptable – for example if you are being taken somewhere you are unlikely to be able to escape from – then resistance may be your only option.

POINT IT THE OTHER WAY

You cannot be shot by a gun that is not pointed at you. Even if you are shot, this will not necessarily be lethal. A good rule to have in your mind is – if a gunshot wound does not immediately put you down, it is not going to put you down. Many people panic and fall down upon being shot, more out of fear than actual injury.

Any gunshot wound can be lethal, and certainly you will need urgent medical attention, but if you are running away or wresting with a gunman and you are hit, carry on if you possibly can and worry about the injury once you are safe. Giving up means death. Carrying on offers a chance at survival.

....

Left: If threatened with a firearm, you have nothing to lose. Defend yourself with total commitment.

12

Consider tackling an armed opponent only if your life is in imminent danger.

In Action
Defeating Firearm Threats

TIP:
FIGHTING FOR A GUN

If you grab a firearm and pull it towards you, you will pull it against the user's trigger finger and cause it to discharge. It may well go off, intentionally or unintentionally, while you are disabling the gunman. No matter where the bullet goes, the weapon will make a huge noise and the barrel will become very hot.

Be prepared for this and do not freeze. Even if you are wounded, a gunshot that does not put you down immediately is not going to stop you unless you panic or give up. Once you are fighting for a gun, to stop or give up means almost certain death. Finish what you have started then worry about whether you are wounded, deafened, dazed, or unhurt but scared half to death.

Being scared half to death is a certainty. All else depends upon what you do and how determinedly you do it.

GUN THREATS VS GUN ATTACKS

Much as with knives, someone who shows you a firearm wants something. If the intent is to cause harm then an attack will likely take the form of an assassination attempt. The gunman in this case is likely to conceal the weapon and his intent. One example of this is a drive-by shooting. The gunman is driven past the target by a comrade, takes his shot, and then escapes quickly.

If an attack is already underway, your best chance is to take cover and escape as quickly as possible. The same applies to gun-threat situations if you judge that the gunman (or gunmen) are likely to start killing people. Note that there is nothing cowardly about fleeing while others are captured. If you can raise the alarm quickly and provide details of the situation to the authorities, you are helping the hostages far more than by heroically tackling a gunman and being killed.

If There is No Alternative
If you can escape, do so. If there is a negotiated outcome that

guarantees your safety, then this is usually a better option than tackling a weapon. But if you think you are going to be killed, you might as well fight for your life.

If you are close to a gunman, you will need to disable him. Trying to run when very close to an armed opponent makes you an easy target. An all-out assault is the only chance, though you need to remember your goal is to escape and to take an opportunity if it arises.

No half-measures are possible when dealing with a firearm. If you do attack an armed opponent and later discover that his weapon was not loaded, or was a replica, you will not have acted unlawfully. So long as you believed the weapon was real at the time, virtually any action you could take would be lawful.

HANDGUN THREATS

A handgun pointed at the chest is difficult to counter due to the width of the torso. It must be deflected a considerable distance before the defender is safe, and all the attacker has to do is pull the trigger. Whatever you do must be fast and, far more important, sudden.

Push the weapon aside so that it is not pointed at you. It will almost certainly go off at this point, but do not stop no matter how shocked you are by the noise. If you can, grab the weapon so that no part of your hand is in front of the muzzle and twist it to

TIP: COVER AND CONCEALMENT

It is vital to understand the difference between cover and concealment.

- Concealment will hide you but will not stop a bullet. Smoke, foliage, most internal walls and most parts of a car offer concealment but not cover.

- Cover will hide you and stop a bullet. A car engine block, a thick wall or a tree trunk will offer cover. Note that some weapons penetrate better than others. Pistol rounds will often bounce off things that a rifle bullet will rip straight through.

the side. Be brutal; the gunman's finger will be trapped in the trigger guard and you may have to twist hard enough to break it. Twisting up or down can also work, but be sure not to point the weapon at yourself.

Handgun threat to back of head

Raise your hands as if in surrender, then spin to knock the weapon aside. Wrap the weapon arm and deliver strikes to the head, then use an outer reap takedown to dump the opponent. Keep control of the weapon arm as you finish off the attacker with a knee drop and strikes to the head.

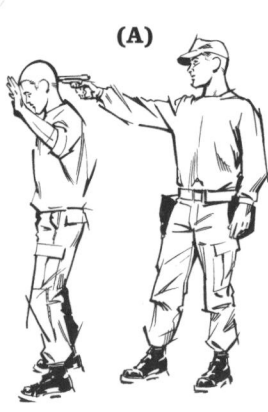

(A)

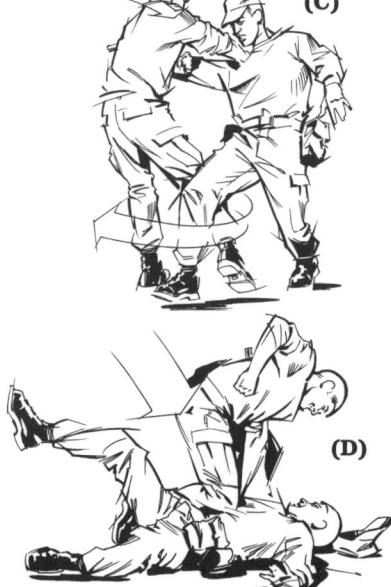

(C)

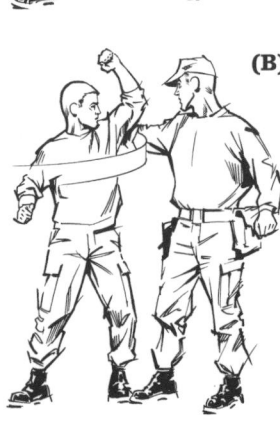

(B)

(D)

TIP:
SHOTGUNS

Shotgun cartridges generally contain several small projectiles. These spread out in a cone when the gun is fired and can hit multiple targets. Shotguns are especially deadly at close range where the shot is concentrated, but their effective range is quite short. If the barrel is sawn off, this reduces the range but spreads the shot out more, making it hard to miss with a sawn-off shotgun at close range.

Most sporting shotguns have two barrels, which are loaded separately each with a single cartridge. Thus a gunman armed with a double-barrelled shotgun has at most two shots before he must reload by breaking the weapon and inserting new cartridges.

Pump-action and semi-automatic shotguns can carry several rounds, usually in an internal magazine. Pump-action shotguns are reloaded after each shot by operating the 'pump'; semi-automatics reload themselves. Both types allows the user to take several shots in rapid succession.

TIP:
SUB-MACHINE GUNS

Sub-machine guns sometimes resemble overgrown handguns and sometimes small rifles. They use pistol-type ammunition with a relatively short range (compared to a rifle) and which does not penetrate cover very well.

Sub-machine guns are fed from a detachable magazine that can hold 30, 50 or even more rounds. Most can fire single shots or fully automatically, allowing the user to spray a room or group of targets.

TIP:
SECURE THE WEAPON

Unless you are familiar with firearms there is little point in trying to use a gun you have grabbed as anything but a club. Fumbling about looking for a safety catch or checking if the weapon is loaded will give the assailant a chance to attack you. But do secure the weapon as soon as you can. Disabling the gunman takes precedence, but as soon as you get the chance, grab the weapon and make sure he or his comrades cannot use it.

However, be aware that if a hostage-rescue team sees you with a weapon they may open fire in the belief that you are one of the bad guys. If appropriate, put the weapon somewhere inaccessible, e.g. drop it down a drain or kick it under a low and heavy piece of furniture.

If you lose control of the weapon or cannot grab it, move in close and keep the gunman's arm pushed away from you. Keep striking to stop him bringing his weapon into play, and get control of it as soon as you can.

Handgun Threat to Forehead
Although the consequences of a bullet in the head are even worse than being shot in the body, it is actually simpler to deal with this threat since the head is smaller and more mobile than the torso. However, the noise and muzzle blast from a discharge that misses you, so close to your head, is considerable.

Bring up your hands in a typical 'surrender' position, then sharply knock the weapon aside. Move in the opposite direction as you do so. Grab the weapon and twist it out of the gunman's hand, striking him repeatedly to keep him defensive.

Handgun Threat from Rear
Raise your arms slowly as if surrendering, then turn rapidly and use your arm to sweep the weapon aside. Depending on which way you turn, your response will be slightly different.

If you find yourself 'inside' the weapon, trap it by wrapping the gunman's weapon arm with your arm, and deliver a palm strike under the chin. Follow up with a barrage of knee strikes, blows and headbutts. The attacker will almost certainly try to pull his weapon free as a first response, giving you a couple of free shots. Take them for all you can get.

If you find yourself 'outside' the weapon, this is a better position. Keep turning until you are facing the same way as the attacker, and pull his arm across in front of you, twisting the weapon out of his hand. Keep turning and drop your weight,

dragging the gunman down. If you cannot twist the weapon free, it may be possible to bash the gunman's arm down onto your knee to break it or jerk the weapon out of his hand.

Handgun Threat to Back of Head
For a weapon to the back of the head, it is necessary to raise your arms higher before beginning to turn. A 'surrender' position is a good starting point. As before, turn and knock the weapon aside, trapping it and delivering strikes to disable the

TIP: HANDGUNS

Handguns are relatively small and easily carried. They can usually be concealed under clothing without much difficulty. Few handguns or handgun-sized weapons are capable of full-automatic fire, i.e. they fire one shot at a time and cannot spray a room. Most people are not capable of accurate fire with a handgun except at very short ranges. However, this does not mean they are not highly dangerous.

There are two general types of handgun. Revolvers carry their ammunition – usually six rounds – in a revolving cylinder that swings out to reload. They are slower to load than semi-automatic pistols and usually cannot be fired quite as quickly.

Semi-automatic (or self-loading) pistols carry their ammunition in a detachable magazine, which might hold 17 or more rounds. Reloading is thus much quicker and the user has more shots available. Even if a semi-automatic has no magazine in place, it may still have a single round in the firing chamber and is thus still dangerous.

Rear handgun threat to body (1)

Turn and sweep the weapon to the 'outside'. Wrap the weapon arm and deliver a barrage of strikes to the attacker's head.

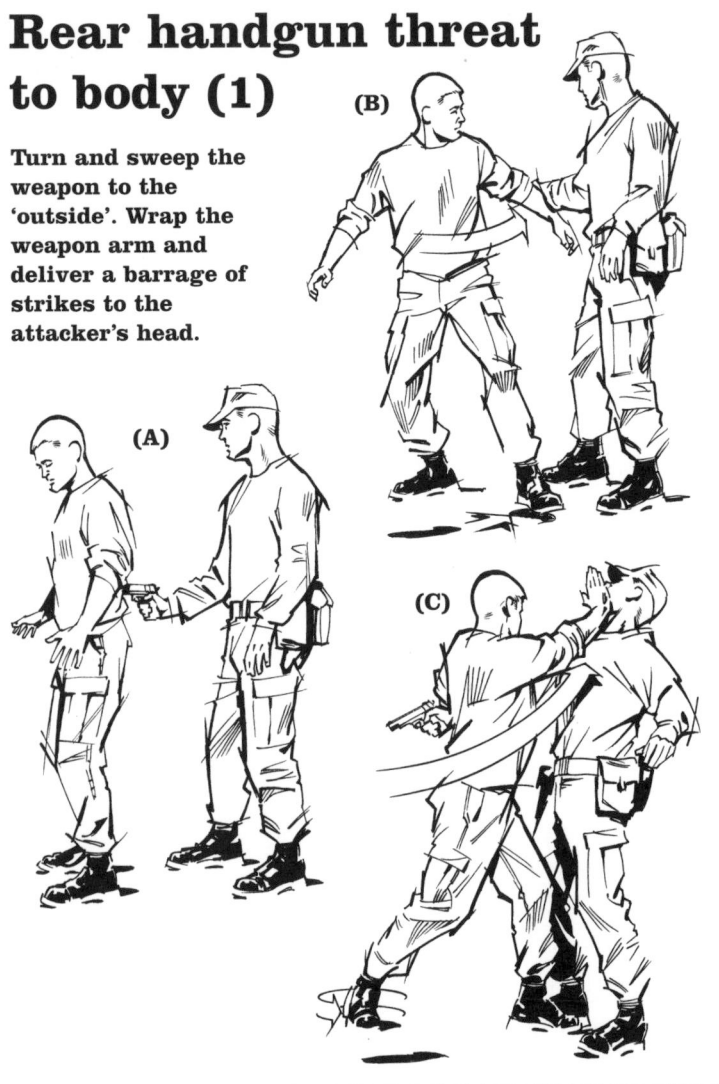

(A)

(B)

(C)

Rear handgun threat to body (2)

Alternatively, turn and sweep the weapon to the 'inside', pulling the weapon arm out straight. Yank it out and up, slamming your shoulder into the opponent's armpit to drive him down. By dropping to one knee you can sweep his foot away, making him fall harder.

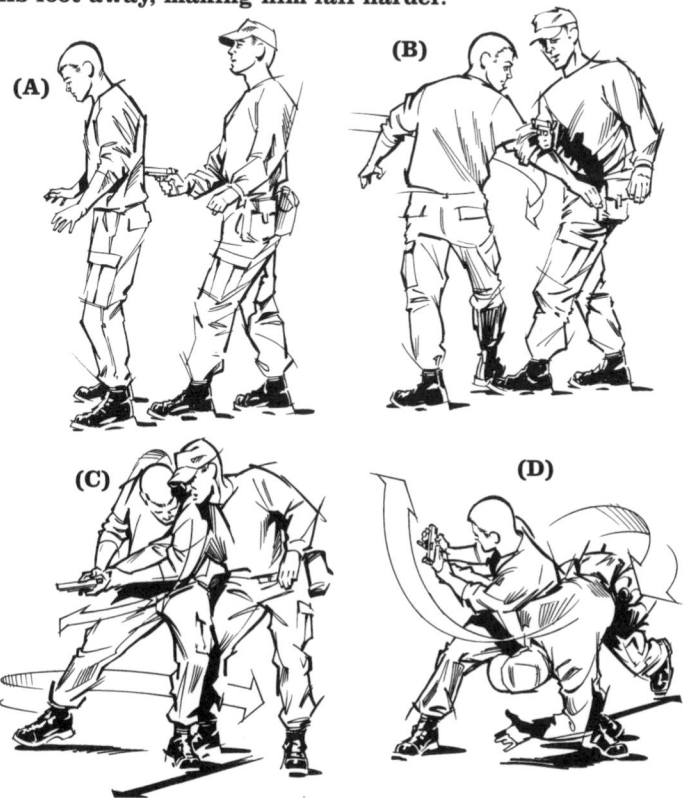

Tackling a rifleman from the rear

Take hold of the weapon arm as you grab the head, pulling the latter up and back. This exposes the throat for an edge-of-hand strike. Take the opponent down and choke him before he can recover from the blow.

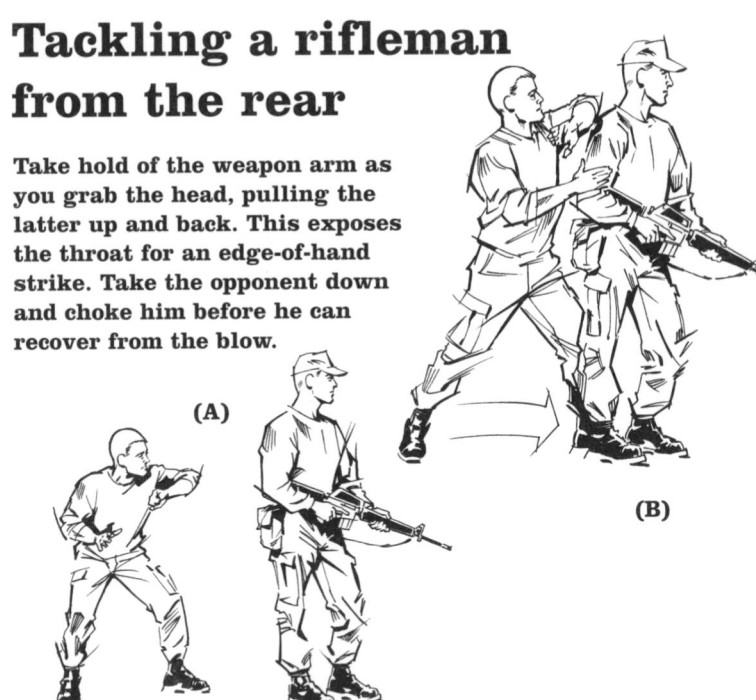

(A)

(B)

opponent. If you can, take him down and deliver a knee drop to the ribs, then strike the head and throat to finish him off.

THE 'LONGARM' THREAT

In this context, a 'longarm' is any two-handed firearm, such as a rifle or shotgun. Knock the barrel aside and close in, trapping the weapon by wrapping it with your arm. Deliver strikes to the throat, head or groin. The gunman will likely cling to his weapon and try to pull it free, which gives you a chance to hit him hard and repeatedly before he switches tactics.

Tackling a Gunman from the Rear

Generally speaking, it is better to take the opportunity to escape from a

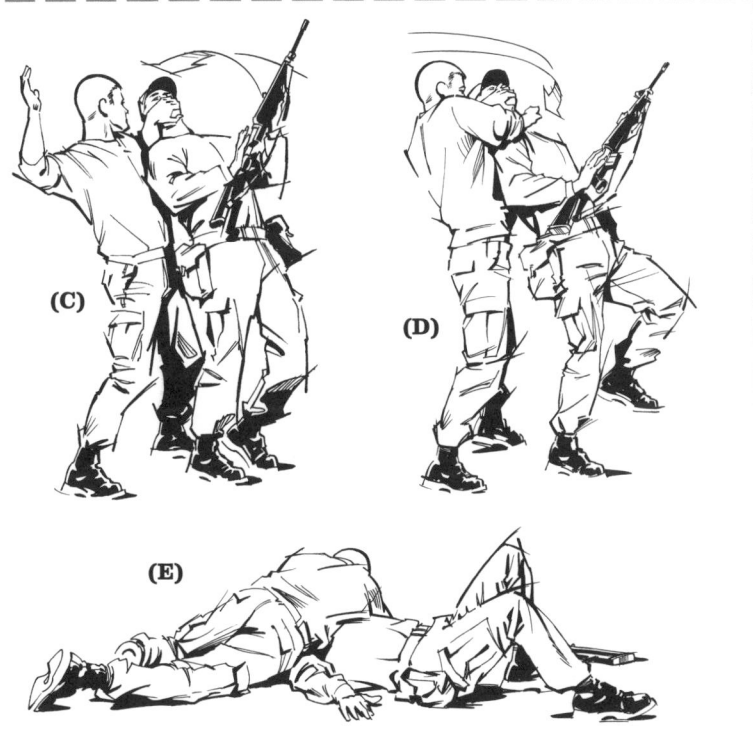

gunman who is unaware of your presence. However, if you have to tackle him for some reason, approach stealthily and grab his head from behind, pulling his chin up and back to take him off balance.

If noise is an issue, a hand clamped over the mouth can stifle any cry for help, but if the opponent's weapon goes off this then becomes academic.

With his throat exposed, smash him in the larynx with the edge of your hand or the inside of your forearm and drag him over backwards. Slam his head into the ground. One option is to follow him down and finish off with a choke. As an alternative, dump him on his back and stamp on his trigger hand or head. Make sure the weapon does not point at you at any time.

TIP: ESCAPING A GUNMAN

Most people are very poor shots. Even trained military personnel find accuracy under stress to be a major challenge. Thus if you are more than a few metres from a gunman and are moving, you are quite unlikely to be hit. Your best option is to flee, ideally changing direction and putting obstacles between you and the gunman. Even if these will not stop a bullet, they will obscure you and make you harder to hit.

Despite what we see in the movies, most gunshot wounds do not immediately disable or kill the victim. A lethal injury is much less likely if you are moving, and even if you are hit you may still be able to escape. Rapid movement and intelligent use of cover offers a good chance of escape.

TIP: RIFLES

Rifles shoot a powerful bullet that can pass through a lot of objects used as cover and are accurate at long range. Most rifles are limited by the skill of their user rather than their intrinsic accuracy. Many civilian hunting-type rifles are bolt-action weapons, which hold several rounds of ammunition but must be readied by manually working the bolt after each shot. Military rifles are often capable of full-automatic fire and are fed from a magazine containing about 30 rounds. Some civilian rifles look like military weapons but are semi-automatic, firing one shot and reloading themselves each time the trigger is pulled.

Rifle threat from the front

Bat the weapon aside with your lead hand and close in, wrapping your arm around the weapon barrel to immobilize it. If the muzzle is behind you, you cannot be hit. Strike the head and groin to disable the attacker.

(A)

(B)

(C)

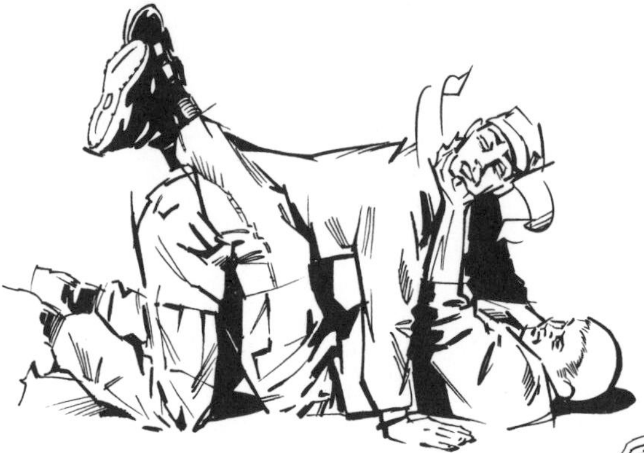

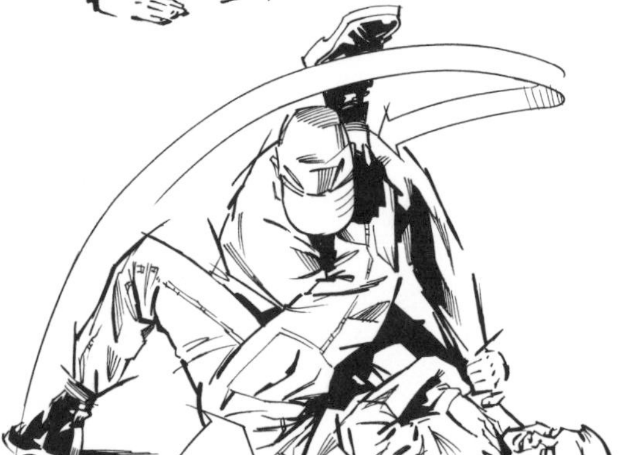

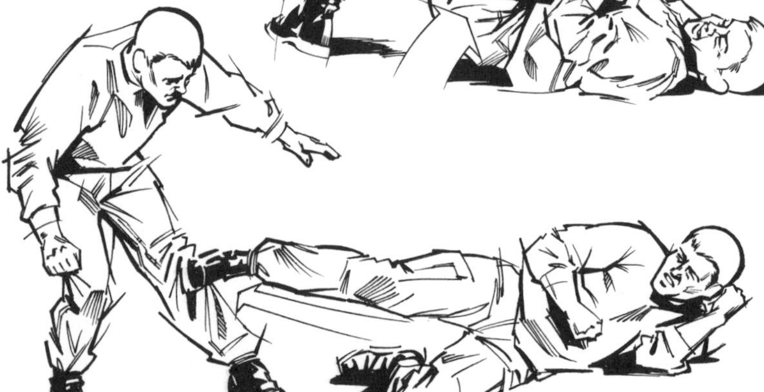

Military training is designed to prepare troops for combat, giving them the tools, tactics and mindset to deal with whatever might happen. Nothing ever goes exactly to plan, but good training allows soldiers to adapt to changing circumstances. So it is with unarmed combat; if you encounter difficult circumstances you can give up or you can find a way to struggle through. Training can only help so much; in the end it is down to you.

Groundfighting is a huge subject. Some martial arts are almost entirely devoted to this one aspect of combat. However, there is a considerable difference between being taken to the ground by a superbly conditioned athlete trained in groundfighting and falling over while wrestling with a drunk outside a kebab shop.

Everyone who intends to learn to defend themselves should learn some elementary groundfighting, but it is not necessary to go into the intricacies of sporting technique, nor is it desirable to fixate on groundfighting. True, many situations do go to the ground but they usually start standing up – and it is rare for a fight to go to the ground while both parties still have a good chance to win.

. . . .

Left: It should never be your intention to go to the ground, but you can end up there for all kinds of reasons.

13

Being able to fight on the ground is an essential survival skill.

In Action

Fighting on the Ground

TIP:
REASONS FOR
GROUNDFIGHTING

There are all kinds of reasons why you might end up on the ground. Attempted rape, a deliberate takedown, a sort of mutual drag-down … you might simply fall over something.

The reason does not matter. If you are on the ground with an opponent then you will need to fight from there until you can get up. The important thing is not to panic. Being down is a disadvantage but it can be overcome.

On the ground

If you are knocked down, you need to get back up as soon as possible. However, your first priority is to protect yourself against being kicked. Defend your vital organs and head with your arms and legs, and position yourself to kick out at the attacker.

has a big advantage, and if you are on the ground while an assailant is still upright, you are in serious trouble. Thus the key to winning a ground fight is the ability to get out of a difficult position and into an advantageous one. This is practised best by 'rolling', i.e. friendly competitive groundfighting.

Positional skills are vital even if all you want to do is hit, headbutt and bite the opponent into submission. Whoever can get the best position will usually win.

TECHNIQUES

Most of the techniques used standing up will also work on the ground. You can strike, knee and elbow, choke, strangle and lock joints. Biting and 'shutdown techniques' also work well. The mechanics are a bit different but the tactics are much the same.

The key to groundfighting is position. Normally, whoever is on top

POSITIONS AND COUNTERS

The commonest groundfighting position is what some people call an 'FUT' – we'll say that stands for Fouled-Up

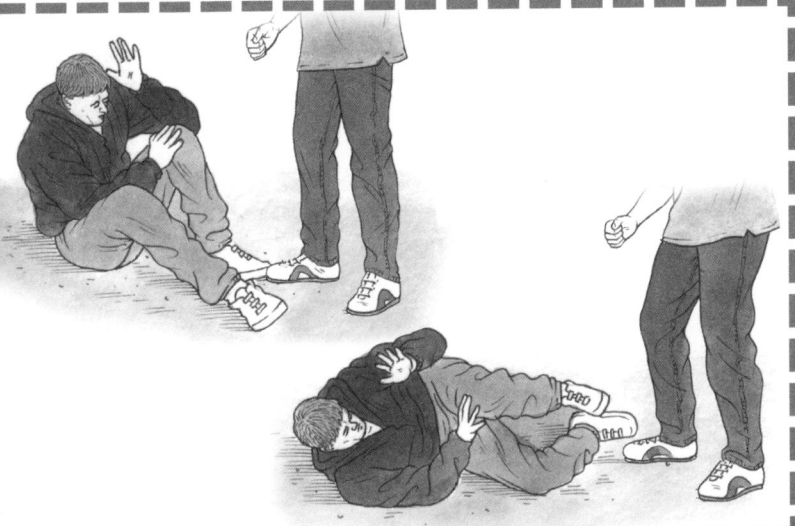

Tangle, though the military might use a slightly different term. An FUT is, as the name suggests, a tangled mess of limbs, generally resulting from two or more people grabbing at one another as they fall. However, certain positions naturally suggest themselves and quite often the tangle will resolve itself into a variant of one of the following. Even untrained people will usually find one of these positions as they instinctively see the advantages they offer.

There are many ways to counter each position. Brute force can work, as can causing the opponent pain by biting him or squeezing his testicles. The counters shown below are applicable to other positions. Experience gained in 'rolling' helps in choosing the best option for any given circumstance.

Downed with Standing Opponent

If you go down, get your feet towards the opponent and kick out at his knees or groin. A side kick is one option, or you can kick from your back. If he runs in to kick you, you may have to 'cover up' for lack of a better option, but you cannot stay in this position. You will have to grab his leg and either pull him down, or climb up him to regain your feet.

The Mount

This is the dominant position sought by almost all untrained fighters intent on inflicting harm. The assailant straddles you and either strikes downwards or attempts to choke you with a two-handed strangle or a forearm across the throat. Clothing chokes from this position are an option but are unlikely for an untrained opponent.

Most untrained fighters will rear up to get as much force behind their blows as possible. It is possible to 'bump' someone who does this off you by driving your knee into his lower back and pushing up with your hips while you grab him and pull him over your head.

Alternatively you can protect yourself by pulling him down on top of you, then induce him to roll to one side by jamming a thumb into his eye socket. As he flinches away, roll him off you. Trap his arm on the side you are rolling him towards to prevent him using it for support.

The Guard

Being on your back is never a good position, but you can gain control of an assailant by using the 'guard'. This basically means wrapping your legs around him and locking your ankles together and pulling him in close. This will stop him hitting you, if nothing else. Once he is under control you can begin working towards an escape.

This position is very similar to one that an assailant intent on rape would want you in. However, he cannot do anything if he cannot move, especially if he needs to get clothing out of the way. The guard is a starting point for your efforts to escape. You cannot stay there.

One good option is to grab the assailant around the chin and back of the head and twist. He will roll to the side to relieve the pressure. Go with him; you will end up in a 'mount' position from which you can subdue him or begin your escape.

Alternatively, place your foot on the assailant's hip and push hard, wriggling away from him to make some room to scramble out. If you can get your knees in between you and his torso, you may be able to push him off you or make enough room to free yourself.

The guard (2)

One way to get an opponent off you is to throw a leg over his head, then use the powerful muscles in your leg to push his head down. His body will follow wherever his head goes – to the side and off you, though you need to unlock your legs at the right moment to let him go.

The guard (1)

You can control an attacker who is on top of you by wrapping your legs around him. This prevents him from sitting up to rain down blows on you. Twisting his head violently will encourage him to roll to the side and off you.

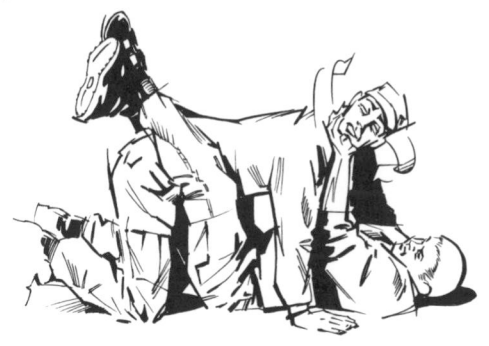

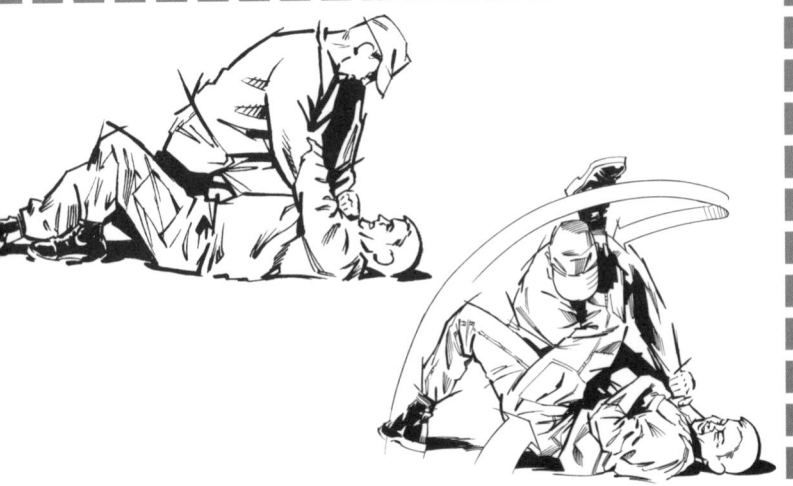

TIP:
GROUNDFIGHTING PRINCIPLES

Trained martial artists have many more options of course, but the typical opponent will rely on his instincts to suggest what to do. He will generally try to get on top and rain down blows (martial artists call this 'Ground and Pound'), or choke, or attempt rape. He will probably not roll around looking for joint locks or complex techniques. He will know that his weight can be used to hold you down, but may not use it very efficiently.

Your basic gameplan should be: get out from underneath, get a dominant position, hurt the assailant enough that he cannot stop you getting up, get up and away. Trying to shortcut this by just wriggling out and running away can result in you being dragged back down.

Thrust kick from the ground

A sideways kick at the knees will stop any attacker in his tracks, and may take him right out of the fight. The kick is executed in much the same way as a standing side kick.

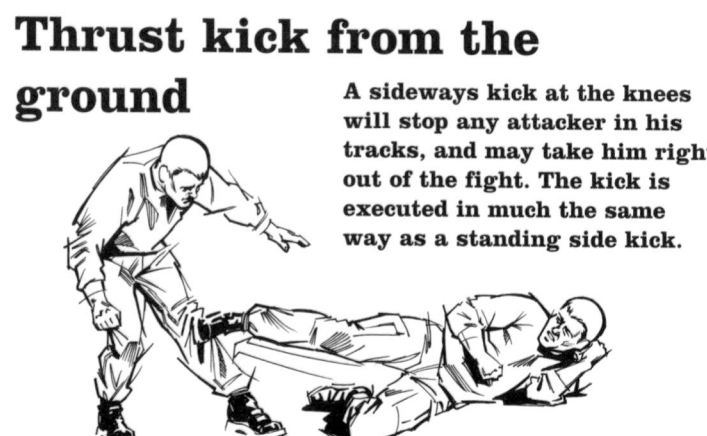

TIP: GROUNDFIGHTING TACTICS

In a 'street' situation, your goal must always be to get back to your feet and to end the situation. Do not go to the ground if you can avoid it, and get up as soon as you can. You are simply too vulnerable on the ground to risk staying there. If you have to disable an aggressor to get back up, do so. As always, this is not a goal but a means to an end.

Getting Up

Even from a dominant position, if you simply try to get up off an opponent who is still in the fight, you will fail. You will be pulled back down or tripped up as you try to move away. It is necessary to make an escape route.

Obviously, an opponent who is stunned by heavy blows to the head will be unlikely to interfere in your escape. Another alternative is the 'tactical dismount'. Push the opponent down by the head or throat, ideally turning his head away from you, and move away in the direction of his head rather than to the side where he can grab you.

Thrust kick to the groin

If the attacker is a bit closer, it is possible to kick up at his groin. It is important to drive him back with this kick, or he may fall on you.

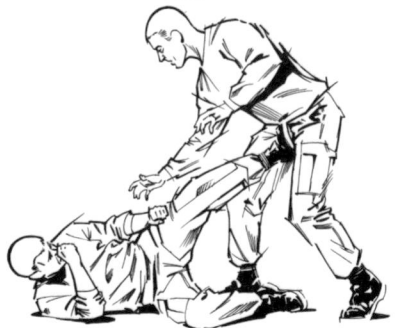

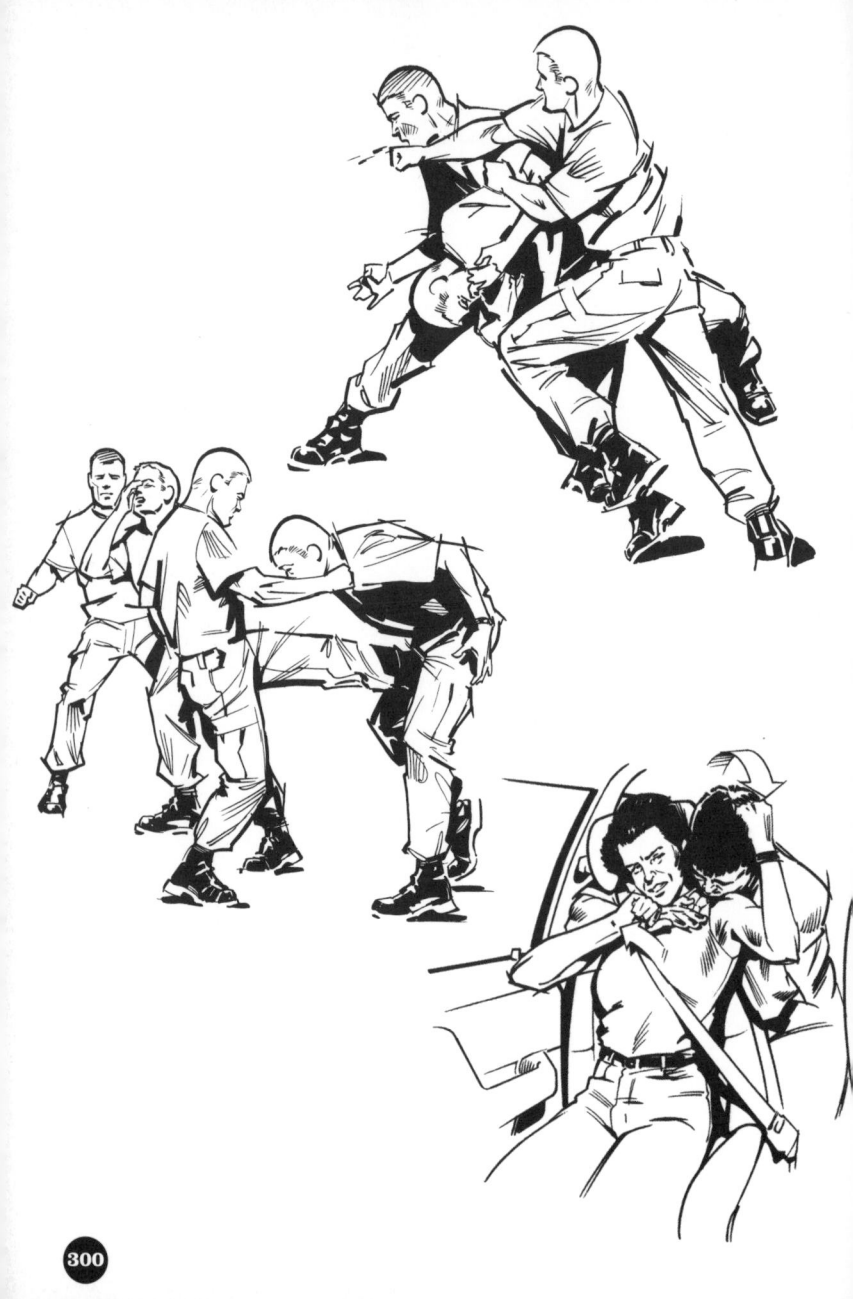

I t is an old military axiom that all battles take place at the junction of four map sheets, in the dark, uphill, in the rain … and in truth any fight can be considered an adverse situation. However, some situations are particularly difficult. The key, as always, is not to panic. Work out a gameplan and implement it with determination.

FIGHTING IN A CAR

Ordinarily, you should be safe in a car. Its structure will protect you somewhat and its mobility allows you to escape from most situations. Many problems can be avoided by driving sensibly, avoiding obviously 'bad' neighbourhoods and routes, and so forth. Wherever possible, slow down early so that you can keep moving as you approach traffic lights. Keep your doors locked and windows only open a little. However, sometimes the unexpected happens. Any fight in an enclosed space such as a car will involve awkward positions, so it is necessary to learn to strike at extreme close quarters with short, hard blows to vulnerable points. You will almost certainly have to grapple, and 'shutdown techniques' will be useful for gaining an advantage.

....

Left: In truth, all fights take place under 'adverse conditions', but some situations are worse than others. You may have to fight a group or in a confined space.

14

Good basic skills and an aggressive mindset will get you through most situations.

In Action
Fighting
Under Adverse
Conditions

TIP: AGGRESSORS IN CARS

Someone who is intending to get out of his car and attack you will take his seatbelt off and will probably stop the engine. An aggressor who rolls down his window and shouts abuse or threats at you but does not do these things will probably content himself with posturing from the safety of his vehicle unless you give him a reason to get out and fight you, say by becoming involved in a shouting match. The aggressor will probably drive off once he has satisfied his ego. If he does get out of his car, assume that he probably means to assault you.

Tactics for Fighting in a Car

Since your car represents an escape route, in most situations your goal will be to create an opportunity to drive away. Obviously, you will need to get an assailant out of the car one way or another if he is already in it. If you can get him out and lock the doors, you will gain time to escape. An attacker may try to smash his way in through the windows or kick the bodywork, but rather than worrying about this you should concern yourself with making an escape.

If the attacker is already in the car, you may have to subdue him to get him out, or to enable you to get out yourself and escape another way. In any case, take your seatbelt off as it will get in the way of any attempt to fight or flee.

Fighting a Driver or Front-Seat Passenger

If you are being forced to drive somewhere, crash your car. This sounds extreme but these are extreme circumstances. Obviously, do not do this at a suicidal speed, but hitting an obstruction will make it impossible for the attacker to take you somewhere in the car, which could save your life. It will also attract attention and, since you are likely to be more ready for the impact than the passenger, give you a chance to fight or escape.

If you are the passenger, yank the handbrake on, ideally on a corner, to cause a skid or force the driver to fight for control of the vehicle. You can also shove the gear lever into neutral to interfere with driving or slow down the car as you prepare to jump out.

An aggressor sitting beside you can be attacked with an edge-of-

Edge-of-hand-strike

An edge-of-hand strike to the throat is effective against a passenger in the seat alongside you. At closer quarters you can use your elbow instead, which is effective against a wider range of targets.

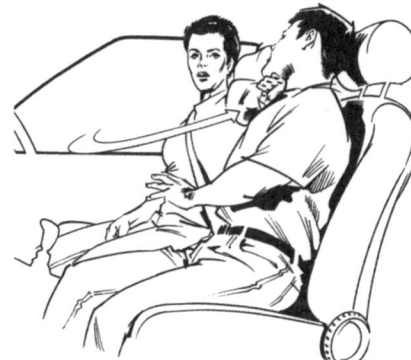

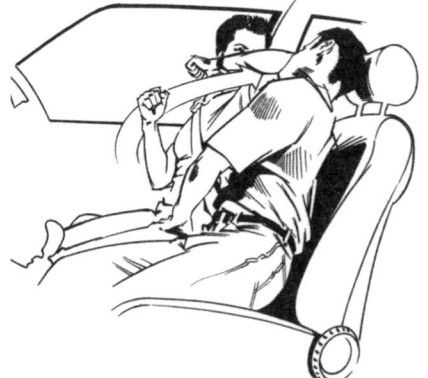

hand strike or an elbow, depending on how close he is. Be prepared to strike several times. If he seems inclined to scramble out of your car, drive off as soon as you can. If he wants to fight you, getting out of the car is probably your best option, especially if he is stronger than you. In a close-quarters environment, strength is even more of an advantage than elsewhere.

If you end up in a grappling match with an aggressor, use 'shutdown techniques' to make him want to get out of your car. Thumbs in eye sockets, biting, tearing at flesh and raking with nails can all be used to make your car an unpleasant environment that he will want to vacate as quickly as possible.

Fighting a Rear-Seat Passenger

There is little that someone in the rear seat can do the driver except choke them or grab them from behind. Do not worry about keeping control of the car; if it hits something while you are fighting for your life, so be it. Stamping on the brakes might cause the attacker to lose his grip or fall forward, which may help. However, it is critical to pull any choke off your throat as fast as possible. Grab and break fingers if you can. It may also be possible to reach back and grab the assailant by the collar or hair, and pull him forward. If you can make him fall into the gap between the front seats you can hold him down while you get your seatbelt off and prepare to escape from the vehicle.

Removing an Intruder from a Vehicle

The most effective way to remove someone who is clinging on to the steering wheel is to drag and twist his head. Use his eye sockets or nostrils to grip, which will inflict pain if he resists. If you cannot drag him out, use a series of sharp yanks to wrench his head about. He may well decide to let you pull him out in order to protect his neck.

Be careful that he does not come loose suddenly and fall on top of you; again, sharp jerks delivered from a good, well-balanced posture are a good idea. Short, hard elbow and knee strikes can also assist in the process.

Aggressor Outside Your Car

It is very difficult to fight someone who is leaning in through a window, and virtually impossible to push him out. Instead, grab him and pull him in, using your elbow or opposite hand to strike

Fighting a rear-seat passenger

Once you have dealt with the initial attack, you need to get your seatbelt off as quickly as possible so that you can turn around or get out of the car.

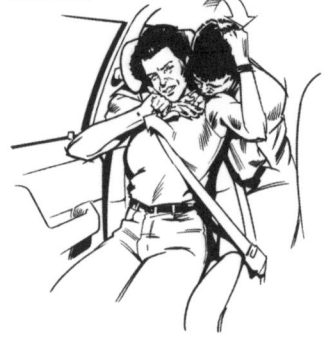

with. 'Shutdown techniques' such as biting or eye-poking will encourage him to pull himself back out of your car. You may be able to escape by driving off, or you may have to get your seatbelt off quickly and continue fighting under less awkward circumstances.

FIGHTING IN A CLUTTERED ENVIRONMENT

The main danger in a cluttered environment is the possibility of falling over something or being jammed up against a wall or other obstruction by an attacker. However, obstructions can be used to your advantage. For example, if you can put the corner of a table between you and the opponent by stepping around it or pulling it in the way, you will know where he has to move in order to hit you. It may be possible to intercept him or escape as he changes position.

You can make use of your surroundings in various ways. Normally, shoving an opponent is of little use. However, if he can be pushed into something or caused to trip this can inflict injury or at least delay him. If you are skilled it may be possible to

Removing an intruder

If you can get a door open and drag the intruder out, this is a reasonable option. But you should never jump on the bonnet or put yourself in the path of a car; many attackers will quite happily drive over you.

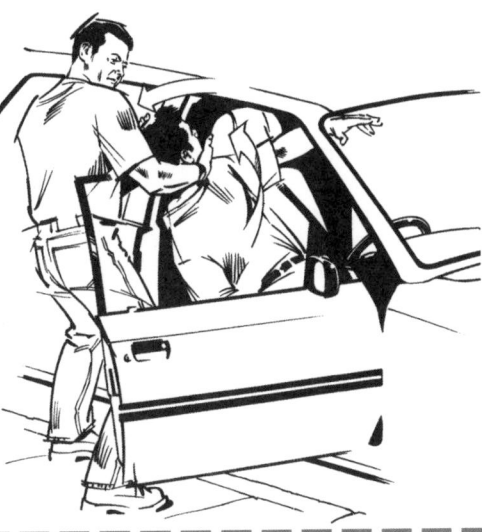

magnify the effects of a throw or hard takedown by sending the assailant crashing into something that will hurt him more than the floor.

Your habitual appraisal of the surroundings in the moments before violence breaks out is of paramount importance here. If you are at least vaguely aware of the environment around you, your chances of avoiding disaster and using the conditions to your advantage are far greater.

FIGHTING A GROUP

It is virtually impossible for one person to successfully fight several if they are well coordinated, but most of the time a group of assailants will be a mob rather than an organized force. Highly trained military units can overcome much larger enemy forces by coordinating their actions to defeat the enemy one at a time. It is also possible to do this when fighting a group.

If you can prevent the opposition from acting in concert, it is possible to defeat them in a series of small fights rather than one huge one against massive odds. This is a daunting task but it can be done.

Sometimes it is possible to take the fight out of a group by dealing with one of their number in a manner that gives the others pause. This is best done by taking the initiative and attacking suddenly, demolishing one opponent before the others are physically and mentally ready to attack.

Tactics for Fighting a Group

When dealing with a group, it is vital to keep moving and, if possible, to make opponents get in one another's way. If you are fighting three people you are in real trouble. However, if you can shove one opponent away and move so that another cannot get to you because his friend is in the

Fighting a group: Part 1

The defender does not wait to be attacked. Instead he seizes the initiative to take one of the assailants out of the fight.

(1)

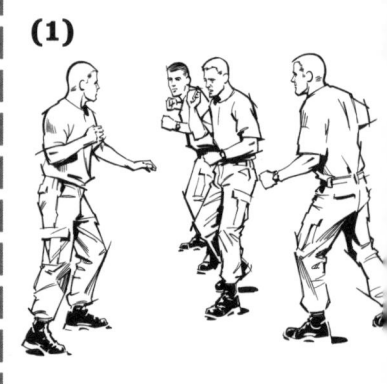

way, then for a moment you are only fighting one man.

The key is to hit–move–hit and not get bogged down. Often an opponent who is part of a group can be taken out of the fight with less effort than if he was alone. He can rely on the protection of the group and thus has less at stake than if he was alone, so might back off with a lesser injury than would otherwise be needed. You, on the other hand, have everything at stake and are totally committed.

Example of Anti-Group Tactics

Any combat against a group is a desperate affair in which you must take any opportunity that presents itself.

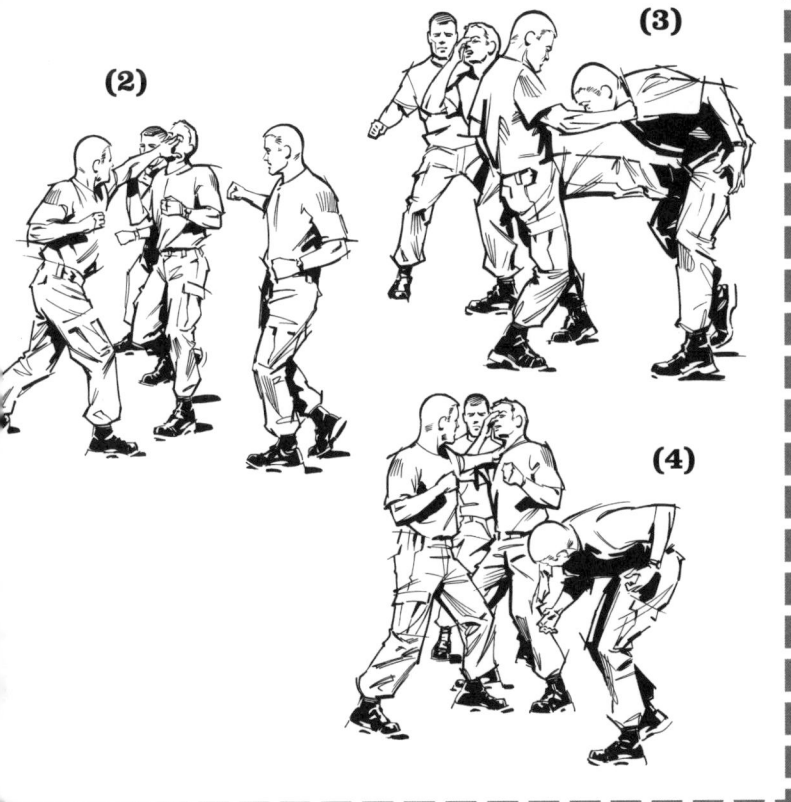

In this example, a lone man is confronted by three opponents. (1)

Taking the initiative, he chooses a target and throws an eye jab. This is unlikely to put the opponent out of the fight completely, but it will stop him for a moment. The movement also causes the eye-jabbed opponent to recoil into the path of the man beside him. (2)

For the next couple of seconds, the defender is just facing one opponent. This one had begun an attack but is now hesitating. This may be due to surprise at seeing his friend poked in the eyes, or perhaps it is because the intended victim did not wait to be punched but has moved and thus changed the tactical situation. As this attacker reorients himself, the defender launches a groin kick which will hopefully put him right out of the fight. (3)

Not waiting to see if he has defeated his opponent or merely bought some time, but sure that he has at least neutralized him for a moment, the defender turns back to the other two and shoves the man he eye-jabbed, establishing the range for a strike as well as pushing him into his companion as a shield. (4)

The defender punches the nearest attacker in the throat (5) and shoves him into his companion (6), making it impossible for that attacker to get into the fight. Meanwhile the kicked attacker stumbles away. He is out of it, but the defender does not know

that for sure. He thus needs to deal with the others quickly in case there is an active opponent behind him.

With one opponent still coughing from the throat blow, the defender keeps pushing him into his companion and delivers a punch to the face. (7)

With two men down, the defender goes after the kicked opponent, who

Fighting a Group: Part 2

With one assailant out of it, the defender moves so that the others get in one another's way and hits 'targets of opportunity' as they present themselves.

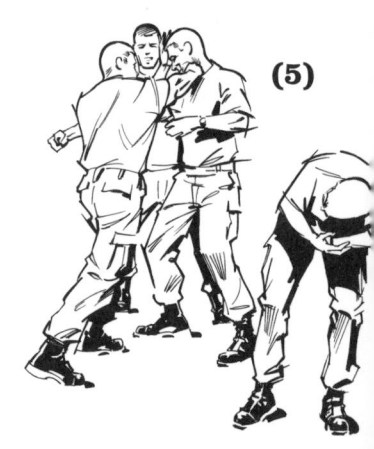

(5)

is starting to recover. Giving him no chance to rejoin the fight, the defender takes him out with a kick to the face. (8)

FIGHTING WITH IMPROVISED WEAPONS

Even in countries where it is not permitted for civilians to go armed, self-defence laws allow you to arm yourself with an improvised weapon if you need to. Thus, if you are in serious danger and grab something to use to protect yourself then provided what you do is reasonable, you will not have acted unlawfully.

This is subject to the same common-sense interpretation as any

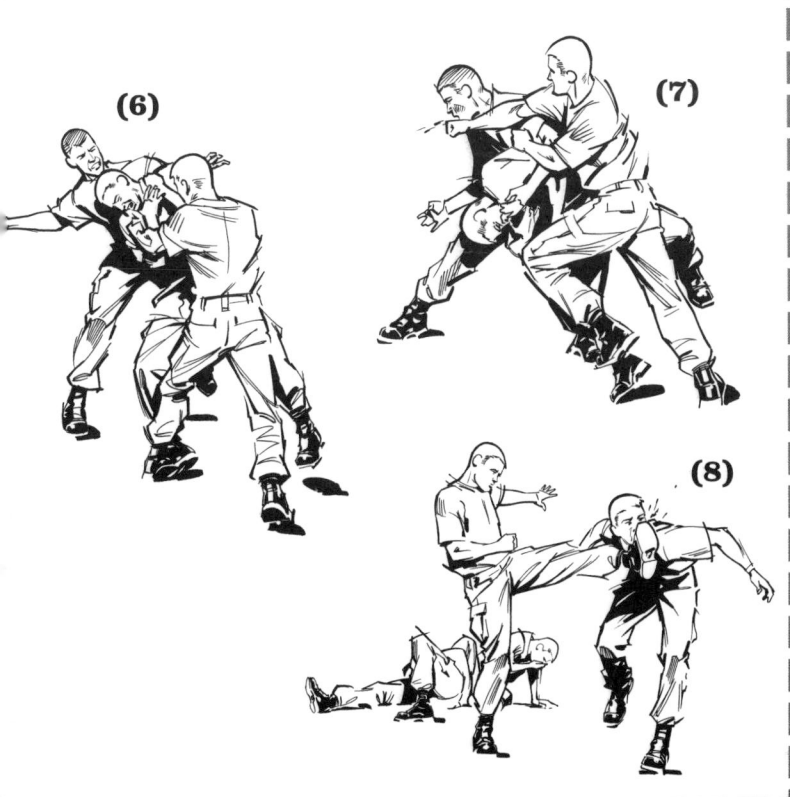

(6)

(7)

(8)

TIP:
DON'T KNOW WHAT TO DO?

If you are ever in a fight and do not know what to do for the best, hit the other guy in the head as hard as you can and keep doing it. You cannot go far wrong that way.

other self-defence issue; if you grabbed a kitchen knife to defend yourself against a big, strong man who had broken into your house and was ferociously attacking you, this would seem reasonable.

On the other hand, if he ended up dead with two dozen stab wounds in the back then you would have to show that you needed to inflict those injuries.

Sharp and Pointed Weapons

Sharp and pointed weapons are not ideal for self-defence, though they are excellent for killing people. In a military context, that is usually the intent, but for self-defence such weapons create an all-or-nothing situation. It is actually quite hard to wound someone in the chaos of a fight without endangering their life.

That might be fine if you are fighting for your life, but it does make the use of knives and other blades problematical for self-defence under other circumstances.

A sharp or pointed weapon is an excellent threat and may cause an aggressor to back off, but only if he believes that you will actually use it. If he does not believe this, or attacks anyway, then you have to make the choice whether to use your weapon or not. If you are not willing to use it, all you have done is brought a lethal implement into the equation and made it potentially available to the aggressor.

Blunt Weapons

Blunt instruments are much better for self-defence. They still make a decent deterrent and can be used to cause pain and injury with a much smaller chance of permanent consequences. This is not to say that blunt weapons cannot kill, especially if the skull is struck, but the chance of accidental lethality is smaller.

Blunt weapons can be used to strike targets that it would be foolish to hit with a fist, such as the forearm or shin. A badly hurt or broken limb will stop most people from making an attack. Blunt weapons can also be used to apply pressure in order to cause pain. All manner of locks and holds can be applied with a weapon, but for the purposes of self-defence there is no need for anything so complex. Instead, the weapon can be dug into the aggressor almost anywhere to cause pain, but ideally where there are bones close to the surface such as the face, hands, collar-bones and so forth.

Small Batons

Any short, hard rodlike object can be used for self-defence. A specialist variety, called a kubotan, is advocated by many martial artists. Kubotans are useful for training purposes but they have one problem associated with them – they are recognized as weapons by most police forces. This does not matter if local laws permit weapons to be carried, but in areas where this is not the case (e.g. Britain) then carrying a kubotan is an offence.

The reason for this is that it is an offence to carry a weapon or to carry anything specifically for the purposes of using it as a weapon. Since the kubotan is sold as a weapon and recognized as one, it is hard to justify carrying it. However, it is perfectly legal to use as a weapon an object that you happen to be carrying anyway, if you need to do so. Thus if you have trained with a kubotan you can use the same techniques with, say, a pen.

Using the Kubotan or Small Baton

Unless you have received specialist training, do not try to be clever and apply complex locks with a kubotan. Nor should you change your grip on

TIP: DON'T FIXATE

When fighting or confronting more than one opponent, try not to fixate on any one of them. There is little to be gained in battering one assailant into submission if you are then hit from behind and taken out. Attack one opponent, hurt him, then break off before his mates can gang up on you. Keep moving, hit anything that comes within reach, and sooner or later the mob will begin to thin out as individuals are taken out or decide they have had enough.

it mid-fight. There is a whole body of martial arts technique surrounding this weapon, but for self-defence it is wise to stick to the least complicated options.

The simplest technique is to grip it in your fist and punch normally. Having something in your hand helps support the hand and wrist. With the end of the kubotan sticking out of the

TIP:
WEAPONS FOR SELF-DEFENCE

It is an offence in many countries to carry anything specifically for use as a weapon. It would be illegal to carry something as innocent as a pair of socks or even a kitten if you were doing so because you had somehow contrived a way to use it as a weapon. However, it is perfectly acceptable to arm yourself if this is necessary and reasonable under the circumstances, which usually means pressing into service an object that you would normally have with you or to hand.

What this amounts to is that you have the right to do what you have to in order to protect yourself, including arming yourself, but not to carry a weapon 'just in case'. Thus if you were in the kitchen and grabbed a knife normally kept there, or you were in the car and you grabbed a spanner from the toolbox that you always carry, then providing it was not unreasonable to use these items in self-defence, no offence would be committed.

bottom of your hand, you can hammerfist an assailant to potent effect. The kubotan can also be used to release a grab by grinding it into the bones of the assailant's hand.

Alternatively, hold the kubotan in your hand with the end sticking out in the direction of your thumb. This end can be used to jab or grind into an assailant. The neck and face are good targets but, unlike an empty-handed blow, hitting almost anywhere will hurt.

Larger Batons
Virtually any reasonably dense, lengthy object can be used as a baton or club, though some are clumsier than others. Spanners, sticks, rolled-up newspapers … weapons can be improvised from whatever is to hand.

Most people will swing with a baton or club, usually at the head. However, it is often better to jab instead. Not only is this difficult to defend against, but it also keeps the weapon between you and the assailant as a barrier.

A baton can be used in one or both hands as necessary. A walking-stick, for example, is best used much like a rifle with a bayonet on the end. Even though the hooked end offers all manner of intriguing possibilities for tripping an assailant up or entangling their limbs, it is best to restrict yourself to simple jabs to avoid leaving yourself open to counterattack.

OTHER IMPROVISED WEAPONS

It is possible to use almost any object to gain an advantage in a fight. A handful of coins can be thrown in an attacker's face as a distraction, or you can spray deodorant or hairspray for the same purpose. A cup of coffee can be used as a weapon or a distraction, depending upon temperature. A faceful of liquid will cause most people to pause while you hit them; if it is hot then you might not need to follow up.

You can also use any heavy object you pick up, from a rock to a can of beer, to add weight to a blow. Alternatively, you could throw it. Lighter but hard objects such as combs or pens can be used to rake with, causing pain if not usually much harm. Once you start looking, you will be surprised at just how many ordinary items can be pressed into service as weapons.

FINAL NOTES

The most vital weapons at the disposal of a special forces soldier are his intellect and his mental toughness. Sometimes it all comes down to 'who wants it most', i.e. whoever is more willing to keep fighting and trying to survive. Being able to keep your head and look for advantages or escape routes is a big plus too.

Getting into 'survival mode' requires shifting mental gears when you need to. Good training helps with this as well as giving you the skills you need, but ultimately the will that drives your bid to survive is yours.

If you give in to fear or go into denial, pretending that it is not happening, then you will fail. Instead you must accept that it IS really happening and deal with it. So if you find yourself thinking, 'What's he going to do to me?', you have to force yourself to answer, 'Nothing. I'm not going to let him.'

If you have done all you can to avoid trouble and it finds you anyway, then it is down to you to make a way out of the situation with as little harm to yourself as possible. Yes, you will be scared. Yes, you might indeed get hurt. Yes, it is possible that you could fail to defend yourself … but not for lack of trying. If the bad guy will not let you withdraw or de-escalate the situation, if he insists on fighting then he has decided that someone is going to get hurt. But it is you, not him, that gets to decide who.

Index